Tutorial Topics in Infection for the Combined Infection Training Programme

Tutorial Topics in Infection for the Combined Infection Training Programme

Cheuk Yan William Tong[†]
Consultant in Clinical Virology
Department of Infection
Barts Health NHS Trust
London, UK

Caryn Rosmarin
Consultant in Medical Microbiology
Department of Infection
Barts Health NHS Trust
London, UK

Armine Sefton
Emerita Professor of Clinical Microbiology
Barts and the London School of Medicine and Dentistry
Queen Mary University of London
London, UK

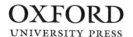

OXFORD
UNIVERSITY PRESS

OXFORD
UNIVERSITY PRESS

Great Clarendon Street, Oxford, OX2 6DP,
United Kingdom

Oxford University Press is a department of the University of Oxford.
It furthers the University's objective of excellence in research, scholarship,
and education by publishing worldwide. Oxford is a registered trade mark of
Oxford University Press in the UK and in certain other countries

© Oxford University Press 2019

The moral rights of the authors have been asserted

First Edition Published in 2019

All rights reserved. No part of this publication may be reproduced, stored in
a retrieval system, or transmitted, in any form or by any means, without the
prior permission in writing of Oxford University Press, or as expressly permitted
by law, by licence or under terms agreed with the appropriate reprographics
rights organization. Enquiries concerning reproduction outside the scope of the
above should be sent to the Rights Department, Oxford University Press, at the
address above

You must not circulate this work in any other form
and you must impose this same condition on any acquirer

Published in the United States of America by Oxford University Press
198 Madison Avenue, New York, NY 10016, United States of America

British Library Cataloguing in Publication Data
Data available

Library of Congress Control Number: 2018949670

ISBN 978–0–19–880174–0

Printed and bound by
CPI Group (UK) Ltd, Croydon, CR0 4YY

Oxford University Press makes no representation, express or implied, that the
drug dosages in this book are correct. Readers must therefore always check
the product information and clinical procedures with the most up-to-date
published product information and data sheets provided by the manufacturers
and the most recent codes of conduct and safety regulations. The authors and
the publishers do not accept responsibility or legal liability for any errors in the
text or for the misuse or misapplication of material in this work. Except where
otherwise stated, drug dosages and recommendations are for the non-pregnant
adult who is not breast-feeding

Links to third party websites are provided by Oxford in good faith and
for information only. Oxford disclaims any responsibility for the materials
contained in any third party website referenced in this work.

This book is dedicated to our colleague and friend Dr Cheuk Yan William Tong,
whose knowledge, humility and love for his work continues to inspire us all.

Acknowledgment

Thank you to Dr Maximillian Habibi and Dr Mark Hopkins, who reviewed Dr William Tong's chapters. We are grateful for your help.

Contents

Abbreviations

+ve	positive
-ve	negative
A&E	Accident and emergency
ACDP	Advisory Committee on Dangerous Pathogens
ACT	Artemisinin combination therapy
ADEM	Acute disseminated encephalomyelitis
AFB	Acid fast bacilli
AHA	American Heart Association
AMR	Antimicrobial resistance
AMS	Antimicrobial stewardship
ANTT	Aseptic non-touch technique
APC	Antigen-presenting cells
API	Analytical profile index
ART	Antiretroviral therapy
ASOT	Antistreptolysin O Titer
AST	Antimicrobial susceptibility test
ATLL	Adult T cell leukaemia/lymphoma
ATP	Adenosine triphosphate
ATS	American Thoracic Society
BAL	Broncho-alveolar lavage
BBV	Blood-borne virus
BCG	Bacillus Calmette-Guérin
BDG	Beta-D-glucan
BNF	British National Formulary
BP	Blood pressure
BSAC	British Association of Antimicrobial Chemotherapy
BSC	Biological safety cabinet
BSE	Bovine spongiform encephalopathy
BSI	British Standards Institution
CA-MRSA	Community-acquired MRSA
CAP	Community-acquired pneumonia
cART	Combination anti-retroviral therapy
cccDNA	Covalent-closed-circular DNA
CCG	Clinical Commissioning Groups
CCHF	Crimean/Congo haemorrhagic fever
CDC	Centers for Disease Control
CDI	*Clostridium difficile*

cDNA	Complementary DNA
CFS	Chronic fatigue syndrome
CJD	Creutzfeldt-Jakob disease
CL	Containment level
CLO	Campylobacter-like organism
CMV	Cytomegalovirus
CN V	Trigeminal nerve
CNS	Central nervous system
CNS	Coagulase-negative staphylococci
COPD	Chronic obstructive pulmonary disease
COSHH	Control of Substances Hazardous to Health
CPA	Clinical Pathology Accreditation
CPE	Cytopathic effect
CPE	Carbapenemase-producing Enterobactericeae spp.
Cq	Quantification cycle
CQC	Care Quality Commission
CRE	Carbapenem-resistant enterobacteriacae
CRO	Carbapenem-resistant organisms
CRP	C-reactive protein
CSF	Cerebrospinal fluid
CSF	Colony stimulating factor
CT	Computed tomography
Ct	Crossing threshold
CTLA-4	Cytotoxic T lymphocyte-associated protein 4
CVC	Central venous catheter
CVID	Combined variable immune deficiency
DAIR	Debridement and retention of implant
DALY	Disability-adjusted-life-years
DHFR	Dihydrofolate reductase
DHR	Dihydrorhodamine
DIC	Disseminated intravascular coagulation
DIF	Direct immunofluorescence
DIPC	Director of Infection Prevention & Control
DMSA	Dimercaptosuccinic acid
DNA	Deoxyribonucleic acid
DoH	Department of Health
DTP	Diphteria, tetanus, and polio
DVT	Deep venous thrombosis
EBV	Epstein-Barr Virus
EFI	European Federation of Immunogenetics
EIA	Enzyme immunoassay
ELISA	Enzyme-linked immunosorbent assay
ELISPOT	Enzyme-linked immunospot
EM	Electron microscopy
EORTC	European Organisation for Research and Treatment of Cancer
EPI	Expanded Programme on Immunisation
EPP	Exposure-prone procedure
ESBL	Extended spectrum betalactamase
ESC	European Society of Cardiology
ESIMS	Electrospray ionization-mass spectrometry
ESR	Erythrocyte sedimentation rate

EVD	External ventricular drain
EWD	Endoscope washer-disinfector
FBC	Full blood count
FITC	Fluorescein isothiocyanate
GAS	Group A strep
GBS	Group B strep
GCS	Glasgow Coma Score
GCSF	Granulocyte Colony Stimulating Factor
GDH-EIA	Glutamate dehydrogenase enzyme immunoassay
GIT	Gastro-intestinal tract
GM	Galactomannan
GMC	General Medical Council
GPEI	Global polio eradication initiative
GPEI	Glycopeptide-resistant enterococci
GUM	Genito-urinary medicine
GVHD	Graft versus host disease
H&E	Haematoxylin and Eosin
HAART	Highly active anti-retroviral therapy
HACEK	Haemophilus, Aggregatibacter, Cardiobacterium, Eikenella, Kingella
HAP	Hospital-acquired pneumonia
HBIg	Hepatitis B immunoglobin
HBV	hepatitis virus B
HCAI	Healthcare-associated Infection
HCC	Hepatocellular carcinoma
HCCA	Alpha-4-cyano-4-hydroxy cinnamic acid
hCMV	Human cytomegalovirus
HCV	hepatitis virus C
HCW	Healthcare worker
HEPA	High-efficiency particulate air
HFMD	Hand, foot, and mouth disease
hGISA	heterogeneous glycopeptide-intermediate S. aureus
Hib	Haemophilus influenzae type b
HICPAC	Hospital Infection Control Advisory Committee
HII	High-impact interventions
HIV	Human immunodeficiency virus
HLIU	High Level Isolation Unit
HNIg	human normal immunoglobulin
HPT	Health protection team
HRIg	Human rabies immunoglobin
HSE	Health and Safety Executive
HSE	Herpes simplex encephalitis
HSV	Herpes simplex virus
HTA	Human Tissue Authority
HTIg	Human tetanus immunoglobin
HUS	Haemolytic uraemic syndrome
IA	Invasive aspergillosis
ICED-IE	ICED-infective endocarditis
ICED-LI	ICED lead infections
ICP	Intracranial pressure
ICPT	Infection Control and Prevention Team
ID	Infectious diseases

IDSA	Infectious Diseases Society of America
IE	Infective endocarditis
IFD	Invasive fungal disease
IFU	Instructions for use
IgG	Immunoglobulin G
IgM	Immunoglobulin M
IGRA	Interferon Gamma Release Assay
IPC	Infection prevention and control
IRIS	Immune reconstitution inflammatory syndrome
ISAGA	Immunosorbent agglutination assay
ISO	International Standards Organization
ITN	Insecticide-treated bed nets
ITP	Idiopathic thrombyocytopenic purpura
IUGR	Intrauterine growth restriction
IV	Intravenous(ly)
IVDMDD	In Vitro Diagnostic Medical Device Directive
IVDU	Intravenous drug use
IVIg	Intravenous immunoglobulin
JCVI	Joint Committee on Vaccines and Immunisation
KOH	Potassium hydroxide
KPC	Klebsiella pneumoniae carbapenemase
KS	Kaposi's sarcoma
LAIV	Live attenuated intranasal influenza vaccine
LDH	Lactate dehydrogenase
LDT	Laboratory developed test
LFT	Liver function test
LP	Lumbar puncture
LPS	Lipopolysaccharide
LRINEC	Laboratory Risk Indicator for Necrotizing Fasciitis
LTBI	Latent TB infection
MAC	Membrane attack complex
MAG3	Mercapto acetyl tri-glycine
MALDI-ToF	Matrix-assisted laser desorption/ionization-Time of Flight
MAP	Mean arterial pressure
MASPs	Mannose-binding lectin-associated serine proteases
MAT	Microscopic agglutination test
MBL	Mannose-binding lectin
MBL	Metallo-beta-lactamases
MC&S	Microscopy, culture, and sensitivity
MDR	Multi-drug resistant
MDR-TB	Multidrug-resistant tuberculosis
MDT	Multidisciplinary team
MHC	Major histocompatibility complex
MHRA	Medicines and Healthcare Products Regulatory Authority
MIC	Minimum inhibitory concentration
MLSB	Macrolides, lincosamides (clindamycin), and streptogramin B
MMR	Measles, mumps, rubella
mRNA	Messenger RNA
MRSA	Meticillin-resistant Staphylococcus aureus
MS	Mass spectrometry
MSM	Men who have sex with men

MSU	Midstream specimen of urine
MTB	Mycobacterium tuberculosis
NAAT	Nucleic acid amplifying test
NaTHaC	National Travel Health Network and Centre
NBT	Nitroblue-tetrazolium
NEC	Necrotizing enterocolitis
NETs	Neutrophil extracellular traps
NEWS	National early warning score
NGS	Next-generation sequencing
NICE	National Institute for Health and Care Excellence
NNRTI	Non-nucleoside reverse transcriptase inhibitor
NPV	Negative predictive value
NRTI	Nucleoside reverse transcriptase inhibitors
NTM	Nontuberculous mycobacteria
NVE	Native valve endocarditis
OCT	Outbreak control team
OI	Opportunistic infection
OLM	Ocular larva migrans
OPAT	Outpatient parenteral antimicrobial treatment
OPV	Oral polio vaccine
PAMPs	Pathogen-associated molecular patterns
PAN	Polyarthritis nodosa
PAS	Periodic acid shift
PBP2a	Penicillin-binding protein
PCP	Pneumocystis jiroveci pneumonia
PCR	Polymerase chain reaction
PD	Pharamcodynamic
PD-1	Programmed cell death protein 1
PEG	Polyethylene glycol
PEP	Postexposure prophylaxis
PET	Positron emission tomography
PHI	Primary HIV infection
PHT	Public health team
PI	Protease inhibitor
PICC	Peripherally inserted central catheter
PII	Periods of increased incidence
PIR	Post-infection review
PIS	Post-infection syndrome
PJI	Prosthetic joint infection
PK	Pharamcokinetic
PLHIV	People living with HIV
PML	Progressive multifocal leukoencephalopathy
PMR	Polymyalgia rheumatica
PMTCT	Prevention of mother-to-child transmission
PNA FISH	Peptide nucleic acid fluorescence in-situ hybridization
PPD	Purified protein derivative
PPE	Personal protective equipment
PPV	Positive predictive value
PPV23	Pneumococcal polysaccharide vaccine
PR	Rectal examination
PrEP	Pre-exposure prophylaxis

PRRs	Pathogen recognition receptors
PTFE	Teflon
PTLD	Post-transplant lymphoproliferative disease
PUO	Pyrexia of unknown origin
PVE	Prosthetic valve endocarditis
PVL	Panton-Valentine leucocidin
PWID	People who inject drugs
QA	Quality assurance
QC	Quality control
QMS	Quality management system
qSOFA	Quick Sequential Organ Failure Assessment
RA	Rheumatoid arthritis
RBC	Red blood cells
RCA	Root cause analysis
rCTB	Recombinant cholera toxin B
RDT	Rapid diagnostic test
RIPL	Rare and Imported Pathogens Laboratory
RITA	Recent infection testing algorithm
RMP	Registered medical practitioner
RNA	Ribonucleic acid
RPR	Rapid plasma reagin
RR	Respiratory rate
RSV	Respiratory syncytial virus (or bronchiolitis)
RT	Reverse transcriptase
S	Svedberg units
S/CO	Signal-to-cutoff ratio
SAPO	Specified Animal Pathogens Order
SARS	Severe Acute Respiratory Syndrome
SCT	Stem cell transplant
SD	Standard deviation
SDGs	Sustainable Development Goals
SFTS	Severe fever with thrombocytopaenia syndrome
SIGN	Scottish Intercollegiate Guidelines Network
SIRS	Systemic Inflammatory Response Syndrome
SIV	Simian immunodeficiency virus
SLE	Systemic lupus erythematosus
SNHL	Sensorineural hearing loss
SOFA	Sequential Organ Failure Assessment
SOP	Standard operating procedure
SPE	Streptococcal pyrogenic exotoxin
SSI	Surgical site infection
SSPE	Subacute sclerosing panencephalitis
SSTI	Skin and soft tissue infection
SUI	Serious untoward incident
SVR	Sustained virological response
TB	Tuberculosis
TBE	Tick-borne encephalitis
TCR	T cell receptor
Th	T-helper
TOE	Transoesophageal echocardiogram
ToF	Time of flight

TORCH	Toxoplasma, rubella, cytomegalovirus, and herpes simplex virus
TPPA	Treponema pallidum particle agglutination
TSI	Triple sugar iron
TSS	Toxic shock syndrome
U&E	Urea and electrolytes
UKAS	UK Accreditation Service
ULN	Upper limit of normal
URT	Upper respiratory tract
UTI	Urinary tract infection
UV	Ultraviolet
VAP	Ventilator-associated pneumonia
VDRL	Venereal disease research laboratory
VFR	Visiting friends and relatives
VHF	Viral haemorrhagic fever
VIP	Visual Infusion Phlebitis
VISA	Vancomycin-intermediate Staphylococcus aureus
VP	Ventriculoperitoneal
VRE	Vancomycin-resistant enterococci
VZIG	Varicella-Zoster immunoglobulin
VZV	Varicella-zoster virus
WBC	White blood cells
WCC	White cell count
XDR-TB	Extensively drug-resistant TB
XLD	Xylose lysine deoxycholate
ZN	Ziehl-Neelsen

Contributors

Fatima Ahmad, Biomedical Scientist, Department of Infection, Barts Health NHS Trust, London, UK

Sarfaraz Ameen, Anti-Microbial Pharmacist, Barts Health NHS Trust, London, UK

Gurtan Atamturk, Biomedical Scientist, Department of Infection, Barts Health NHS Trust, London, UK

Zahir O. E. Babiker, Assistant Professor and Consultant in Infectious Diseases, College of Medicine and Health Sciences, United Arab Emirates University, Al Ain, United Arab Emirates

Marina Basarab, Consultant, Department of Infection, Barts Health NHS Trust, London, UK

Ruaridh Buchanan, Specialist Registrar in Microbiology and Infectious Diseases, Barts Health NHS Trust, London, UK

Duncan Clark, School of Life Sciences, University of Glasgow, Glasgow, UK

Martina N. Cummins, Clinical Director Infection Prevention and Control, Barts Health NHS Trust, London, UK

Subathira Dakshina, Specialist Registrar in Genitourinary Medicine, Barts Health NHS Trust, London, UK

Satya Das, Consultant, Barts Health NHS Trust, London, UK

Jayshree Dave, Consultant Microbiologist, HPA Specialist Microbiology Network (SMN), Public Health England

Heather Dolphin, Chief Biomedical Scientist, Barts Health NHS Trust, London, UK

Rohma Ghani, Specialty Trainee, Infectious Diseases, Barts Health NHS Trust, London, UK

Jennifer Henderson, Biomedical Scientist, Department of Infection, Barts Health NHS Trust, London, UK

Desmond Hsu, Specialist Registrar in Microbiology, Barts Health NHS Trust, London, UK

Mark Hopkins, Consultant Clinical Scientist, Department of Infection, Barts Health NHS Trust, London, UK

George Jacob, Consultant in Medical Microbiology, Royal Berkshire NHS Foundation Trust, Berkshire, UK

Angelina Jayakumar, Specialist Registrar in Infectious Diseases, Barts Health NHS Trust, London, UK

Anna Jeffery-Smith, Infectious Diseases and Virology Registrar, Barts Health NHS Trust, London, UK

Steve Kempley, Clinical Senior Lecturer in Paediatrics, Blizard Institute, Barts and The London, School of Medicine and Dentistry, London, UK

Palwasha Khan, Clinical Epidemiologist, Department of Infectious Disease Epidemiology, London School of Hygiene & Tropical Medicine, London, UK; Interactive Research and Development, Karachi, Pakistan

Jonathan Lambourne, Consultant in Infectious Diseases, Department of Infection, Barts Health NHS Trust, London, UK

Tim Linehan, Biomedical Scientist, Department of Infection, Barts Health NHS Trust, London, UK

Rohini J. Manuel, Consultant Medical Microbiologist, National Infection Service, Public Health England, London, UK

Sylvia Martin, Decontamination Lead, Barts Health NHS Trust, London, UK

Mark Melzer, Consultant in Microbiology and Infectious Diseases, Department of Infection, Barts Health NHS Trust, London, UK

Michael Millar, Consultant, Department of Infection, Barts Health NHS Trust, London, UK

Caoimhe NicFhogartaigh, Consultant in Infectious Diseases and Microbiology, Barts Health NHS Trust, London, UK

Anthony R. Oliver, Programme Manager at CliniSys, Chertsey, UK; Formerly Advanced Practitioner, Virology, Barts Health NHS Trust, UK

Chloe Orkin, Consultant Physician, Barts Health NHS Trust, London, UK

Sarah Parry, Specialist Registrar in Genitourinary Medicine and HIV, Department of Infection and Immunity, Barts Health NHS Trust, UK

Lynette Phee, Clinical Research Fellow, Blizard Institute, Queen Mary University of London; Specialist Registrar in Medical Microbiology and Virology, Barts Health NHS Trust, London, UK

Anna Riddell, Specialist registrar in Infectious Diseases and Virology, Barts Health NHS Trust, London, UK

Caryn Rosmarin, Consultant in Medical Microbiology, Department of Infection, Barts Health NHS Trust, London, UK

Marta Gonzalaz Sanz, Specialist Registar in Medical Microbiology, University College London Hospitals, Barts Health NHS Trust, London, UK

Shila Seaton, Bacteriology Scheme Manager, UK NEQAS for Microbiology, National Infection Service, PHE, Colindale, London, UK

Armine Sefton, Emerita Professor of Clinical Microbiology, Barts and the London School of Medicine and Dentistry, Queen Mary University of London, London, UK

Gee Yen Shin, Consultant Virologist, Public Health Laboratory London, Public Health England, London, UK

Stephanie J. Smith, Specialist Registrar in Medical Microbiology, Department of Infection, Barts Health NHS Trust, London, UK

Sherine Thomas, Consultant in Infectious Diseases, Department of Infection, Barts Health NHS Trust, London, UK

Simon Tiberi, Consultant, Department of Infection, Barts Health NHS Trust, London, UK

Cheuk Yan William Tong †, Consultant in Clinical Virology, Department of Infection, Barts Health NHS Trust, London, UK

Robert Serafino Wani, Consultant in Infectious Diseases and Microbiology, Department of Infection, Barts Health NHS Trust, Royal London Hospital, London, UK

David Wareham, Clinical Senior Lecturer/Honorary Consultant in Microbiology, Queen Mary University of London, Barts Health NHS Trust, London, UK

Mark Wilks, Clinical Scientist, Department of Microbiology, Barts Health NHS Trust, London, UK

Elizabeth Williams, Consultant in Sexual Health and HIV, Homerton Sexual Health Services, Homerton University Hospital NHS Foundation Trust, UK

Emily Zinser, Specialist Registrar in Immunology, Department of Immunology, Barts Health NHS Trust, London, UK

BASIC BIOLOGY OF BACTERIA, VIRUSES, FUNGI, AND PARASITES; HOST-PATHOGEN RELATIONSHIPS

CHAPTER 1

The biology of bacteria

Armine Sefton

CONTENTS

1.1 Organisms that cause infection in man

Bacterial infections and infestations of man can be caused by both microbes and non-microbes. Microbes include bacteria, viruses, fungi, and protozoa. Non-microbes include worms, insects, and arachnids. This chapter concentrates on the basic biology of bacteria.

1.2 What determines pathogen, pathogenicity, and virulence?

A pathogen is an organism that is able to cause disease in its host and the pathogenicity of any organism is its ability to produce disease. Microbes express their pathogenicity by means of their virulence. The virulence of any pathogen is determined by any of its structural, biochemical, or genetic features that enable it to cause disease in the host.

The relationship between a host and a potential pathogen is non-static; the likelihood of any pathogen causing disease in its host depends both on the virulence of the pathogen and the degree of resistance or susceptibility of the host, due mainly to the effectiveness of the host's defence mechanisms. Two of the main factors influencing a bacteria's pathogenicity are its ability to invade and it ability to produce toxins—either exotoxins or endotoxins.

1.3 The basic structure of bacteria

Bacteria are unicellular prokaryotic micro-organisms, unlike human cells, which are eukaryotic. Fungi, protozoa, helminths, and arthropods are also eukaryotic. Prokaryotic organisms contain both DNA and RNA, but their genetic material exists unbound in the cytoplasm of the cell as, unlike eukaryotic cells, they have no nuclear membrane. Sometimes bacteria contain additional smaller circular DNA molecules, called plasmids.

The main features of a bacterium are the cell wall, cytoplasm, and cell membrane. However, some bacteria have additional features such as spores, capsules, fimbriae (pili), and flagellae. The construction of the cell wall is different in different bacteria, but all cell walls contain peptidoglycan. The structure of the cell wall determines the staining characteristics when stained using the Gram stain. Although its first use was over a hundred and fifty years ago, is still the standard method for primary classification of bacteria. Occasionally, bacteria do not have a cell wall.

Gram staining of a fixed smear of bacteria is used to separate bacteria into Gram positive or Gram negative, and also to demonstrate their shape. Bacteria with a thick peptidoglycan layer but with no outer membrane stain purple and are called Gram positive. Bacteria with a thinner peptidoglycan layer but with an outer membrane stain pink and are called Gram negative. The cell wall is rigid, and imposes shape on the bacterium.

1.3.1 The Gram stain

The Gram stain has four stages.

1. A slide: containing a fixed smear of bacteria, it is initially covered with crystal violet for thirty seconds to a minute, which penetrates the cell wall and plasma membrane and stains the cells purple.
2. A mordant: Gram's iodine is added for about the same period and forms a complex with the crystal violet.
3. The slide: it is rinsed briefly with acetone, which interacts with the cell membrane lipids and removes the outer layer, exposing the peptidoglycan layer. As this layer is very thin in gram-negative bacteria, the crystal violet/iodine complex is easily washed away and the purple stain is removed, whereas the multilayered structure of gram-positive bacteria retains the purple stain.
4. A pink/red counterstain: neutral red or carbol fuchsin is applied to the slide for about a minute and gives a pink/red colour to the decolourized gram-negative bacteria, but the gram-positive bacteria retain their purple colour.

It is important to note that some bacteria, e.g., mycobacteria, also have fatty acids and waxes within the cell walls, making it very difficult for materials to pass through the wall and making them resistant to Gram staining. Hence, special stains e.g., the Ziehl–Neelsen stain are required.

1.3.2 The cell wall

This important structure surrounds the bacterium outside the plasma membrane. As human cells do not have cell walls, antimicrobials which work at this site, e.g., beta-lactams, are likely to have good selective toxicity, i.e., be much more toxic to bacteria compared to human cells. Different groups of bacteria have differently shaped walls. The main shapes are:

- Spherical (cocci): which may occur in pairs (diplococci) or clusters like grapes (staphylococci), or in long chains (streptococci);
- Rod shaped (bacilli);
- Comma shaped (vibrios); and
- Spiral (spirochaetes).

1.3.3 The cytoplasm

Within the bacterial cytoplasm are other structures, which include:

- the genome: a single circular chromosome. The genetic material is coiled and supercoiled under the control of the enzymes DNA gyrase and DNA topoisomerase;
- Bacterial mRNA: transcribed from DNA as in animal cells;
- Ribosomes: both bacteria and eukaryotic organisms have ribosomes. However, bacterial ribosomes are smaller than eukaryotic ribosomes. Bacterial ribosomes are 70 S ('S' refers to

Svedberg units, which is how a particle behaves under ultracentrifugation) and are composed of two sub-units—a 30s sub-unit, which contains 16S sRNA, and a 50 S sub-unit. Eukaryotic organisms are 80 S: they contain a 40 S sub-unit, which contains 18S RNA, and a 60 S sub-unit;

- Granules: some bacteria have granules containing stored nutrients;
- Mesosome: an invagination of the cell membrane, involved in cell division;
- Other constituents: proteins, carbohydrates, messenger and transfer RNA, amino acids, etc; and
- plasmids: these structures, which occasionally appear, are independently replicating fragments of circular double-stranded DNA.

1.3.4 The cell membrane

This is a phospholipid bilayer with embedded protein molecules and structures and is similar to that of eukaryotic membranes. Entry and exit of molecules through the membrane is controlled by permeases through a variety of mechanisms. The membrane has several important features:

- Pores to control the entrance and exit of substances, such as nutrients, waste products and toxins;
- Respiratory enzymes on its inner surface;
- Enzymes involved in cell wall synthesis on the outer surface; and
- Is involved in binary fission.

1.3.5 Other features present in some bacteria

- Endospores: tough, spherical forms that resist extremes of temperature. Spore formation is triggered by adverse environmental conditions. In this form they remain dormant, with the ability to survive for many years.
- A capsule: it is outside the cell wall in gram-positive bacteria or outside the outer membrane in gram-negative bacteria. The capsule is composed of carbohydrates and/or proteins and helps hide the antigenic proteins, making the bacteria more resistant to host cell phagocytosis.
- Flagella: whip-like structures that move, making the bacterium motile.
- Pili (fimbriae): long, thin, stiff structures that enable bacteria to adhere to the cells of the host through specialized molecules called adhesins.

1.3.6 Unusual types of bacteria

- *Chlamydia* spp.: small, difficult-to-see, gram-negative bacteria, which can only divide within host cells. They have a 'lifecycle' with two forms: the elementary body and the reticulate body. Both forms have a cell wall and an outer membrane. They are similar to viruses in that they have to replicate in a host cell, but they encode all of their own materials, except ATP which they cannot produce and obtain from the host.
- Rickettsia: only replicate within a host cell, but they lack the special structures and lifecycle of chlamydia. They are just small, fastidious bacteria with a gram-negative structure.
- *Mycoplasma* spp.: have no cell wall, are very small, and of no definite shape. As they have no cell wall, they are resistant to antibiotics such as the penicillins, cephalsosporins, carbapenems, and glycopeptides that act at this site.

1.4 Other basic ways of categorizing bacteria

- Microscopy (see 1.3.1): shape and staining characteristics. Most bacteria are gram-positive cocci or bacilli, or gram-negative cocci or bacilli, but some do not fit into either category.
- Growth characteristics, e.g., haemolysis, lactose fermentation, aerobic/anaerobic growth.
- Motility.
- Other tests include biochemical tests, antigen detection, toxin demonstration, or molecular techniques. Tests commonly used in the laboratory include:
  - Catalase test: used for gram-positive organisms only. Gram-positive cocci are divided into streptococci and staphylococci by catalase test. Staphylococci are catalase positive whereas streptococci are catalase negative.
  - Coagulase test for gram-positive organism only. Staphylococci are divided into coagulase positive (*S. aureus*) and coagulase negative by coagulase test.
  - Oxidase test, urease, etc.

1.5 How bacteria multiply

The rate at which bacteria grow and divide depends mainly on their nutritional environment. Bacteria divide by binary fission. The circular chromosome replicates by using a DNA-dependent DNA polymerase, with the help of DNA gyrase and DNA topoisomerase to facilitate uncoiling. When placed in a new environment, they undergo four sequential main phases.

1. Lag phase.
2. Exponential phase—with rapid growth and constant doubling rate.
3. Stationary phase—induced as nutrients are depleted and toxic products accumulate.
4. Death phase—cell growth declines and the cells die.

1.6 DNA exchange between bacteria

DNA can be exchanged between bacteria by various methods.

1. Conjugation: a conjugation tube forms between two bacteria, made by an outgrowth of the cell wall. Plasmids pass from one bacterium to the other along the tube.
2. Transduction: bacteriophage viruses infect bacteria and replicate. The new virions may incorporate bacterial genes from the chromosome or from plasmids, and transfer them to other bacteria.
3. Transformation: bacteria can pick up exogenous bacterial DNA.

1.7 What we need to know about each pathogen we study

Information you should know on each pathogen you study includes its:

- Ecology;
- Epidemiology;
- Structure and function;
- Virulence mechanisms;
- Effects on man; and
- Diagnosis, therapy, and prevention.

1.8 Assessment questions

1.8.1 Question 1

Bacterial cells are significantly different from human cells.

Which of the following is the most correct description of the differences between human and bacterial cells?

A. Bacteria are multicellular eukaryotes with a nuclear membrane and differently sized ribosomes to humans.
B. Bacteria are multicellular prokaryotic micro-organisms with no nuclear membrane and similarly sized ribosomes to humans.
C. Bacteria are unicellular eukaryotic organisms with a nuclear membrane and similarly sized ribosomes to humans.
D. Bacteria are unicellular prokaryotic micro-organisms with a nuclear membrane and differently sized ribosomes to humans.
E. Bacteria are unicellular prokaryotic micro-organisms with no nuclear membrane and differently sized ribosomes to humans.

1.8.2 Question 2

Staphylococcus aureus is a common cause of wound infection. The Gram film, catalase, and coagulase tests are commonly used to help identify infections caused by this organism in the laboratory.

Which of the following is the most accurate description of the properties of *Staphylococcus aureus*?

A. Gram-negative coccus, which is catalase negative, coagulase negative.
B. Gram-negative coccus, which is catalase negative, coagulase positive.
C. Gram-positive coccus, which is catalase negative, coagulase negative.
D. Gram-positive coccus, which is catalase positive, coagulase negative.
E. Gram-positive coccus, which is catalase positive, coagulase positive.

1.8.3 Question 3

Some, but not all, bacteria possess a capsule, which is generally regarded as a virulence factor.

Which of the following best describes the main pathogenic function(s) of a bacterium's capsule?
A. Induction of antibodies.
B. Mediation of detachment from host cell surface.
C. Prevention of bacteriophage-induced cell lysis.
D. Prevention of desiccation of bacterium.
E. Prevention of phagocytosis and complement-mediated cell lysis.

1.9 Answers and discussion

1.9.1 Answer 1

E. Bacteria are unicellular prokaryotic micro-organisms with no nuclear membrane and differently sized ribosomes to humans.

Bacteria are unicellular prokaryotic organisms with no nuclear membrane, unlike fungi, helminths, arthropods, protozoa, and human cells, all of which are eukaryotic. Bacteria also have smaller sized ribosomes (70 S) compared to eukaryotic organisms, which have 80 S ribosomes. In the diagnostic laboratory for important specimens, when an infective aetiology is thought likely but standard culture has been negative, the samples can be sent for sequencing of the 16 S gene (for bacteria) or 18 S for fungi to try and determine the infective cause. Additionally, the prokaryotic organisms have a cell wall, which the eukaryotic cells do not. These differences are important when trying to find an antimicrobial agent with good selective toxicity (selective toxicity means that the antimicrobial should be highly effective against the microbe, but have minimal or no toxicity to humans). The selective toxicity of antimicrobials is brought about by finding vulnerable targets for the drug in the microbe that either do not exist in humans or are dissimilar, e.g., differently sized ribosomes. As a general rule it is easier to do this for agents effective against the prokaryotic bacteria than against the eukaryotic fungi, helminths, arthropods, and protozoa.

1.9.2 Answer 2

E. Gram-positive coccus, which is catalase positive, coagulase positive.

The two most common types of aerobic/facultatively anaerobic gram-positive cocci are streptococci and staphylococci, and both can cause cellulitis and wound infections. Staphylococci can be differentiated from streptococci by a simple catalase test. In this test staphylococci are catalase positive whereas streptococci are catalase negative. Streptococci will then be further identified by whether or not they cause beta, alpha, or no haemolysis on blood agar plates. The beta-haemolytic streptococci, Groups A–G, especially Group A beta-haemolytic streptococci, are the most likely streptococci to cause cellulitis and wound infections. *Streptococcus pneumoniae* is the most well-known alpha-haemolytic streptococci and is a common cause of both community-acquired pneumonia and bacterial meningitis.

Staphylococci are identified further by a rapid test called the coagulase test; *S. aureus* are coagulase positive, whereas other staphylococci are coagulase negative. Both *S. aureus* and coagulase-negative staphylococci may be present on a person's skin. However, whereas *S. aureus* is a common cause of skin and soft tissue infections and can also cause severe bacterial endocarditis, osteomyelitis, sepsis, and pneumonia, coagulase-negative staphylococci generally only cause infection if people have prosthetic material in situ.

1.9.3 Answer 3

E. Prevention of phagocytosis and complement-mediated cell lysis.

For bacteria to cause disease in a host they need to escape phagocytosis by macrophages or polymorphonuclear phagocytes, and having a capsule is a common way they do this. If a capsule is removed from a normally capsulated bacterium it becomes much less pathogenic. The capsule has many pathogenic functions. It helps the bacteria to adhere to the host surface prior to invasion, The capsule prevents opsonization and prevents phagocytes adhering to and then engulfing the bacteria. It also deters neutrophil killing of engulfed bacteria. Additionally, the capsule helps shield the bacterium from desiccation and helps protect anaerobes from oxygen toxicity.

Induction of antibodies by the capsule is not one of it pathogenic functions. However, it is important in medicine because it is the basic of the serological diagnosis of infections caused by some capsulated bacterium. It is also the basis for vaccine production against some infections, e.g., the polyvalent (twenty-three serotypes) polysaccharide vaccine of the *Streptococcus pneumoniae* capsule.

CHAPTER 2

The biology of viruses

Anna Jeffery-Smith and C. Y. William Tong

2.1 What is a virus?

In order to be classified as a virus, certain criteria have to be fulfilled. Viruses must

- Be only capable of growth and multiplication within living cells, i.e. obligate intracellular parasite. Host cells could include humans, animals, insects, plants, protozoa, or even bacteria.
- Have a nucleic acid genome (either RNA or DNA, but not both) surrounded by a protein coat (capsid).
- Have no semipermeable membrane, though some have an envelope formed of phospholipids and proteins.
- Be inert outside of the host cell. Enveloped viruses are susceptible to inactivation by organic solvents such as alcohol.
- Perform replication by independent synthesis of components followed by assembly (c.f. binary fission in bacteria).

Viruses are considered as a bundle of genetic programmes encoded in nucleic acids and packaged with a capsid +/- envelope protein, which can be activated on entry into a host cell (compare this with computer viruses packaged in an enticing way in order to infect and take over control of your PC).

2.2 Why mycoplasma and chlamydia are not viruses

Although they share some similarities in their properties, mycoplasma and chlamydia are true bacteria (Table 2.1).

Table 2.1 Differences between mycoplasma/chlamydia and viruses

	Mycoplasma	Chlamydia	Viruses
Size	0.15–0.3 μm	~ 0.3 μm	0.017–1μm
Number of species	> 100 species	3 species of chlamydia (C. trachomatis, C. suis, C. muridarum) and 3 species of chlamydophila (C. psittaci, C. pneumoniae, C. pecorum)	Numerous (> 300,000 infecting mammals)
Semipermeable membrane	Has cell membrane but no cell wall	Has cell membrane but no cell wall	No, some virus have a lipid envelope containing viral proteins
Shape	Variable—spherical to filamentous	Spherical elementary bodies and larger intracellular reticulate bodies	Spherical (icosahedral), helical or complex (e.g., poxvirus, rabies virus)
Genome	Chromosomal DNA +/- plasmids	Chromosomal DNA +/- plasmids	Either DNA or RNA
Requires a living cell for growth and multiplication	No—can grow in tissue fluids	Obligatory intracellular, energy parasite as cannot produce ATP	Obligatory intracellular
Cytopathic effect (CPE)	No CPE, but can contaminate cell culture	Inclusion bodies identified by staining with Giemsa, iodine (if glycogen positive), or monoclonal antibodies	Variable—some viruses are cytocidal, others are not
Require cholesterol for membrane function and growth	Yes	Yes	No
Mode of replication	Binary fission	Binary fission	Independent synthesis of components and assembly
Susceptibility to antibiotics	Yes	Yes	No

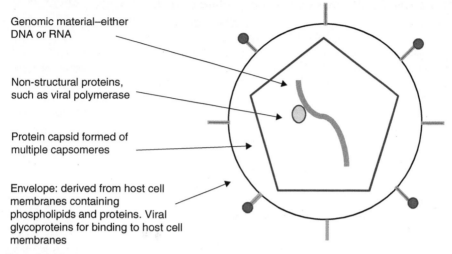

Genomic material–either
DNA or RNA

Non-structural proteins,
such as viral polymerase

Protein capsid formed of
multiple capsomeres

Envelope: derived from host cell
membranes containing
phospholipids and proteins. Viral
glycoproteins for binding to host cell
membranes

Figure 2.1 Virus structure.

2.3 The structure of a typical virus

The virion (assembled infectious particle) consists of viral nucleic acid and capsid (Figure 2.1).

The nucleic acid of a virus can either be ribonucleic acid (RNA) or deoxyribonucleic acid (DNA), and the amount of genetic material varies widely, with some viruses able to encode a few proteins and others having genetic material that encodes hundreds of proteins. In association with the nucleic acid there may be non-structural viral proteins, such as a viral polymerase. The nucleic acid and non-structural proteins are protected by a surrounding layer of capsid proteins. The capsid includes proteins which can attach to host cell receptors. The proteins and the cell receptors to which they bind determine a virus' tropism, i.e., the ability to bind to and enter different cell types. The term nucleocapsid refers to the nucleic acid core surrounded by capsid protein.

Some viruses also have an envelope made up of phospholipids and proteins surrounding the nucleocapsid. This envelope can be formed by the host cell membrane during the process of a virus budding from a cell during replication. Protein spikes from the envelope can also attach to cell receptors.

2.4 Virus classification

Viruses are grouped into families with similar properties based on morphology, chemical composition, and mode of replication.

2.4.1 Morphology

- Protein capsid shape: capsomeres form capsids of differing shapes—helical, icosahedral, or complex
- Presence or absence of an envelope

2.4.2 Chemical compositions and method of replication

The chemical composition of the genome, i.e., RNA or DNA, determines the mode of replication, i.e., the route to obtaining mRNA for translation of viral proteins.

DNA is single stranded, double stranded, or partially double stranded. RNA is single or double stranded. Single-stranded RNA genomes can be positive sense or negative sense, depending on whether the RNA genome is the same as the mRNA coded (positive sense) or forms the complementary strand to mRNA (negative sense).

Some viruses have a segmented genome with multiple pieces of nucleic acid, e.g., influenza viruses, rotavirus.

Viruses in the same family share a common morphology, genomic structure, and replication mechanism, e.g., all herpesviruses are composed of double-stranded DNA genome surrounded by an icosahedral protein capsid and a phospholipid envelope. However, modern taxonomy of virus is based on the degree of nucleic acid homology, rather than morphology. As a result, many viruses have been reclassified, e.g., echovirus 22 and 23 have been reclassified as parechovirus type 1 and type 2 based on their genetic differences from enteroviruses.

2.5 The Baltimore classification system and its use

The Baltimore classification system uses the nucleic acid composition and mechanism of replication to separate viruses into seven groups (Figure 2.2).

Coding +mRNA is the central point as this is the template from which viral proteins are translated by the host cell apparatus. The route to obtaining +mRNA is determined by the original nucleic acid composition of the genome. Viruses within a group all behave in a similar way during the process

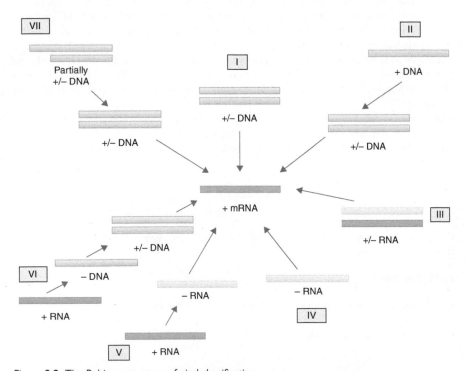

Figure 2.2 The Baltimore system of viral classification.

Table 2.2 The Baltimore system of classification of viruses

Baltimore group	Genome	Examples
I	dsDNA	Adenoviruses, herpesviruses, poxviruses
II	ssDNA	Parvoviruses
III	dsRNA	Reoviruses
IV	(+)ssRNA	Picornaviruses, togaviruses
V	(−)ssRNA	Orthomyxoviruses, rhabdoviruses
VI	(+)ssRNA RT	Retroviruses
VII	Partially dsDNA RT	Hepadnaviruses

ds: double stranded; ss: single stranded; (+) positive sense; (-) negative sense; RT: reverse transcriptase.

of replication, and so understanding of the virus and research into targets for antiviral medications can be based on this information. Grouping of viruses by disease phenotype or morphology does not guarantee this due to the diversity of viruses and similarities of infectious presentations. Table 2.2 gives examples of the viruses in each Baltimore group.

2.6 The life cycle of a virus

The main stages in the life cycle of a virus can be separated into attachment, penetration, uncoating, replication, assembly, and release (Figure 2.3).

1. Attachment: The virus attaches to the target cells occurs through specific binding between proteins on the viral surface and receptors on the host cell surface. The specificity of the viral surface protein determines the cell types to which the virus can bind, and therefore, which hosts and tissues it can infect.

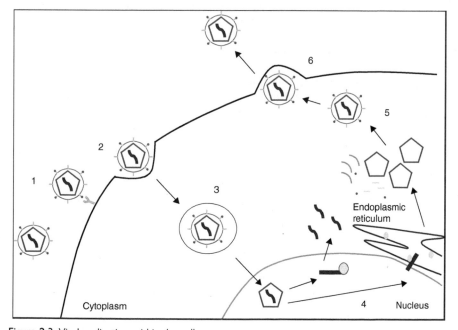

Figure 2.3 Viral replication within the cell.

2. Penetration: The viral particle is engulfed by the cell membrane.
3. Uncoating: Cellular lysosymes remove the viral envelope if one is present. The capsid is often removed following trafficking of the viral genomic material to the nucleus.
4. Replication: The components required to assemble new viral particles are produced by the infected cell. Copies of the viral genome are made using the cell's nucleotides. Viral proteins are translated from viral mRNA using the cell's ribosomes on the endoplasmic reticulum.
5. Assembly: Virions are assembled from viral nucleic acid and viral proteins. This can occur in the cell nucleus or cytoplasm.
6. Release: Assembled virions are released from the cell, either by budding from the cell membrane, which for enveloped viruses contributes to the formation of the envelope, or by cell lysis, whereby the cell dies during the release of viral particles.

2.7 The importance of the cellular receptor

The cellular receptor determines which cells a virus can enter—the tissue tropism of the virus (Table 2.3). The proteins within the capsid or envelope of a virus determine to which host cell receptors the virus can bind, and therefore, which cells it can enter and replicate. Some viruses have widespread host tissue tropism, i.e., their receptors result in an ability to bind and enter multiple cell types. Other viruses are very limited in which cells they can bind to and enter.

Cellular receptors are also important as a potential therapeutic target. If the binding between viral surface proteins and cellular receptors can be blocked the virus will not be able to enter and replicate within the cell.

2.8 The effects of selection pressure on a virus

Natural selection determines that individuals most suited phenotypically to the environment are more likely to survive and reproduce. Phenotypic variation in viruses determined by genetic variation means that some viruses will be better adapted to the changing host environment during the course of infection, and more likely to survive to perpetuate infection and be transmitted to others.

During the course of viral infection the environment of the host can change in multiple ways, e.g., through host immune system formation of antibodies in response to infection and development of specific cytotoxic T cells targeting viral epitopes on infected cells. External factors like antiviral

Table 2.3 Examples of viruses and their cellular receptors

Virus	Cellular receptor	Cell type
HIV	CD4 + co-receptor (CCR5 or CXCR4)	CD4+ cells including T lymphocytes and macrophages
Hepatitis B virus	Sodium taurocholate co-transporting polypeptide	Hepatocytes
Hepatitis C virus	CD81	Hepatocytes
Primate erythroparvovirus 1 (formerly Parvovirus B19)	Erythrocyte P antigen	Erythroid progenitor cells
Rabies	Acetylcholine receptor	Neurons
Rhinovirus (major group)	Intercellular adhesion molecule 1 (ICAM-1)	Respiratory epithelial cells

medications will also apply selection pressure. Features favouring survival in the face of these pressures arise from genetic mutations during viral replication that cause phenotypic differences in viral progeny. Mutations occur naturally during virion production in the host cell, and are more likely to occur in some viruses, e.g. HIV and hepatitis B, than others due to the nature of the enzymes involved in replication. The majority of mutations arising through this route will be lost due to reduced viral fitness, but some will become fixed in the population due to advantages such as resistance to anti-viral medications. In the face of anti-viral selection pressure virus with the anti-viral resistance mutation will become the dominant viral population.

2.9 Outcomes for a cell infected with a virus

The outcome of a cell infected with a virus depends on both the cell type and the virus. Infected cells that support viral replication are called permissive. Cells that do not support the virus infection—and so cannot be used to produce viral progeny—result in abortive infection.

Alterations to a cell following infection with a virus can be morphological, physiological, and biochemical, and can include toxic effects on the genetic composition of the cell. Combined, these effects can result in one of three outcomes for the cell—cell death, persistent infection, or transformation of the cell. Within an infected individual the virus can demonstrate all of these effects on host cells, e.g., Epstein-Barr Virus (EBV) can cause an acute infection with cytocidal effects in some infected cells, resulting in the symptoms of glandular fever syndrome. In other infected cells the virus can become latent, with the ability to reactivate in the future, and in some cells, transformation can occur resulting in an EBV-related malignancy (Table 2.4).

2.9.1 Cell death

Infection results in the hijacking of cellular machinery to produce viral progeny. This can cause death of the cell by the following routes:

- Immune killing of the cell—the host immune system recognizes the cell as being infected and it is destroyed.
- Direct viral effects—the effects of viral production cause changes in the cell such that cellular apoptosis occurs when the cell is unable to fulfil its usual functions, e.g., by damage of cellular DNA during viral replication causing genetic instability and cell death.

Table 2.4 Examples of malignancies associated with viruses

Virus	Associated malignancy
Epstein–Barr Virus	Nasopharyngeal carcinoma Burkitt's lymphoma EBV-associated B cell lymphoma
Hepatitis B virus	Hepatocellular carcinoma
Hepatitis C virus	Hepatocellular carcinoma Lymphoma
Human T cell lymphotropic virus type 1 (HTLV-1)	Adult T cell leukaemia/lymphoma (ATLL)
Human Herpes Virus 8	Kaposi's sarcoma Primary effusion lymphoma Castleman's disease
Human papillomavirus	Cervical cancer Ano-genital cancer Oropharyngeal cancer

2.9.2 Persistent infection

The virus remains in some of the host's cells following an initial acute infection, often with minimal detectable changes in the host. This can occur with chronic infection, latent infection, and transforming infections:

- Chronic infection—e.g., hepatitis B. After initial infection some host cells remain infected and actively synthesize viral particles, continuing to release viral progeny but with minimal resulting cell death. Virus and viral proteins continue to be detectable in laboratory testing, but the infection appears to be kept in check by host immune system factors such that damage to the host through viral replication is not detectable, or appears to be minimal. These hosts remain infectious to others.
- Latent infection—e.g. herpesviruses. All herpesviruses are characterized by the ability to remain latent in their target cell. In latent infection the viral genome persists in certain host cells and retains the ability to reactivate and utilize cellular machinery to produce virus and cause cytopathic effects in the future. Between episodes of reactivation viral replication is restricted and viral nucleic acid cannot be detected. Reactivation can occur as a result of effects on the immune system reducing immune surveillance. Environmental stressors causing immunosuppression include infection with another virus (e.g. HIV), stress to the host caused by bacterial sepsis or organ dysfunction due to non-infectious causes, or iatrogenic immunosuppression as a result of chemotherapy. Between episodes of reactivation the patient is not infectious.

2.9.3 Transformation

The cell develops the potential to become cancerous after viral infection. In such cases the virus causes alterations to the cellular DNA such that the cell becomes immortal, usually by incorporation of the viral genetic material into that of the cell. Following immortalization viral proteins acting as transcription factors can inactivate tumour suppressor genes resulting in impaired cell cycle regulation. During unregulated cellular replication, mutations in other cellular genes are likely to develop, resulting in cumulative genetic changes and highly abnormal malignant cells with the ability to invade tissues (Table 2.4).

2.10 Assessment questions

2.10.1 Question 1

A patient known to have long-standing, well-controlled HIV on combination anti-retroviral therapy (cART) with undetectable plasma viral load presents with new onset confusion. A contrast CT scan of the head shows volume loss, but no focal lesions. Lumbar puncture is performed and the following results are obtained:

	Plasma	Cerebrospinal fluid (CSF)
HIV viral load ($\log^{10}$ copies/ml)	Not detected	4.7

What mechanism is the most likely to explain these discordant results between plasma and CSF?
A. Elite controller.
B. Failure of drug penetration to central nervous system (CNS).
C. Poor adherence to cART.
D. Progressive multifocal leucoencephalopathy (PML).
E. Switching co-receptor usage to CXCR4.

2.10.2 Question 2

A patient is immunosuppressed following chemotherapy for lung cancer. She subsequently presents to hospital with a unilateral vesicular rash on her trunk, associated with burning pain. She is diagnosed and commenced on anti-viral medication.

In which cell type does the causative virus lie dormant?
A. Astrocytes.
B. B lymphocytes.
C. Dorsal root ganglion cells.
D. Hepatocytes.
E. Purkinje cells.

2.10.3 Question 3

A patient who is co-infected with HIV and hepatitis B virus is started on a regimen that contains tenofovir and emtricitabine (Truvada).

What is the target of this drug combination?
A. Cellular RNA polymerase II.
B. DNA-dependent DNA polymerase.
C. DNA-dependent RNA polymerase.
D. RNA-dependent DNA polymerase.
E. RNA-dependent RNA polymerase.

2.11 Answers and discussion

2.11.1 Answer 1

B. Failure of drug penetration to CNS.
Certain anatomical sites in the body, such as the CNS and the genital tract, are identified as sanctuary sites whereby the selection pressure on the virus could be different from other parts of the body. This could result in compartmentalization with a different rate of virus replication and development of drug resistance. One of the mechanisms that leads to compartmentalization is the restriction of penetration of certain antiretroviral agents into CNS. This patient probably has good adherence to cART as the plasma viral load is undetectable. Nevertheless, the antiviral agents for this patient need to be reviewed. CNS HIV are often R5 in tropism but a tropism test will be required if CCR5 entry inhibitors are to be used for intensification.

2.11.2 Answer 2

C. Dorsal root ganglion cells.
Varicella-zoster virus as the causative agent of shingles lies dormant in the dorsal root ganglia. Immunosuppression, as in the case of this patient, can result in the virus reactivating and the patient developing shingles. The vesicular rash typically arises in a dermatomal distribution, reflecting the sensory nerve root from which the virus has reactivated. In those who are heavily immunosuppressed, reactivation of varicella can become widely disseminated. In addition, viral shedding from lesions will persist for far longer periods than from immune-competent individuals with the concomitant infection control concerns.

2.11.3 Answer 3

D. RNA-dependent DNA polymerase.
RNA-dependent DNA polymerase is reverse transcriptase, which is used in the replication cycle of both HIV and hepatitis B virus. Tenofovir and emtricitabine are nucleos(t)ide analogues

that target reverse transcriptase encoded by the virus. Neither HIV nor HBV uses host polymerase enzymes. RNA-dependent RNA polymerase enzymes are commonly carried by RNA viruses; DNA-dependent DNA polymerase can be viral (in DNA virus) or host. DNA-dependent RNA polymerases (transcriptase) are used by viruses and host to transcribe DNA into RNA.

CHAPTER 3

The biology of fungi

Stephanie J. Smith and Rohini J. Manuel

3.1 Fungi and how they are classified

Fungi are found ubiquitously in the environment such as soil, water, and food. There are an estimated 1.5 million fungal species worldwide, although this number is felt to be grossly underestimated and is regularly updated. Of these vast numbers, around 500 fungi to date have been implicated in human disease.

As opposed to bacteria, which are prokaryotes, fungi are eukaryotes, meaning they have a well-defined nucleus and have membrane-bound organelles in the cytoplasm, including an endoplasmic reticulum and a golgi apparatus.

In 1969, the scientist R. H. Whittaker first proposed that organisms be classified into five kingdoms: *Monera* (Bacteria), *Protista* (Algae and Protozoans), *Plantae* (Plants), *Mycetae* (Fungi), and *Animalia* (Animals). Since then, there have been dramatic changes to the classifications of fungi, largely due to the appliance of phylogenetic molecular techniques. This has resulted in variances to the number of phylums, and the species assigned to them.

Table 3.1 shows the seven phyla of the Fungi Kingdom.

The majority of fungi pathogenic to humans inhabit the Ascomycota and Basidiomycota phyla.

Fungi used to be dually named if they had a pleomorphic life cycle with sexual/asexual stages (*teleomorph/anamorph*, respectively), which meant that fungi often had two names and were classed differently. This practice was discontinued in January 2013 after the International Commission on the Taxonomy of Fungi decided that a 'one fungus, one name' approach should be followed.

3.2 The fungal structure and its notable organelles

Fungi can be unicellular (yeast) or multicellular (fungi). Yeasts may look globose in nature when grown, whereas multicellular fungi grow as tubular, filamentous material called *hyphae* that can create a branching, hyphal network called a *mycelium*. Hyphae may have septa that cross their walls or be nonseptate, which is a method of differentiating fungi. An early hyphal outgrowth from a spore is called a *germ tube*. The germ tube test can be used to differentiate the yeasts *Candida albicans* and *Candida dubliniensis* from other *Candida* species.

Table 3.1 Kingdom Fungi and examples

Ascomycota	Largest phylum in the kingdom Examples: *Candida* spp., *Fusarium* spp., *Aspergillus* spp., *Saccharomyces* spp., *Penicillium* spp.
Basidiomycota	Second-largest phylum in the kingdom. This group and the Ascomycota make up the *Dikarya* subkingdom Example: *Cryptococcus* spp.
Glomeromycota	Example: *Rhizopus* spp.
Chytridiomycota	The Chytridiomycota are unique among all fungi in having motile stages in their life cycles; no other fungi have this trait Example: *Rhizophidium* spp.
Microsporidia	Once considered protozoans. Lack mitochondria and can produce spores Example: Toxospora
Blastocladiomycota	Example: *Coelomomyces spp.*
Neocallimastigomycota	Anaerobic fungi commonly found in animal digestive tracts Example: *Piromyces* spp.

The fungal cell wall is composed of chitin and glucans, which are different components to the human cell wall. This means that they can be an effective target for antifungal therapy.

Some fungi grow solely as *yeasts*, which undergo asexual reproduction by budding (budding yeasts) or binary fission (fission yeasts). An example is *Saccharomyces cerevisiae,* a budding yeast.

Some types of fungi are able to exist in both yeast and mould forms (depending on environmental temperature and conditions), and these are called *dimorphic fungi*. Examples include *Histoplasma* and *Coccidioides* species.

Candida albicans is a polymorphic fungus that can grow either as an ovoid-shaped budding yeast, as elongated ellipsoid cells with constrictions at the septa (pseudohyphae), or as parallel-walled true hyphae.

Spores can be produced by fungi, and vary in size and structure.

Some fungal structures are characteristic of a particular species. For example, *Aspergillus* and *Penicillium* species have multiple-branched hyphae with flask-shaped phialides and conidial spores at the end, which are released to disseminate in the environment (Figure 3.1)

Fungi can be described as being *heterotrophic*, meaning that they use organic carbon for growth. They can be further divided into *photoheterotrophs* and *chemoheterotrophs*.

Fungi generate energy from a variety of methods (Table 3.2).

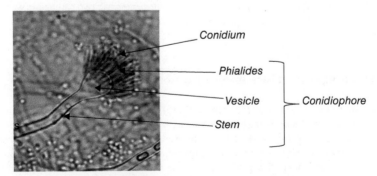

Figure 3.1 Conidiophore of *Aspergillus* spp.
Reproduced courtesy of UK NEQAS.

Table 3.2 Methods of fungal energy production

Biotrophs	Receive nutrients from a living host
Saprotrophs	Derive nutrients from dead plants/animals
Chemoheterotrophic	Utilization of organic carbon sources in the environment and subsequent energy produced from these to make further compounds grow
Photoheterotrophic	Fungi that use light for energy, but cannot use carbon dioxide as their sole carbon source

Smaller compounds, like amino acids, can be absorbed via the cell wall. Larger proteins must be broken down first by extracellular enzymes to allow for absorption.

3.3 The key elements of the fungal reproductive cycle

Reproduction in fungi can either be asexual or sexual, the latter being a more complicated process (Figure 3.2 and 3.3).

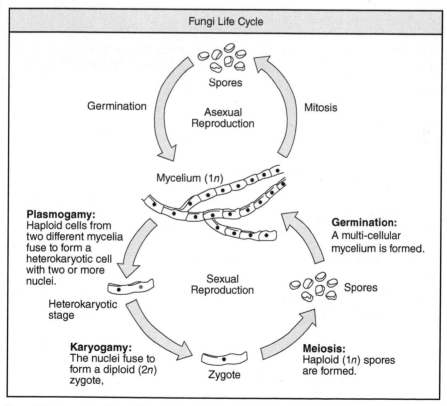

Figure 3.2 Asexual and sexual fungal reproduction.

Reproduced from Boundless Biology. *Fungi Reproduction.* Boundless Biology and Lumen. Copyright © 2016 Boundless Biology. Available at: https://www.boundless.com/biology/textbooks/boundless-biology-textbook/fungi-24/characteristics-of-fungi-149/fungi-reproduction-591-11810/

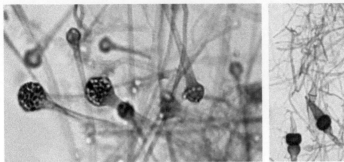
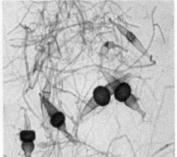

Figure 3.3 Mucoraceous mould structures of asexual and sexual spores.
Reproduced with permission from Wahlert, J. H. et al, *Laboratory Notes for BIO 1003*. Copyright © 1999 John H. Wahlert & Mary Jean Holland. Available at: http://faculty.baruch.cuny.edu/jwahlert/bio1003/fungi.html

3.3.1 Asexual reproduction

Asexual reproduction occurs via *spores*. The resulting offspring are genetically similar to the parents and are produced by mitosis. Spores may be endogenous or exogenous in nature (*sporangium* and *conidia*, respectively). Different genera may be identified by the characteristics of their conidia, such as their shape, size, and pigmentation. The sporangium is essentially an enclosed ball of spores that may be released to disseminate freely in the environment.

Asexual reproduction can also occur via a process termed *fragmentation*. The ends of hyphae may break to produce fragments (arthrospores) that can develop into new individuals. The hyphae may also detach via *fission* or *budding*. An example of budding occurs in *Saccharomyces* species.

3.3.2. Sexual reproduction

Sexual reproduction has a *haploid* and *diploid* phase. The haploid phase (*One set of chromosomes*) possesses the (n) number of chromosomes in the nucleus, whereas this number becomes (2n) in the diploid phase (*two homologous copies of each chromosome, usually one from the mother and one from the father*).

The gametes are haploid (n) and, by sexual reproduction, become diploid (2n) sexual spores. To become haploid (n) cells once more, meiosis occurs and the number of chromosomes halves. The fusion of the plasma of the gametes is called *plasmogamy*, which is usually followed by the nuclear fusion called *karyogamy*.

Examples of sexual spores include *zygospores* and *basidiospores*.

When both the gametes occur on the same mycelium, the fungus is said to be *homothallic*, and when they are found on different mycelia, the fungus is called *heterothallic*.

3.4 The structures of a spore and why they are important for the survival of fungi

Spores are specialized structures of a fungus that function as an effective dispersal method to allow for spread of a species, further reproduction, and provide dormancy in unfavourable environmental conditions for a prolonged period of time. After they are produced they can be easily dispersed in the environment, permitting transportation to areas that may potentially be more nutritionally beneficial to the spore.

Fungal spores can be produced via asexual or sexual reproduction—(see Section 3.3).

Spores may be unicellular or multicellular. They are composed of an outer exosporium surrounding an inner core. The cell wall is very resistant to any adverse conditions, including extreme cold, heat, desiccation, and pH changes. The inner core contains a nutrient source of glycogen and lipids that allows for nourishment, although the spore itself decreases its metabolic actions during the dormant phase. Spores are capable of germinating to produce new hyphae when environmental conditions improve, which could be days to years.

Of note, fungal spores may present a challenge to hospital infection prevention and control teams, as they require specific methods of sterilization to ensure they are effectively killed.

3.5 Assessment questions

3.5.1 Question 1

A forty-two-year old HIV-positive man presents acutely to hospital with confusion and photophobia. He is poorly compliant with his anti-retroviral medications, and his most recent CD4 count is 10/µl. An India ink-positive organism is found on microscopic examination of cerebrospinal fluid.

Which fungal kingdom does the likely pathogen belong to?
A. Ascomycota.
B. Basidiomycota.
C. Chytridiomycota.
D. Glomeromycota.
E. Neocallimastigomycota.

3.5.2 Question 2

A thirty-five-year old woman is admitted to the ITU of a busy district general hospital with oro-pharyngeal candidiasis. Culture of a mouth swab isolates *Candida albicans*.

Which of the following is characteristic of *Candida albicans*?
A. It cannot be stained by Calcofluor white.
B. It gives a positive germ tube test result after 2–4 hours.
C. It belongs to the phylum Basidiomycota.
D. It produces a late hyphal outgrowth from a spore after incubation for 1 day.
E. It undergoes both asexual and sexual reproduction.

3.5.3 Question 3

The structural components of which fungus is typified in Figure 3.4?
A. Aspergillus.
B. Fusarium.
C. Mucor.
D. Penicillium.
E. Rhizopus.

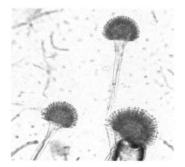

Figure 3.4 Fungal Microscopy.

3.6 Answers and discussion

3.6.1 Answer 1

B. Basidiomycota

Cryptococcus species belong to the second largest phylum in the fungal kingdom. This group, together with the Ascomycota, make up the Dikarya subkingdom.

3.6.2 Answer 2

B. It gives a positive germ tube test result after 2–4 hours.

Candida albicans (*Candida* species) belongs to the largest phylum in the fungal kingdom, along with other fungi such as *Aspergillus* species, *Fusarium* species, *Penicillium* species, and *Saccharomyces* species. *Candida albicans* produces an early hyphal outgrowth from a spore, called a germ tube. A positive germ tube test result may be used to identify *Candida albicans* (and *Candida dubliniensis*).

3.6.3 Answer 3

A. Aspergillus

Aspergillus spp. have characteristic conidiophores which are short and smooth walled, and have flask-shaped terminal vesicles that support a series of spore-bearing cells called phialides. Repeated mitotic division yields a chain of asexual spores called conidia. Conidia are extremely hydrophobic and easily dispersed by air.

Parasites and worms

Robert Serafino Wani

4.1 Why parasites and worms are important?

A parasite is an organism that lives on or in a host and gets its food from or at the expense of its host. Worms or helminths either live as parasites or free of a host in aquatic and terrestrial environments. Parasites and worms are found worldwide but mainly in the tropics. It is estimated that 20% of immigrants from endemic countries may have helminthic infections at their arrival to the UK. These people could be asymptomatic, but tend to present with unexplained symptoms, especially gastrointestinal in nature or eosinophilia. Travellers to endemic countries tend to be newly infected and have greater immune response and pronounced eosinophilia in some but not all parasitic infections.

Parasites that can cause disease in humans fall under three classes: protozoa, helminths, and ectoparasites

4.2 What are protozoa?

Protozoa (Table 4.1) are microscopic, one-celled organisms that can be free living or parasitic in nature. Transmission of protozoa that live in a human's intestine to another human typically occurs through a faeco-oral route (for example, contaminated food or water, or person-to-person contact). Protozoa that live in the blood or tissue of humans are transmitted to other humans by an arthropod vector (for example, through the bite of a mosquito or sand fly).

4.3 What are helminths?

Helminths are large, multicellular organisms that are generally visible to the naked eye in their adult stages. Like protozoa, helminths can be either free living or parasitic.

There are three main groups of helminths that parasitize humans: cestodes, trematodes, and nematodes.

Table 4.1 Examples of protozoa that infect humans.

Intestinal protozoa	Extra-intestinal protozoa
Balantidium coli	Amoebic meningoencephalitis e.g. *Naegleria fowleri*
Cryptosporidum parvum	*Babesia microti* (Babesiosis)
Blastocystis hominis	*Leishmaniasis* species
Cyclspora cayetensis	Malaria *Falciparum* species
Dientamoeba fragilis	*Toxoplasma gondii*
Entamoeba histolytica	*Trichomonas vaginalis*
Giardia lamblia	Trypanosomiasis (*Trypanosoma brucei rhodesiense, Trypanosoma brucei ghambiense, Trypanosoma cruzii*)
Isospora belli	
Microsporidium species	
Non pathogenic: *Entamoeba dispar*	

Table 4.2 Examples of nematodes that infect humans.

Intestinal nematodes	Extra-intestinal nematodes
Anisakis simplex (Anisakiasis)	*Ancylostoma braziliense, caninum* (Cutaneous larva migrans)
Ascaris lumbricoides	*Dracunculus medinensis*
Enterobius vermicularis	*Toxocara canis/catis*
Capillaria philippinensis	Filariasis
Hookworms (*Necator americanus, Ancyclostoma duodenale*)	*Gnathostoma spinigerum*
Strongyloides stercoralis	*Trichinella spiralis*
Trichurus trichiura, whipworm	

A. Cestodes (tapeworms)

These are flat worms that comprise *Echinococcus* species: intestinal tapeworms and neurocysticercosis (*Taenia solium*)

B. Trematodes (Flukes)

These are leaf-shaped, and they vary in length from a few millimetres to 8 cm. They include:
- Liver fluke: Clonorchis sinensis, *Fasciola hepatica*
- Intestinal fluke: *Fasciola buski, Heterophyes heterophyes,*
- Lung fluke: *Paragonimus westernmani*
- Blood flukes: Schistosoma species

C. Nematodes (roundworms)
These are cylindrical in structure (see Table 4.2).

4.4 What are ectoparasites?

Blood-sucking arthropods such as mosquitoes are considered as ectoparasites because they depend on blood meal for their survival. Narrowly speaking, ectoparasites include organisms like ticks, fleas, lice, and mites (scabies) that attach or burrow into the skin and remain there for relatively long periods of time (e.g. weeks to months).

4.5 The epidemiology of parasitic infections

Parasitic infections cause a tremendous burden of disease in both the tropics and subtropics as well as in more temperate climates (Tables 4.3, 4.4, and 4.5). Of all parasitic diseases, malaria causes the most deaths globally (interested readers are referred to Chapter 57 for more information).

4.6 How parasitic infection should be investigated?

Table 4.6 listed the diagnostic tests for some common parasitic infections.

4.7 Further reading and useful resources

http://www.cdc.gov/parasites/about.html
https://www.gov.uk/guidance/helminth-infections-migrant-health-guide
Arosemena, R., Booth, S. A., Su, W. P., 'Cutaneous Myiasis', *Journal of the American Academy of Dermatology*, 28 (1993), 254.
Checkley, A. M., Chiodini, P. L., Dockrell, D. H., Bates, I., Thwaites, G. E., Booth, H. L., Brown, M., Wright, S. G., Grant, A. D., Mabey, D. C., Whitty, C. J. M., Sanderson, F., 'Eosinophilia in Returning Travellers and Migrants from the Tropics: UK Recommendations for Investigation and Initial Management', *Journal of Infection*, 60/1 (2009), 1–20.

4.8 Assessment questions

4.8.1 Question 1

A fifty-year-old female presents with fever, rigors, and right upper quadrant pain. Liver ultrasound is suggestive of a liver abscess. She has had no change in bowel habits in her recent past. She moved to the United Kingdom from Pakistan forty years ago. Despite five days of intravenous antibiotics (coamoxiclav and gentamicin) she continues to feel unwell and has a sustained fever of > 38 degrees.

What is the most appropriate antimicrobial agent to add to the current regimen?
A. Amikacin.
B. Amphotericin B.
C. Clindamycin.
D. Meropenem.
E. Metronidazole.

4.8.2 Question 2

A sixty-year-old female Afro-Caribbean woman is referred by her GP to the infectious disease clinic for investigation of an eosinophilia of 0.8 which was found after a routine blood check. Her strongyloides serology is found to be positive.

What viral infection is the most likely to predispose to disseminated strongyloidiasis in this patient?
A. HHV-6.
B. HHV-8.
C. HIV-1.
D. HIV-2.
E. HTLV-1.

Table 4.3 Global distribution and clinical manifestations of common protozoal infections.

Geographical area	Parasite	Common syndrome, name	Mode of transmission	Clinical features	Treatment
Worldwide	Entamoeba histolytica	Amoebiasis	Faeco-oral	Dysentery Abdominal pain Liver abscess	Metronidazole/Tinidazole (Trophozoites) Diloxanide furaote/Paromomycin (cysts)
	Giardia lamblia	Giardiasis	Faeco-oral	Bloating Flatulence Abdominal pain	Metronidazole/Tinidazole
	Cryptosporidium Parvum C. hominis	Cryptosporidiosis	Faeco-oral	Diarrhoea Abdominal pain Cholecystitis Cholangitis Pancreatitis	Nitazoxanide Paromomycin
	Balantidium coli	Balantidiasis	Faeco-oral	Diarrhoea Abdominal pain Dysentry	Tetracycline Metronidazole Tinidazole Paraomomycin
South Asia, East Africa, Mediterranean, The Middle East, South Europe, Latin America	Leishmania donovani L. infantam	Visceral leishmaniasis Kala-azar (Black fever)	Sand fly bite	Fever Malaise Weight loss Splenomegaly	Amphotericin B Sodium stibogluconate Miltefosine
Old World Africa	L. major L. tropica L. ethiopica	Cutaneous leishmaniasis	Sand fly bite	papule painless ulcer	Spontaneous healing Intralesional sodium stibogluconate Miltefosine
New World South and Central Americas	L. mexican L. venezuelensis L. amazonensis L. brazilensis L. paruviana L. gayanensis L. panamensis	Cutaneous and mucocutaneous leishmaniasis	Sand fly bite	Multiple skin ulcers, erosion of mucosal surfaces Nasal septum deformity	Miltefosine Systemic sodium stibogluconate Amphotericin B

Table 4.4 Global distribution and clinical manifestations of common helminthic infections.

Geographical area	Parasite	Common syndrome, name	Mode of transmission	Clinical features	Treatment
Worldwide	Ancylostoma duodenale	Hookworm	Larva penetrate the skin while walking barefoot or lying on affected soil	GI: nausea, vomiting, diarrhoea Cutaneous: transient itch, maculopapular rash Other: fever, dry cough (Loeffler's syndrome)	Albendazole
	Ascaris lumbricoides	Roundworm	Faeco-oral	GI: Abdominal pain, diarrhoea, biliary obstruction Respiratory: Wheeze, dry cough (Loeffler's syndrome)	Albendazole or mebendazole
	Echinococcus granulosus	Cystic hydatid	Ingestion of eggs from canine faeces or via contaminate vegetable matter	Asymptomatic, GI: right upper quadrant pain Respiratory: cough, pleuritic pain, breathlessness Other: anaphylaxis	Praziquantel (Abendazole—post-operatively)
	Enterobius vermicularis	Pinworm, threadworm	Faeco-oral	GI: diarrhoea, abdominal pain, weight loss Cutaneous: pruritus ani Other: vaginal discharge	Albendazole or mebendazole
Worldwide	Fasciola hepatica	Fascioliasis	Consumption of vegetation contaminate with encysted intermediate stage metacercariae	Fever GI: upper abdominal pain, biliary obstruction, and hepatic abscesses	Triclabendazole
	Necator americanus	Hookworm	Larva penetrate the skin while walking barefoot or lying on affected soil	GI: nausea, vomiting, diarrhoea Cutaneous: transient itch, maculopapular rash Other: fever, dry cough (Loeffler's syndrome)	Albendazole
	Strongyloides stercoralis	Strongyloidiasis	Larva penetrate the skin while walking barefoot or affected soil	Respiratory: Wheeze, dry cough (Loeffler's syndrome), hyperinfestation syndrome (paralytic ileus and gram-negative septicaemia with pulmonary involvement) GI: diarrhoea, abdominal pain, bloating, hyperinfestation syndrome Cutaneous: itchy urticarial rash (larva currens)	Ivermectin or Albendazole

Table 4.4 Continued

Geographical area	Parasite	Common syndrome, name	Mode of transmission	Clinical features	Treatment
	Taenia saginata	Beef tapeworm	Consumption of undercooked beef	GI: abdominal pain, diarrhoea, segments expelled in faeces	Praziquantel
	Toxocara canis *Toxocara catis*	Visceral larva migrans	Ingestion of soil containing larva or through eating raw meat	Respiratory: wheeze Gastrointestinal: abdominal pain, hepatosplenomegaly CNS: meningoencephalitis	Albendazole plus steroids and antihistamines for hypersensitivity reactions
	Trichuris trichiura	Whipworm	Faeco-oral	GI: diarrhoea, dysentery	Albendazole or Mebendazole
	Trichinella spiralis	Trichenellosis, trichinosis	Consumption of raw or undercooked meat, usually pork	GI: Upper abdominal pain, fever, vomiting, diarrhoea Dysphagia CNS: meningo-encephalitis Cutaneous/muscle: periorbital oedema, urticaria, myalgia, muscle weakness Others: myocarditis, cardiac conduction disturbances	Albendazole plus Prednisolone (severe disease)
Worldwide, tropical only	*Ancylostoma* species	Cutaneous larva migrans	Larva penetrate the skin while walking barefoot or lying on affected soil	Cutaneous: serpiginous rash	Ivermectin or Albendazole
	Hymenolepis nana	Dwarf tapeworm	Faeco-oral	GI: diarrhoea, abdominal pain	Praziquantel
	Taenia solium	Pork tapeworm	Consumption of undercooked beef	GI: abdominal pain, diarrhoea, segments expelled per rectum CNS: usually space occupy lesions, meningoencephalitis	Praziquantel
	Wuchereria bancrofti	Lymphatic filariasis, tropical pulmonary eosinophilia	Mosquito borne	Respiratory: Dry cough, wheeze, breathlessness, and fever (tropical pulmonary eosinophilia) Cutaneous: lymphadenitis, lymphoedema	Diethylcarbamazine

Region	Organism	Disease	Transmission	Clinical features	Treatment
Africa	Loa loa	Eye worm, Calabar swelling	bite from Chrysops fly	Calabar swelling Eyes: conjunctival worm migration	Diethylcarbamazine
Africa (predominantly central and western)	Onchocerca volvulus	Onchocerciasis, river blindness	Simulium black fly bite	Cutaneous: nodules, pruritic dermatitis, hypopigmented patches, limb swelling Eyes: keratitis, anterior uveitis, choroidoretinitis, blindness	Ivermectin
Africa, Yemen, and India	Dracunculus medinensis	Dracunculiasis or Guinea worm	Consumption of unfiltered water containing copepods (small crustaceans) infected with larvae	Cutaneous: papule, pruritus Worm can migrate to ectopic sites (lung, eye, pericardium, or spinal cord) and can produce abscesses	Worm extraction Wound care
South Asia Oceania	Brugia malayi	Lymphatic filariasis	Mosquito-borne	Respiratory: Dry cough, wheeze, breathless (Tropical pulmonary syndrome)	Diethylcarbamazine (DEC)
Middle East, Central Asia, Africa, South America	Schistosoma haematobium	Bilharzia Katayama syndrome	Cercariae penetrate the skin during fresh water exposure	Cutaneous: urticarial rash Respiratory: dry cough, haematuria, haematospermia, paraplegia, spinal cord syndromes	Praziquantel
	Schistosoma mansoni	Bilharzia Katayama syndrome	Cercariae penetrate the skin during fresh water exposure	Cutaneous: urticarial rash GI: abdominal pain, diarrhoea, hepatosplenomegaly, portal hypertension CNS: Paraplegia, spinal cord syndromes	Praziquantel
South-East Asia, South and Central America, Caribbean	Anisakis species	Fish tapeworm	Larva in raw or pickled fish	GI: Severe abdominal pain, diarrhoea	Albendazole Endoscopic or surgical removal of the worm
	Gnathostoma Spinigerum	Gnathostomiasis	Ingestion of larva in undercooked fish, frog, snake, or chicken	Cutaneous: intermittent subcutaneous nodules, pruritus GI: abdominal pain CNS: meningo-encephalitis and myelitis, focal neurology, subarachnoid haemorrhage	Albendazole plus Prednisolone
	Paragonimus westermanii	Paragonimiasis	Ingestation of intermediate stage metacercariae in raw fresh-water crab and crayfish	Respiratory: Pleuritic chest pain, pleural effusion, cough, haemoptysis Abdominal pain CNS: meningo-encephalitis, transverse myelitis, myelopathy Cutaneous: subcutaneous nodule	Praziquantel or Triclabendazole
Siberia	Clonorchis sinensis Opisthorchis species	Clonorchiasis Opisthorchiasis	Ingestion of intermediate stage metacercariae in raw fish	GI: Abdominal pain, hepatomegaly, biliary obstruction, Cholangiocarcinoma Cutaneous: urticarial rash Other: fever	Praziquantel

Table 4.5 Global distribution and clinical manifestations of common ectoparasitic infections.

Geographical area	Parasite	Common syndrome, name	Mode of transmission	Clinical features	Treatment
Worldwide, tropical	*Dermatobia hominis* (botfly) *Cordylobia anthropophaga* (tumbufly)	Myiasis	Arthropod bite	Insect bite that slowly enlarges into a painful nodule, producing serosanguinous discharge	Occlusion of the opening with petroleum jelly and extraction of the worm
	Tunga penetrans	Tungiasis	Sand flea penetrating the skin, usually feet	Single or multiple nodules with black colour centrally	Extraction of flea
Worldwide	*Pediculus humanus humanus*	Pediculosis corporis	Direct contact	Itch; Excoriation of trunk and neck areas	Topical: Permethrin or Malathion Ivermectin Clothing should be heat washed
	Pediculus humanus capitis	Pediculosis capitis	Direct contact	Itch of scalp, neck and post-auricular areas	Topical: Permethrin or Malathion Ivermectin
	Phthirus pubis (crab louse)	Pediculosis pubis	Sexually	Itch in pubic areas Lymphadenopathy may occur	Topical: Permethrin or Malathion Ivermectin
	Sarcoptes scabiei	Scabies	Direct contact	Small erythematous papules, generalized urticaria Burrow marks	Topical: Permethrin or Malathion

Table 4.6 Investigations of parasitic infections

Infection	Diagnostic test
Ascaris lumbricoides	Concentrated stool microscopy
Enterobius vermicularis	Perianal sellotape
Fasciola hepatica	Concentrated stool microscopy Serology
Ancyclostoma duodenale/Necator americanus	Concentrated stool microscopy
Echinococcus granulosus/Echinococcus multilocuralis	Serology
Loa loa	Day blood microscopy Serology
Onchocerca volvulus	Skin snips, filarial serology Slit lamp
Schistosoma haematobium	Microscopy of nitrocellulose-filtered terminal urine serology
Schistosoma mansoni	Concentrated stool microscopy
Strongyloides stercoralis	Concentrated stool microscopy Serology Stool culture
Taenia solium *Taenia saginata*	Concentrated stool microscopy
Trichuris trichiura	Concentrated stool microscopy

4.8.3 Question 3

A thirty-year-male entomologist returns from field research in Guyana and develops a papule in the back of his neck which enlarges over eight weeks as shown in Figure 4.1.

What is the most likely diagnosis?

A. Chancre.

B. Cutaneous leishmaniasis.

C. Infected insect bite.

D. Myiasis.

E. Pyoderma gangrenosum.

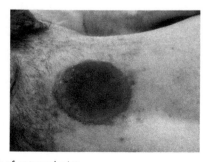

Figure 4.1 Lesion on neck of entomologist

4.9 Answers and discussion

4.9.1 Answer 1

E. Metronidazole

The most common causes of liver abscess are either bacterial or parasitic infections. *Entamoeba histolytica*, enterobacteriaceae, streptococci of the *anginosus/milleri* group, and other anaerobic bacteria are typical organisms causing liver abscess. Co-amoxiclav and gentamicin would cover the bacterial causes, whereas metronidazole is recommended for possible amoebic liver abscess that can be diagnosed serologically as well as through microscopy of the pus drained from the liver abscess. Finding of amoebic cysts in stool will necessitate further treatment with diloxonate furoate or paromomycin.

4.9.2 Answer 2

E. HTLV-1

Patients from or travellers to endemic areas are not uncommonly infected with more than one parasitic or helminth infections, and therefore will need stool microscopy for ova, cyst, and parasites, plus other serological tests to exclude other parasitic infections. *Strongyloides stercoralis* is associated with a significant risk factor for disseminated strongyloidiasis and treatment failure in patients with depressed T cell mediated immunity, as in HTLV-1, which is endemic in southern Japan, the Caribbean, South America, the Melanesian islands, Papua New Guinea, the Middle East, and in West, Central, and Southern Africa. Patients with HTLV-1 will require intense treatment with ivermectin.

4.9.3 Answer 3

B. Cutaneous leishmaniasis

This patient had a lesion with rolled up edges that started as a papule. The most likely aetiological agent is *Leishmania*, given the country he visited. The diagnostic test is biopsy of the lesion taken from the rolled up edges. This is sent for histopathology as well as microscopy, culture, and molecular testing.

CHAPTER 5

The host-parasite (microbe) relationship

Caryn Rosmarin

5.1 Are humans sterile?

No and yes. The skin, oropharynx, upper airways, gastrointestinal tract, and lower female genital tract are full of bacteria, with the highest concentration being in the colon and in dental plaque. Overall, humans are made up of slightly more bacterial cells than human cells; about 40 versus 30 trillion respectively. Although much less prominent, fungi and viruses are also present.

In addition to these endogenous microbes, humans come into contact with numerous others on a daily basis—they are inhaled, ingested with food and drink, and picked up on the skin from the environment. Some of these remain in and on the human body for periods of time, while others slough off or die.

In contrast to this, there are certain areas of the body where microbial agents are not expected to occur under normal circumstances. These are called sterile sites and include: major organs and their surrounding fluids and capsules; blood and body fluids other than faeces and saliva (yes, including urine!); bone, bone marrow, and joint fluid; subcutaneous tissue, fat, muscle, and tendons; the lower respiratory tract; and some of the genital tract. Microbes only enter these protected sterile sites through various breaches in physical and immunological defences.

5.2 Are the bacteria found on our body harmful to us?

Again—no and yes. This is a question that has posed much debate over the centuries and seems to evolve as understanding of both humans and microbes expands. Early understanding of infectious diseases was based on the idea that the microbe was an aggressor and the host a passive victim. Currently there is a better understanding of the relationship between microbe and host, which is more of a dance than a war.

In order to express an understanding of the relationships between host humans and microbes, a language is required that describes this confusing and complex interaction, especially considering that knowledge in this field is still evolving.

The bacteria that reside in or on human bodies on a semi-permanent basis are called *normal flora*, or *indigenous microbiome*. Each person has a relatively unique set of fairly stable microbes likely determined by early experience, and continued exposures and diets. Humans live with their bacteria in ecological symbiotic relationships, which are defined as being the close associations between two or more organisms of different species. There are three common types of *symbiotic* relationships we have with our normal flora.

1. *Commensalism*: an almost inconsequential association between the microbe and human, in which the microbe benefits from having a place to call home, but the host is neither helped nor harmed, e.g. *Staphylococcus epidermidis* that live on the skin.

2. *Mutualism*: where the relationship is beneficial to both microbe and host. Examples include;
   a. *anaerobic bacteria in the gut* that benefit from the environment, temperature, and supply of nutrients found in the colon while benefiting the host in a number of ways—from fermenting dietary fibre into forms that can be absorbed, aiding in the synthesis of vitamins B and K, helping eliminate toxins, and playing a role in the host inflammatory and immune system.
   b. *lactobacilli of the vaginal epithelium* benefit from a stable temperature and supply of nutrients in exchange for production of lactic acid. This lowers the pH to around 4–5, which is optimal for the lactobacilli but inhibitory for the growth of many other bacteria, thus protecting the vagina from overgrowth of yeast and other potentially harmful microbes.

3. *Parasitism*: While parasites are usually considered only in the biological sense of infection with macro-organisms such as protozoa or helminths, parasitism in the ecological sense refers to any microbe where the relationship is beneficial to the microbe and potentially harmful to the host, in that the microbe may cause disease in the host. It is unusual for our normal flora to cause us harm without an additional contributing host factor, such as an alternation of our gut flora or an immune impairment. The harm caused may be directly related the microbe itself and lead to an infectious disease, or may be caused more indirectly, e.g. harm in some dietary patterns leading to a changed gut microbiome pattern implicated in obesity and metabolic syndrome in the host.

There will, at certain times, be additional transient host-microbe interactions with non-resident flora. This temporary association is termed <u>colonization</u> or <u>carriage</u>, and classically is thought to have the same relationship characteristics as commensalism where there is no harm to the host. It occurs under circumstances such as exposure to infectious individuals or hospital environments, after a course of antibiotics, or after recovery from an infectious disease when the host continues to harbour the microbe.

There is lack of agreement as to whether the terms colonization and carriage mean the same thing, and also whether they are always harmless. More recent thought is that colonizers result in a possible continuum of damage to the host; from none to disease, and only those that cause no damage are synonymous with commensals. Some refer to the carrier state as one that is transient, and doesn't result in microbial multiplication, as compared to colonization, where the microbe multiplies and has the possibility to become part of the microbiome.

Colonization is known to be the first step towards potential harm or disease for certain microbes, e.g. throat colonization with *Neisseria meningitides* occurs before invasive disease. Colonizing microbes may be potentially more harmful than our normal flora, in the form of more resistant bacteria, e.g. nasal colonization with methicillin-resistant *Staphylococcus aureus* (MRSA), or gut colonization with carbapenem-resistant enterobacteriaceae (CRE).

Certain individuals may continue to harbour a microbe after clinical recovery from a disease state caused by the microbe in question, and may then serve as carriers of infection that can cause recurrent disease in the host or be transmitted to others. Examples include gut carriage of *Salmonella typhi* (Typhoid Mary), or persistent shedders of Herpes virus. Many viral infections result in a form of carrier state called *viral latency*, where the virus remains in a dormant state (usually at the site of disease) until reactivated.

5.3 The major functions of normal flora

Humans' first exposure to microbes happens as they traverse the birth canal, where the baby is exposed to large numbers of diverse micro-organisms belonging to their mothers' perineal and gastrointestinal flora. These micro-organisms get onto newborn skin and into the newborn gut and nasopharynx. This process is delayed in those born by caesarean section. Further exposures happen through contact with parents, in holding, cleaning, and feeding. Some of these early micro-organisms will stay with the child as resident flora, while some are lost. Determinants of this can include diet (where breastfed neonates have gut flora rich in bifidobacteria, while bottle feeding with formula or cow's milk-based products increases the growth of gram negatives and gas-producing organisms), and antibiotic therapy in the neonatal period that encourages the growth of more resistant organisms, e.g. clostridia and staphylococci, rather than healthy bifidobacteria.

Exposure to micro-organisms (like new dance moves) continues across the lifetime, but it is suggested that the initial exposures determine the first host-microbe interaction, and may set a pattern of host-microbe interactions (and dance styles) to come. They also form the basis of normal flora, and thus have influence over the health of the microbiome.

One of the most important roles of normal flora is to protect the human from pathogenic organisms by providing *competition*. Approximately 10^6 salmonellae need to be ingested to cause disease in a healthy animal, whereas the same disease can be produced by as few as 10^1 organisms when ingested by an animal that has been kept in a completely sterile environment for all its life. Antibiotics that inhibit *Lactobacillus* in the vagina result in overgrowth of resident *Candida* species, causing vulvovaginal candidiasis. Similarly, antibiotics inhibit intestinal flora and allow overgrowth of toxin-producing *Clostridium difficile*.

Another protective effect is in the role of stimulation of the adaptive immune system. Animals reared in microbe-free environments have been shown to have greatly underdeveloped lymphoid tissue. The development of antibodies against normal flora microbes is protective in that these antibodies can bind to pathogens as well. Constant and repeated exposure to microbes in food and in the gut is important in the development of oral tolerance where the immune system learns to lessen its response to these microbes. This tolerance forms the basis of the hygiene hypothesis that proposes a lack exposure to microbes leads to reduced tolerance and the development of allergies.

5.4 When microbes cause harm

Typically, when someone says 'I have an *infection*' what they are really saying is 'I have a *disease* caused by an infectious agent'—an infectious disease.

Infection is the ecological term that describes the process of acquisition of a microbe by a host. In pathogenesis terms, an infection is the invasive state of the microbe-host relationship, which may or may not actually cause harm or the state of disease. It can be used to describe the first step of all forms of host-microbe relationships. *Infectivity* is an epidemiological term used to describe a micro-organisms' capacity for spread among hosts.

Disease, on the other hand, is the physical expression of the harm caused to the host by the microbe. It generally implies a form of damage to the host. Disease can be caused by newly acquired microbes, colonizing microbes, or from our normal flora.

The ability of a micro-organism to cause disease in another organism is termed *pathogenicity*. The higher the pathogenicity, the more likely the host is to develop disease after being infected. For example, HIV has almost 100% pathogenicity. The process of development of disease is termed the *pathogenesis*, and when talking of infectious diseases, the microbe is termed the *pathogen*. However, disease is not an inevitable outcome of the host-pathogen interaction. *Virulence*, a term often used synonymously with pathogenicity, refers to the degree of harm caused by the pathogen. To add to the complexity, pathogens can express a wide range of virulence such that the extent of virulence of an individual pathogen is not fixed but is affected by external factors such as host environment.

5.5 What makes a pathogen pathogenic?

All micro-organisms have the potential to be pathogens (pathogenic potential) under the right circumstances, even normal human flora. Some micro-organisms are better at it, having what is termed a high degree of pathogenicity or virulence ('natural born killers'), while others need a lot of help, relying on a vulnerable host to make their move. These less-pathogenic microbes rely on taking advantage of the opportunity presented by a host vulnerability and are termed *opportunistic pathogens*. Hosts are made vulnerable in a number of ways, including the many forms of immune compromise and suppression, underlying chronic diseases such as diabetes, and compromised defences such as the presence of invasive medical devices, surgery, and trauma.

Virulent pathogens are supplied with an armamentarium of tools for causing disease, called *virulence factors*. These include structural, biochemical, or genetic traits, some of which are part of the chromosome and intrinsic to the microbe (e.g. capsules and endotoxin), while others are obtained from mobile genetic elements like plasmids (e.g. some exotoxins).

Virulence factors work in enabling one or more of the phases of pathogenesis of disease that include attachment, survival and multiplication, invasion and damage. Some pathogens rely on a single virulence factor, such as toxin production, while others use a larger repertoire. The latter are often more able to cause a wider range of diseases in the host.

Adherence or attachment occurs through various adhesion molecules (such as bacterial pili or viral proteins) on the microbe surface to receptors on the host cell surface. Some microbes are able to promote adherence by up-regulating the number of adherence receptors. Adherence and attachment are not limited to pathogens as commensals can also adhere and attach to host cells.

Survival in the host is essential for disease pathogenesis, as microbes need to tolerate the environment and avoid being removed or destroyed by the host defences. Bacteria such as *Helicobacter pylori* can survive and grow in the low pH of the stomach. Staphylococci survive within an extracellular matrix called a biofilm, which hides them from the host immune system. Micro-organisms have many mechanisms of avoiding host immune-mediated killing including the presence of capsules, avoidance of opsonization and phagocytosis, avoidance of recognition by antibodies through antigenic variation and mimicry, serum resistance, the ability to survive inside the host cell and within the phagolysosome, and integration into the host genome by some viruses. In hosts who have no splenic function (either removed or functionally asplenic), defences against encapsulated organisms are lost, which leads to recurrent infections.

Some bacteria can cause disease without *invasion*, but many require entry into deeper tissue to cause disease. Crossing the hosts' natural defences may require a breach such as an insect bite or a medical device; or may occur through hijacking natural systems such as phagocytosis and endocytosis. Certain bacterial enzymes produced may cause damage to host cell structure enhancing invasion and spread, for example, hyaluronidase and streptokinase.

Damage to the host may occur directly due to microbial factors or as a result of the host's own immune response to the microbe. Damage may also help the pathogen to spread further within the host or to leave the host and spread to other vulnerable hosts.

Direct factors for bacterial pathogens are mainly in the form of toxins, broadly grouped as endotoxins and exotoxins. *Endotoxin*, also called lipopolysaccharide or LPS, is an innate part of the gram-negative cell wall. It is released when the bacterial cell is lysed, triggering either a local or systemic inflammatory response ranging from mild to endotoxic shock. Gram-positive cell wall components (peptidoglycans) can cause a similar response.

Exotoxins are those secreted by bacteria, and broadly classified according to their mechanism of action (A-B, membrane disrupting, or superantigens) and the host tissue on which they act, such as neurotoxins (e.g. Botulinum), enterotoxins (e.g. Shiga), and cytotoxins (eg. Diphtheria). Bacteria produce a wide array of these and they can act either locally or systemically.

Direct factors for viruses are mainly in the form of cell lysis or cell transformation.

Indirect damage to the host occurs through a pathogen-induced inflammatory response. While an inflammatory response is a normal and protective mechanism, difficulty in controlling it may end in host tissue damage. This may be in the form of both innate and adaptive immune responses.

5.6 Koch's postulates and their use

The germ theory of disease was proposed in the sixteenth century. It went in and out of favour over the centuries, but with the observations of van Leeuwenhoek, Semelweiss, Lister, and Snow adding to the body of evidence, it wasn't until the research of Louis Pasteur in the 1860s and then Robert Koch in the following decades that provided the scientific proof needed for this concept to take hold.

From his work with tuberculosis, Koch proposed the following postulates in an attempt to devise a standard for identifying whether there was a causal relationship between a particular microbe (the pathogen) and a specific infectious disease. This was both an attempt at convincing sceptics that micro-organisms were pathogenic, as well as a guide to microbiologists in being more rigorous in their claims.

Postulate 1: The micro-organism must be observed in every case of the disease but should not be found in healthy hosts.

Postulate 2: The micro-organism must be isolated from a diseased host and grown in pure culture.

Postulate 3: The micro-organism from the pure culture, when inoculated into a susceptible host, must reproduce the disease.

Postulate 4: The micro-organism must be re-isolated from the inoculated, diseased, experimental host and identified as being identical to the original specific causative agent.

While Koch's postulates formed the basis of the germ theory of disease, there were obvious limitations to these postulates, some of which Koch himself became aware of during his lifetime.

Postulate 1 was abandoned when he discovered that an asymptomatic carrier state of cholera and typhoid fever existed. Modern medicine understands that many microbes can exist in healthy individuals without causing disease.

Postulate 2 was abandoned when it was realized that certain microbes could not be grown (at least easily) in routine pure culture. Included in this group are the atypical bacteria (e.g. rickettsia, chlamydia, mycoplasmas), viruses, and prions. It is also common knowledge that antibiotics might prevent or delay a positive culture.

Postulate 3 was abandoned when Koch discovered that not all hosts exposed to the infectious agent acquired the disease.

Postulate 4 remains partially true, although it is now known that microbes undergo genetic alterations over time or under certain pressures. Bacteria can also acquire additional genetic material in the form of plasmids or bacteriophages.

Over time, the concept of one microbe = one disease has been disproved. It looks more like one microbe = colonization, or carriage, or one of many manifestations of disease. So while Koch's postulates are no longer scientifically as rigorous as when they were conceived, the spirit of understanding pathogenesis of infectious disease lives on.

5.7 Assessment questions

5.7.1 Question 1

A fifty-five-year-old man who suffered abdominal trauma and splenectomy ten years previously is admitted with fever, right-sided chest pain, and a productive cough. On examination he has signs of consolidation in the right lower lobe of the lung (which is confirmed on chest X-ray) and is diagnosed as having community-acquired pneumonia. He says this is the third time this year he has been diagnosed with the same condition. His blood culture grew the organism shown in Figures 5.1, 5.2, and 5.3.

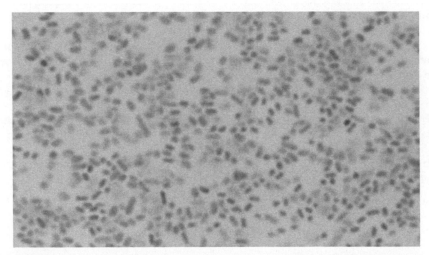

Figure 5.1 Gram stain of organism from blood culture demonstrating small gram-negative rods.

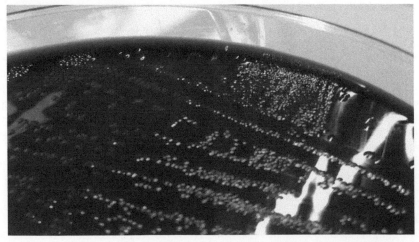

Figure 5.2 Culture on chocolate agar after 24 hours at 37°C in 5% CO_2 demonstrating typical grey, smooth, entire colonies.

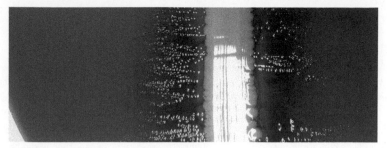

Figure 5.3 Culture (after 24 hours at 37°C) on blood agar with a streak of *Staphylococcus aureus* demonstrating satallitism. No growth present on standard blood agar without the streak of *Staphylococcus aureus*.

What is the most likely cause of his disease?
A. *Streptococcus pneumoniae.*
B. *Haemophilus influenzae.*
C. *Staphylococcus aureus.*
D. *Klebsiella pneumoniae.*
E. *Pseudomonas aeruginosa.*

5.7.2 Question 2

A twenty-eight-year-old male heroin user comes to A&E complaining of severe diplopia. Examination reveals abscesses on his thighs, which he says are due to injecting heroin by skin popping. He is admitted for drainage of the abscesses and investigation of his diplopia. Pus and tissue samples from the abscesses are sent and he is started on IV flucloxacillin. Over the next twenty-four hours his diplopia worsens and he develops slurred speech, difficulty swallowing, and some descending symmetrical weakness. A CT scan of his brain is performed which does not show any abnormalities. Fig 5.4 shows a gram stain of the pus sample.

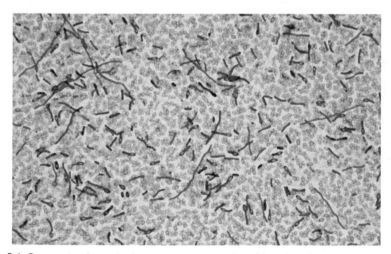

Figure 5.4 Gram stain of sample showing gram-positive/variable rods with spores.

What is the most appropriate next step in managing this patient?

A. Change IV flucloxacillin to IV benzyl penicillin.

B. IV human Immunoglobulin.

C. IV botulinum anti-toxin.

D. IV tetanus anti-toxin.

E. Further surgical debridement of his thigh.

5.7.3 Question 3

A previously healthy three-year-old girl is brought in to hospital by her mother as she has noticed the child looks swollen and has dark urine. Two weeks previously she had suffered a sore throat that improved without any antibiotic. On examination the girl had a raised blood pressure, oedema, and haematuria. What is the most likely cause of these findings?

A. Streptococcal infective endocarditis.

B. Streptococcal myocarditis.

C. Post-streptococcal acute rheumatic fever.

D. Post-streptococcal glomerulonephritis.

E. Streptococcal toxic shock syndrome.

5.8 Answers and discussion

5.8.1 Answer 1

B. *Haemophilus influenzae*

Splenectomized patients are at increased risk of infections caused by encapsulated bacteria, such as *Streptococcus pneumoniae*, *Haemophilus influenzae*, and *Neisseria meningitidis*. The spleen functions to protect the body from infection in two ways: by removing circulating bacteria through its immunological phagocytic filter mechanism, and by producing antibodies when splenic B cells become activated.

While other immunologic mechanisms exist to remove bacteria from the systems of the human body, most of these require the bacteria to be opsonized (coated in antibody) to be recognized by the phagocytic cell. Bacteria that have capsules are not well opsonized as the capsule prevents antibody attachment to the bacterial cell wall. This is one of the immune-evading virulence mechanisms that capsules provide to bacteria. However, the spleen is still able to remove these poorly opsonized encapsulated bacteria, and hence in the absence of a spleen, they can cause overwhelming infections.

Absence of splenic memory B cells results in poor antibody formation and thus poor protection on re-infection with encapsulated bacteria.

5.8.2 Answer 2

C. IV botulinum anti-toxin

Early treatment with anti-toxin is essential and it should be administered as soon as possible after a definite clinical diagnosis of botulism has been made. In addition, antibiotic treatment with IV benzyl penicillin and surgical debridement of infected tissue are also important in patient management in order to avoid ongoing toxin production and relapse after the anti-toxin has been eliminated from the body. Surgery itself may release more toxin and so it should ideally be done after anti-toxin treatment.

Clostridium botulinum is an anaerobic, spore-forming, gram negative bacterium and causes three forms of disease: wound botulism (as in this case), infant botulism, and food-borne botulism. In the

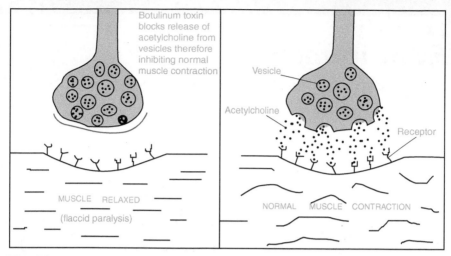

Figure 5.5 Mechanism of action of botulinum toxin.

latter, the toxin is ingested rather than the organism. Disease from all three is caused by botulinum toxin, a neurotoxin that binds to receptors in presynaptic membranes of the neuromuscular junction, inhibiting acetylcholine release and thus neurotransmission, resulting in muscle weakness (Fig 5.5) The latter is typically descending and symmetrical beginning with the small muscles of the face, head, and neck.

There are seven types of botulinum toxin, named type A–G. Human botulism is most frequently caused by toxin types A, B, and E and more rarely by types F and C. Only toxin types A and B have been shown to cause wound botulism to date.

5.8.3 Answer 3

D. Post-streptococcal glomerulonephritis

Streptococcus pyogenes (group A strep or GAS) infection can be complicated by nonsuppurative post-streptococcal sequelae, usually in the weeks following the primary infection. The two most well-described forms of this include rheumatic fever and glomerulonephritis. Rheumatic fever follows a primary streptococcal pharyngitis while glomerulonephritis follows either pharyngitis or skin infection. GAS have antiphagocytic proteins, called M proteins, on their cell wall. These proteins, which form the basis of typing (emm typing), are also important in pathogenesis of post-streptococcal disease. There are over 150 of these proteins; certain M proteins are said to be rheumatogenic and associated with rheumatic fever (M1 and M3), while others are nephritogenic (M12 and M49) and associated with glomerulonephritis. During primary infection, antibodies develop against the M proteins, and these antibodies cause immune-mediated damage of human tissue. In glomerulonephritis the anti-M protein antibodies cross-react with the basement membrane of the glomerulus. In addition, immune complexes formed between antibodies and streptococcal antigens get deposited on the basement membrane. Cross-reacting antibodies against heart tissue are responsible for the damage caused in rheumatic fever.

CHAPTER 6

Basic immunology

Jonathan Lambourne, Ruaridh Buchanan, and Emily Zinser

6.1 The major components of the immune system

There are four major components of the immune system. These include:

1. mechanical barriers to pathogen entry.

2. the innate immune system.

3. the adaptive immune system.

4. the lymphoid organs.

Mechanical barriers include skin and mucous membranes and tight junctions between epithelial cells prevent pathogen entry. Breaches can be iatrogenic, for example, IV lines, surgical wounds, and mucositis, and are a large source of healthcare-associated infections.

The innate immune system provides the first internal line of defence, as well as initiating and shaping the adaptive immune response. The innate system comprises a range of responses: phagocytosis by neutrophils and macrophages (guided in part by the adaptive immune system), the complement cascade, and the release of antimicrobial peptides by epithelial cells (e.g. defensins, cathelicidin).

The adaptive immune system includes both humoral (antibody-mediated) and cell-mediated responses. It is capable of greater diversity and specificity than the innate immune system, and can develop memory to pathogens and provide increased protection on re-exposure.

Immune cells are divided into myeloid cells (neutrophils, eosinophils, basophils, mast cells, and monocytes/macrophages) and lymphoid cells (B, T, and NK cells). These all originate in the bone marrow from pluripotent haematopoietic stem cells. The lymphoid organs include the spleen, the lymph nodes, and mucosal-associated lymphoid tissues—which respond to antigens in the blood, tissues, and epithelial surfaces respectively.

6.2 How phagocytes recognize and respond to pathogens

The three main 'professional' phagocytes are macrophages, dendritic cells, and neutrophils. They are similar with respect to how they recognize pathogens, but differ in their principal location and effector functions.

Phagocytes express an array of Pattern Recognition Receptors (PRRs) e.g. Toll-like receptors and lectins (proteins that bind carbohydrates). PRRs recognize Pathogen-Associated Molecular Patterns (PAMPs)—elements which are conserved across species, such as cell-surface glycoproteins and nucleic acid sequences (Table 6.1). Though limited in number, PRRs have evolved to recognize a huge array of pathogens. Binding of PRRs to PAMPs enhances phagocytosis.

Macrophages are tissue-resident phagocytes, initiating and co-ordinating the local immune response. The cytokines and chemokines they produce cause vasodilation and alter the expression of endothelial cell adhesion factors, recruiting circulating immune cells. This includes monocytes, which differentiate into macrophages once in peripheral tissue. Macrophages also phagocytose and kill pathogens.

Dendritic cells are also tissue-resident phagocytes. However, their main role is the initiation of the adaptive immune response by delivery and presentation of antigens to T- and B-lymphocytes in the regional lymphatic tissue.

Neutrophils usually reside in the circulation, but are drawn by cytokines and chemokines to the tissues, where they undertake phagocytosis and intracellular killing. Neutrophils also release factors into the extracellular environment that damage pathogens. These include neutrophil extracellular traps (NETs), formed of nuclear chromatin, which immobilize micro-organisms; they also release peptides that disrupt pathogen cell membranes (e.g. alpha-defensin, cathelicidin).

Table 6.1 Examples of pathogen-associated molecular patterns (PAMPs) and pattern recognition receptors (PRRs).

PRR	PAMP	PAMP expression
TLR1/2	Triacyl lipopeptides	Bacterial cell wall
TLR2	Zymosan Peptidoglycan Lipoarabinomannan	Fungi Gram-positive bacteria Mycobacteria
TLR3	Double-stranded RNA	Viruses
TLR4	Lipopolysaccharide Mannan	Gram-negative bacteria Candida
TLR5	Flagellin	Flagellated bacteria
TLR6	Diacyl lipopeptides	Mycoplasma
TLR7/8	Single-stranded RNA	Viruses
TLR9	Unmethylated CpG motifs	Bacteria, and DNA viruses
Dectin-1	Beta-glucans	Fungal cell wall
MBL	Repeating mannose and fucose sugars	Bacterial cell membrane and fungal cell wall
NOD-like receptors	Cytoplasmic peptides	Derived from intracellular degradation of bacteria

6.2.1 Phagocytosis

Following phagocytosis, a number of pathways are activated in order to kill the pathogen. These steps include:

1. *acidification of the phagosome*—controlled by the activation of vacuolar ATPase.
2. *fusion of the phagosome with lysosomes*—lysosomes are membrane-bound intracellular granules, containing enzymes (such as *lysozyme*, which hydrolyses peptidoglycan), *anti-microbial peptides*, and compounds which bind metabolic co-factors (such as iron-binding *lactoferrin*).
3. *production of toxic chemicals*—these include *nitric oxide*, hydrogen peroxide, and *reactive oxygen species* (such as the superoxide anion O2-). The latter are produced by NADPH oxidase in the respiratory burst—defects in this pathway underpin the pathophysiology of chronic granulomatous disease.

6.3 Different aspects and functions of the complement cascade

The complement system comprises a collection of plasma proteins that, once activated, initiate a cascade of proteolytic reactions effecting three main functions:

1: *Opsonization*—binding of C3b and C4b renders pathogens more visible to phagocytes, facilitating phagocytosis. Antibody-mediated phagocytosis is also 'complemented' by the system, hence the name.
2: *Chemotaxis*—some complement factors act as chemo-attractants, recruiting phagocytes to the site of complement activation (e.g. C3a, C5a).
3: *Direct pathogen killing*—the terminal complement components (C5–9) form the membrane attack complex (MAC), which creates pores in bacterial cell membranes, leading to leakage of cytosolic contents and bacterial death. Deficiency in any of the terminal complement factors is associated with impaired MAC activity and increased susceptibility to neisserial infection.

The complement cascade can be activated by three distinct mechanisms:

1. *Classical complement pathway*—triggered when the C1 complex binds to antibody-antigen complexes. The C1q portion binds to the immune complex; a conformational change then causes the C1r portion to cleave and activate the C1s portion, which acts as a protease to cleave and active C4 and C2, triggering the cascade.
2. *Mannose-binding lectin (MBL) pathway*—MBL binds to repeating carbohydrate domains found more commonly on bacteria than host cells. It circulates in association with mannose-binding lectin-associated serine proteases (MASPs). In a manner analogous to the classical pathway, MBL binding activates MASPs, which then cleave and activate C4 and C2.
3: *Alternative pathway*—does not require pathogen recognition by antibody or MBL, with complement activation taking place directly on the pathogen cell surface. C3 is abundant in serum, and continuous auto-activation takes place on the surface of host cells and pathogens alike. Host cells possess regulatory factors which curtail C3 activation—pathogen surfaces lack these mechanisms, thus unchecked C3 activation is able to activate the rest of the complement cascade.

6.4 How T cells recognize pathogens

Intracellular pathogens (all viruses, some bacteria and parasites) are 'invisible' to antibodies, and it is the role of T cells to counter these pathogens. This cell-mediated immunity depends on the direct interaction between T cells and the cells expressing the antigen.

6.4.1 Thymic development

T cells begin life in the bone marrow, migrating to the thymus to complete their development. Naïve T cells, expressing a single, specific T cell receptor (TCR) then move into the circulation, travelling to the other lymphoid organs before returning to the circulation via lymphatics. The challenge is creating a diverse library of T cells covering a myriad of pathogens without generating T cells which target host cells. Diversity is attained through DNA recombination, creating billions of TCRs from hundreds of genes—once this process has occurred, the sequence is locked in place, with the lymphocyte and its progeny producing only this sequence. Thymic tissue contains cells that express self-antigens (e.g. thyroglobulin)—any T cell binding too enthusiastically to such an antigen is removed, limiting the self-reactivity of the T cell population. Non-binding T cells are also removed, ensuring there is no waste in the system.

6.4.2 Recognition and maturation

There are two major classes of T cells: CD4+ T helper (Th) and CD8+ Cytotoxic T cells. CD4 and CD8 are important for T cell activation, co-stimulating the T cells when the TCR binds to major histocompatibility complex (MHC) molecules. MHC molecules present peptides for recognition by T cells—MHC-I is expressed by all cells and has affinity for CD8+ cells. By contrast, MHC-II is found only on APCs, including macrophages and B cells, and has affinity only for CD4+ cells.

MHC-I presents proteins from the cell's own cytosol—this will usually be self-peptides, in which case no T cell should exist that recognizes the material. However, it may also present peptides from intracellular pathogens, in which case recognition by a specific T cell will occur. MHC-II presents proteins processed by APCs, derived from extracellular material internalized by APCs by phagocytosis or micropinocytosis. Dendritic cells are the most important APC for T cell activation, residing in the tissues but migrating to local lymphoid tissue following phagocytosis. Once in the lymphatics they release cytokines to attract T cells to their location. Macrophages also perform this role, but less readily, and usually only when containing intracellular pathogens.

T cell activation requires the presentation of the an appropriate antigen along with co-stimulation, both from CD4/CD8 but also from other signals, most commonly the linking of T cell expressed CD28 and APC-expressed B7. TCR stimulation in the absence of co-stimulation results in inactivation of the T cell, the assumption being that the T cell has inappropriately recognized a self-antigen. The threshold for CD8+ cell activation is set higher than CD4+ cells, as inappropriate cytotoxic T cell activity can be hugely destructive. Activation either requires larger quantities of antigen or co-stimulation by an appropriately activated CD4+ cell, for example, mediated via the surface molecule CD40 on CD4+ cells and the corresponding CD40-L (ligand) on the CD8+ cell.

Appropriate activation of naïve T cells results in expression of both interleukin-2 and its receptor—this triggers a positive feedback loop that drives the transition to the activated state. Once fully activated, primed T cells return to the site where the antigen was first recognized. For CD4+ T cells, there are a variety of subsets the cell can differentiate into, which are determined by the local cytokine environment (Table 6.2).

Table 6.2 CD4+ T helper cell subsets.

CD4+ T helper cell 'type'	Cytokine driving differentiation	Intracellular signalling	Transcription factor	Effector cytokines
Th1	IFNg	STAT1, STAT4	T-bet	IFNg
Th2	IL4	STAT6	GATA3	IL4
Th17	TGFb, IL6	STAT3	RORgt	IL17
Treg (regulatory T cell)	IL2	STAT5	Foxp3	TGFb and IL10

There is some suggestion that Th2 is the default phenotype, with differentiation to other phenotypes requiring specific cytokines. It is also suggested that small quantities of antigen may favour Th2, with larger quantities favoring Th1; the rationale here is that small quantities of antigen are more likely to represent product phagocytosed by an APC, with larger quantities suggesting active infection of the APCs.

Following activation, a proportion of T cells remains in the lymphoid tissue instead of migrating back out into the circulation, and mature into T follicular helper cells, which are essential for activation of naïve B cells (see Section 6.6.2).

6.5 How T cells respond to pathogens

6.5.1 Proliferation

As each TCR is unique, there are a limited number of T cells that will respond to any given pathogen—certainly too few to eradicate the infection. It is therefore necessary for activated T cells to undergo clonal expansion to increase the strength of the immune response. As well as proliferation, maturation leads to changes in expression of adhesion markers, which determines where the effector cell will migrate.

6.5.2 Response

Once activated, and expanded, clones of the activated T cell do not need co-stimulation to exert their effect. For CD8+ T cells this means that they are able to respond to cognate antigen presented within MHC-I by any cell type. CD4+ T cells still only respond to antigen bound to MHC-II on APCs but the threshold and nature of the response differs significantly between naïve and activated cells.

When CD8+ cytotoxic T cells recognize an antigen, they kill the cell that is presenting the antigen, the assumption being that the cell is infected with an intracellular pathogen. They do this by a variety of effector mechanisms, including:

1. Releasing cytotoxic molecules into the extracellular environment, including perforin, which perforates the target cell membrane, and granzyme, a serine protease that penetrates the target cell and triggers apoptosis.
2. Cell-cell signalling—activated CD8+ cells express Fas ligand, which can bind Fas on the target cell, initiating apoptosis.

The nature of the CD4+ T helper response depends on which Th cell subtype the cell has differentiated into, the two main subtypes being T helper1 (Th1) and T helper2 (Th2) responses.

Th1 responses drive macrophage activation via secretion of cytokines and growth factors, including IFNg, TNFa, GM-CSF, and by direct cell–cell contact mediated by CD40 on T cells and CD40-L on macrophages. These stimuli alter macrophage function, promoting

- more efficient phagosome/lysosome fusion;
- synthesis of oxygen free radicals and nitric oxide;
- synthesis of antimicrobial peptides and proteases;
- synthesis of TNFα and IL12, which act in a positive feedback loop to drive inflammation;
- up-regulation of MHC-II expression, leading to more efficient antigen presentation; and
- up-regulation of CD40, which allows the macrophage to be more responsive to the stimulatory effects of CD40-L and TNFα.

These changes convert macrophages from phagocytes to antimicrobial effector cells.

Th2 cells activate B cells, secreting cytokines including IL4, IL5, IL13, and directly signalling to B cells via CD40–CD40-L interactions. A Th2-skewed immune response also arises when naïve T cells are activated predominantly by B cells, suggesting an extracellular antigen and thus the need for an antibody mediated response.

6.6 How B cells recognize pathogens

B cells undergo their entire development in the bone marrow. Following ligation of the B cell receptor (and necessary co-stimulation), the naïve B cell is activated and matures into a plasma cell, which produces immunoglobulin of the same specificity as the B cell receptor. Immunoglobulins are soluble antibodies that bind to pathogens in the extracellular space, including the circulation and mucosal surfaces. The receptor diversity and avoidance of self-recognition that apply to T cells also apply to B cells, and B cells use similar mechanisms to achieve both. However, in contrast to T cells, B cells are able to further enhance the diversity of their antigenic repertoire following interaction with cognate antigen. This can occur via isotype switching (e.g. changing from IgM to IgG production) or via somatic hypermutation. This is a process whereby mutations occur in the genes encoding the variable region of the immunoglobulin following initial antigen recognition. These mutations generate a family of closely related antibodies of varying affinity—those with higher affinity are selected for, increasing the efficacy of the response over time—a process referred to as affinity maturation. As the affinity of each individual bond increases, so does the overall strength of binding—referred to as avidity. Antibody avidity measurements can determine how recently an infection occurred, with higher avidity indicating more distant infection.

6.6.1 Structure of the B cell receptor

B cell receptors/immunoglobulins are composed of constant and variable regions—mediating the effector functions following antigen recognition, and recognizing and binding antigens, respectively. Each antibody consists of two identical heavy chains and two identical light chains. The variable regions of light and heavy chains combine to form the antigen-binding site, so both heavy and light chains contribute to the antibody specificity.

6.6.2 Mechanism of antigen recognition

T cells recognize linear peptides, typically consisting of seven to ten amino acids. By contrast, B cell receptors bind conformational epitopes, which are determined by the quaternary structure of the antigen. Altering the quaternary structure of the antigen will significantly alter the repertoire of antibodies that recognize it. Also, antibodies can bind to proteins, carbohydrates, and combinations of the two (glycoproteins), whereas T cells have no way of recognizing carbohydrate antigens. This is significant, as one immune evasion strategy employed by bacteria is to surround themselves with a carbohydrate-rich capsule.

Naïve B cells may meet their cognate antigen in the circulation, or in tissues, but in order to become activated, the majority of naïve B cells must travel to lymphoid tissue and present the peptide portion of their cognate antigen, via MHC-II, to T follicular helper cells. These specialized T cells provide the necessary co-stimulation for B cell activation in the form of CD40-L. All naïve B cells express IgM and IgD, but rapidly undergo isotype switching on activation to produce IgG, IgA, and IgE. Impaired CD40–CD40-L interaction, for example, due to absence of CD40-L on T cells, leads to failure of class switching, e.g. Hyper IgM syndromes.

The small proportion of naïve B cells whose receptors recognize carbohydrate antigens must be activated by T cell independent means, as T cells only recognize peptide antigens. These B cells also require a second signal in order to become activated, which include:

1. Recognition of the same antigen by a separate receptor on the B cell surface, such as one of the TLRs. Antigens able to do this are called T-independent-1 antigens (TI-1).
2. Repeating polysaccharide antigens that cause simultaneous ligation of multiple B cell receptors. These are termed TI-2 antigens.

T-independent antigens can only be recognized by a sub-set of specialized B cells. This population is less efficient at isotype switching, affinity maturation, and memory B cell formation. TI-2 antigens are only recognized by mature B cells, such as B-1 cells (CD5+ B cells) and marginal zone B cells. As it takes some months following birth for B cells to mature, this may explain why young children are particularly susceptible to encapsulated bacteria, including pneumococcus, meningococcus, and *Haemophilus* species.

6.7 How B cells respond to pathogens

Once activated, B cells mature into immunoglobulin-secreting plasma cells. There are five immunoglobulin isotypes, which differ in structure and function. IgG and IgM are most abundant in plasma, IgG and monomeric IgA are found in extracellular fluid, and IgE and dimeric IgA predominate at mucosal surfaces. Through isotype switching, a single B cell is able to generate progeny with the same specificity but at different anatomical locations. IgM is always produced first following activation, as no isotype switch is required—the relatively low affinity of the early response is overcome by the pentameric nature of IgM. Due to its size, IgM is almost exclusively found in the circulation, being too large to migrate out. It is a potent activator of the classical complement cascade. IgG and IgE are always monomeric, and readily diffuse out of the circulation. There are four subclasses of IgG (IgG1–4) with variable capacity for complement activation, opsonization, and crossing the placenta.

Just as there are different antibody isotypes, so are there different Fc receptors. There are at least five Fc receptors that recognize IgG (FcγRI, RII-A, RII-B1, RII-B2, RIII), each with a different series of downstream actions. Most promote phagocytosis and release of pre-formed granules. However, FcγR-IIB is able to negatively regulate neutrophils, mast cells, and macrophages, altering the threshold at which immune complexes activate these cells.

Antibodies exert their effect in three main ways.

1. *Neutralization*—by binding pathogens or toxins, antibodies can protect host cells from their effects. Neutralization is important for preventing viral entry into cells and preventing the actions of bacterial toxins, e.g. Staphylococcal exotoxin. Neutralization cannot prevent bacterial replication.
2. *Antibody dependent cytotoxicity*—phagocytes express receptors for the Fc-portion of antibodies on their cell surface (FcRs)—antibody coating of pathogens is thus a mechanism of opsonization.
3. *Activation of the classical complement cascade*—antibody-antigen complexes activate complement via binding of C1q.

6.8 Immunological memory

Activation of the adaptive immune system following first contact with a pathogen takes approximately seven days, during which time the innate immune system is at the fore of the response. In order to prevent overactivation, the majority of effector T and B cells have a limited life span following activation, undergoing apoptosis. However, a minority of effector cells further differentiate into memory cells, which on re-exposure to antigen can induce a more rapid adaptive response than following primary exposure. Immunological memory underpins the efficacy of immunization. Vaccines expose the immune system to a sub-unit of a pathogen, killed pathogen, or pathogen processed to render it less virulent. The immune system mounts a primary response and establishes immunological memory—thus, when an individual encounters the real pathogen, the adaptive response is much quicker, acting to eradicate the pathogen before infection can occur.

6.9 How the immune system responds to different types of pathogen

The relative importance of different aspects of the immune system for defence against pathogens varies between pathogens, and which niche they occupy (Table 6.3).

Although these principles hold true for most, there are a number of exceptions. For example, among viral infections, hepatitis B and enterovirus species are unusual in requiring humoral immunity for their control.

Table 6.3 The relative importance of different aspects of the immune response varies depending on pathogen location.

Site of infection	Examples of organisms	Examples of relevant immune responses
Extracellular: Epithelial surfaces	Respiratory tract: *S. pneumoniae* GI tract: Shigella Mucous membranes: Candida	Antimicrobial peptides Antibodies (esp. IgA) Th17 response
Extracellular: Blood and interstitial spaces	*Staphylococcus aureus* *Streptococcus pyogenes* *Escherichia coli*	Antibodies Complement Phagocytosis Neutralization
Intracellular: within vesicles	Mycobacteria *Salmonella Typhi* Listeria Cryptococcus and Histoplasma	CD4+ T helper cells Macrophage activation
Intracellular: within cytoplasm	Viruses *Chlamydia sp. & Rickettsia sp.* Some protozoa	CD8+ cytotoxic T cells

6.10 Pathogen mechanisms used to evade the immune system

Pathogens have evolved an array of mechanisms to evade the human immune system. Counter measures to virtually all elements of the immune response have been described. This section provides some common examples.

6.10.1 Antigenic variation

Some pathogens alter the antigens they express. When this occurs, the immune system must respond as if exposed to a novel pathogen. Some pathogens are able to do this during a single infection by altering the composition of their cell membrane (e.g. *Borrelia burgdorferi, Salmonella typhimurium, Neisseria gonorrhoea*, and *Trypanosoma brucei*). For other pathogens there is sufficient antigenic variation within the population that prior infection does not confer immune protection to all members of the species. For example, infection with one 'serotype' of *Streptococcus pneumoniae* does not confer protection to other serotypes.

6.10.2 Latency

Herpes viruses are able to establish latent infection, entering a state within the infected cell where they do not replicate. Because no viral peptides are produced, none are loaded into MHC-I and displayed, so the virus is 'invisible' to cytotoxic T cells. In latency the virus is unable to damage the host cell, but retains the capacity to reactivate, often in the setting of immune suppression.

6.10.3 Signal interference

Some viruses are able to induce host cells to express factors that suppress or misdirect the immune system. For example, viral infection commonly leads to down-regulation of MHC-I expression, reducing presentation of viral peptides to cytotoxic T cells. Some viruses encode homologues of human cytokines. For example, CMV encodes vIL10, which host cells recognize as native IL10, leading to a skew of the immune response towards a more virus-tolerant Th2 phenotype.

6.11 Further reading

Mogensen, T. H. 'Pathogen recognition and inflammatory signaling in innate immune defenses', *Clinical Microbiology Review*, 22/2 (2009), 240–273.

Murphy, K., Weaver, C., *Janeway's Immunobiology* (9th edn, New York, 2016).

Snapshot Archive from CellPress. Contains useful graphics, with succinct explanations of some key areas of basic immunology http://www.cell.com/snapshots

6.12 Assessment questions

6.12.1 Question 1

A twenty-year-old man with a history of recurrent sinopulmonary infections is admitted with meningitis. Enterovirus RNA is detected in CSF.

A defect in which part of his immune system is the most likely responsible for this infection?
A. Cell-mediated immunity.
B. Complement.
C. Humoral immunity.
D. Innate immunity.
E. Neutrophil function.

6.12.2 Question 2

A twenty-four-year-old woman presents with sepsis. *Neisseria meningitidis* is isolated from blood cultures.

Which aspect of immune function would it be most appropriate to investigate?
A. Cell-mediated immunity.
B. Complement.
C. Humoral immunity.
D. Innate immunity.
E. Neutrophil function.

6.12.3 Question 3

A four-year-old male child with a history of recurrent boils and abscesses, mainly with *Staphylococcus aureus*, is admitted with osteomyelitis. Tissue samples grow *Aspergillus nidulans*.

Which aspect of immune function would it be most appropriate to investigate?
A. Cell-mediated immunity.
B. Complement.
C. Humoral immunity.
D. Innate immunity.
E. Neutrophil function.

6.13 Answers and discussion

6.13.1 Answer 1

C. Humoral immunity

The most common manifestation of humoral immunodeficiency, e.g. common variable immunodeficiency, is with recurrent sinopulmonary infections and is associated with susceptibility to invasive enteroviral infection. Assessment of humoral immune response includes checking serum immunoglobulins, serum protein electrophoresis, IgG subclasses, B cell phenotype, and investigating specific antibody levels pre- and post- immunization with polysaccharide and conjugate vaccines (e.g. Pneumovax and Menitorix).

6.13.2 Answer 2

B. Complement

Intact terminal complement pathway leading to formation of membrane attack complex is essential for immune response to *Neisseria sp*. Assessment of complement includes serum levels of C3 and C4, and function of classical and alternative pathways (CH100 and AP100).

6.13.3 Answer 3

E. Neutrophil function

The presentation is most in keeping with chronic granulomatous disease caused by defects in NADPH oxidase, which renders phagocytes unable to destroy certain microbes. Examples of neutrophil function tests include dihydrorhodamine (DHR) flow cytometry test and nitroblue-tetrazolium (NBT) test.

PART TWO

MICROBIOLOGY/ VIROLOGY LABORATORY PRACTICE

The use of the laboratory in the investigation, management, and prevention of infection

Caryn Rosmarin

CONTENTS

7.1 Pre-analytical elements of laboratory practice

The pre-analytical stage is broadly classified into four elements:

1. Appropriate selection and use of diagnostic tests;
2. Proper filling in of request forms (paper or electronic);
3. Collection and transport of specimens; and
4. Checks made when the specimen and request form reach the laboratory to ensure the correct patient, sample, and request have been made.

7.2 The microbiologist/virologist role in influencing the pre-analytical stage

A large part of the laboratory role is to advise on the collection of appropriate samples in order to ensure the best chance of diagnosing a suspected infection syndrome or specific pathogen. This requires having a working knowledge of the range and processes of tests available in the laboratory for each clinical syndrome, and the ability to appreciate their strengths and weaknesses, sensitivities and specificities.

In addition, advice on the sampling technique may need to be provided regarding the timing of the sample, the type of sample, number or volume of samples, and optimal storage and transport conditions that are required for the specific test. Failure to take sufficient amount of the correct sample, at the correct time, and using the correct container, or storing it in a suboptimal manner, may lead to falsely negative or positive results.

Most laboratories have manuals for guidance on sampling details and the tests performed. It is vital that this information is available to clinical staff. Microbiologists and virologists contribute to this guide and assist in ensuring it is communicated to the clinicians taking the samples. This is particularly important for precious samples that cannot easily be repeated, e.g surgical biopsies, CSF from lumbar punctures.

Ensuring the correct completion of the request form is vital. Important clinical details should be included on the request to help guide the most appropriate tests. Examples of important information to be documented on the request include travel history, antibiotic history, immune status, underlying diseases, and site of suspected infection.

7.3 Analytical elements of laboratory practice

The analytical stage consists of the actual testing of the sample. Examples of common tests performed in this stage include microscopy, culture, sensitivity testing, serology, and molecular detection, as well as more novel techniques such as mass spectrometry, bioinformatics, and sequencing.

The analytical stage comprises a mix of both manual and automated testing. While virology has already made the move over the past few decades, there is now a significant move to more automated testing in microbiology as well. This has been driven by both efficiency pressures and technological advances.

This stage of laboratory practice may involve evaluation of new testing platforms and continued monitoring of the quality of current testing methods.

7.4 Knowing which test to perform and how to perform it

Every laboratory test has its benefits and limitations. Understanding the principle behind the tests will help to decide which is most appropriate, and to interpret the result. Unusual test requests and unexplained results may need testing in a reference laboratory. A deeper understanding of the basis of the test and performance of more routine result interpretation corresponds to an increase in the ability to recognize the unusual.

All testing procedures are performed in accordance with standard and best practice. This practice is documented in the laboratory standard operating procedure (SOP), which maintains the quality of laboratory, provides laboratory staff with written instructions on how to perform tests consistently to an acceptable standard, helps avoid short-cuts being taken when performing tests, provides written standardized techniques, and promotes safe laboratory practice.

7.5 Standard operating procedure in the lab

All stages of laboratory practice, not just the analytical stage, should follow standard and best practice procedures to ensure quality, consistency, and safety.

SOPs form the basis of practice against which quality assurance is measured. Monitoring for errors or deviations from SOPs gives laboratory management and external bodies' assurance that the laboratory is of a certain standard. This is essential in accreditation of laboratories with the national and international standards agencies.

7.6 Health and safety in laboratory practice

The laboratory environment poses a risk of exposure to a variety of infectious agents, and hence has a strict code of conduct and behaviours associated with its function. It is essential that anyone working in this environment has an induction regarding local practice, and understands the various risks of the specimens, the processes, and the organisms.

The main risk associated with working with biological agents is the potential for infection. There are three main potential routes of infection to be aware of in the laboratory.

1. Inhalation, e.g. breathing in a fine aerosol or vapour mist which may contain a viable organism.

2. Ingestion, e.g. through poor hygiene practice, mouth pipetting, or eating/drinking in a lab area [the latter two of which should *never* be done]. Remember—chewing gum is considered eating!

3. Skin penetration, e.g. as a result of injury with a contaminated sharp object, contact with mucous membrane of eyes/nose/mouth, or entry via an uncovered wound.

Biologic agents are classified into four hazard groups by the Advisory Committee on Dangerous Pathogens (ACDP) based on their pathogenicity, transmissibility, risk to lab workers, and whether effective prophylaxis is available. (Interested readers are referred to Chapter 13 for more detail).

7.7 Post-analytical elements of laboratory practice

Most clinical microbiologists and virologists are likely to be involved in this stage of laboratory practice on a daily basis, and it requires knowledge of all other stages to be done to the best standard. Once a result has been generated by the laboratory, it then needs to be interpreted and communicated to the requestor, with or without further clinical advice appropriate to the result. The result should be interpreted in the light of the sample type, knowledge of the analytical process, additional investigations, and the patients' clinical condition. It is especially important to understand and convey that a positive microbiology or virology result may not necessarily represent an active infection, but may be the result of contamination, colonization, or past or inactive infection.

All results and the communication that occurs regarding interpretation and advice given need to be accurately documented in an appropriate patient record. Confidentiality should be maintained when communicating results; they should *not* be left on answering machines, faxed, or emailed to non-secure numbers or email addresses.

7.8 Preventing healthcare associated infections

The laboratory contributes to the prevention of spread of infection by diagnosing contagious pathogens in a timely manner from clinical samples, and screening samples from patients at risk of harbouring organisms known to cause healthcare-associated infections (HCAIs), or contacts of those with highly infectious pathogens or HCAIs.

Each of the three stages of laboratory practice provides opportunities to prevent HCAIs.

1. Pre-analytical stage:
   a. Correct filling in of request forms can highlight patients at risk of carrying organisms known to be highly infectious or cause HCAIs, e.g. a history of travel to a high-risk country, recent hospital admission, healthcare in a foreign country, previous antibiotic use, or a history of high-risk behaviours.

b. Requesting the appropriate test can ensure the laboratory performs the correct test for the indication, thus providing a quicker and more accurate result, e.g. requesting an MRSA screen rather than M,C, & S; Hepatitis A IgM, rather than IgG.

c. Taking the correct sample in the correct container and transporting it correctly to the lab ensures a more rapid result, thus limiting the risk of transmission of HCAIs while waiting for results.

2. Analytical stage (priority of accuracy vs speed of the test):

a. Using the test with the highest sensitivity can help to identify all those with the infection will be captured, but may produce some false positives. Therefore, a negative result using a test with a high sensitivity is likely to be a true negative.

b. Using the test with the highest specificity can ensure all those without the infection will be captured, but may produce some false negatives. Therefore, a positive result using a test with a high specificity is likely to be a true positive.

c. Using the test with the most rapid result to ensure rapid isolation of patients with suspected infections is more often highly sensitive, e.g. molecular tests, which if negative are likely to exclude an infection, i.e. have a good negative predictive value.

3. Post-analytical stage:

a. Once the test is complete, delivery of the result in a timely fashion to the correct person/s so action can be taken.

b. Interpretation of the result and institution of isolation and screening procedures based on the result.

7.9 Diagnosing and managing outbreaks

The three stages of laboratory practice each provide opportunities to assist in diagnosis and management of outbreaks.

1. Pre-analytical stage:

a. Correct filling in of request forms can highlight patients at risk of being part of the outbreak, e.g. a history of association with a group or behaviour, or history of contact with someone carrying or suffering from an infectious disease.

b. Requesting the appropriate test can ensure the laboratory tests what is required, e.g. requesting *C. difficile* and typing to facilitate comparison with other cases.

c. Taking the correct sample in the correct container and transporting it correctly to the lab.

2. Analytical stage:

a. Identifying pathogens from patients suspected of being involved the outbreak. This may take the form of culture-based sampling, molecular detection, or seroconversions.

b. Comparing pathogens from patients suspected of being involved the outbreak. The comparison can be made phenotypically and/or genotypically, using (for example) antibiotic sensitivities, protein electrophoresis, gene markers, or more recently, whole genome sequencing.

3. Post-analytical stage:

a. Once the test is complete, delivery of the result in a timely fashion to the correct person so isolation can be undertaken.

b. Recognition of an outbreak by understanding and correctly interpreting results.

7.10 Assessment questions

7.10.1 Question 1

A sixty-four-year old man is admitted to hospital with a one-day history of vomiting and diarrhoea. He is admitted to the acute medical ward in an open bay and receives IV fluids and an antiemetic. He has no further episodes of diarrhoea but vomits twice overnight. A stool sample sent tests positive for norovirus.

The most appropriate course of action is:
A. Isolate the patient in a side room.
B. Barrier nurse the patient in the bay.
C. No isolation precautions are required as the patient had no further diarrhoea.
D. Screen all other patients in the bay for norovirus.
E. Leave the patient in the bay and isolate all the contacts.

7.10.2 Question 2

A thirty-four-year-old woman is seen by her GP and has a stool sample sent to the laboratory. The following clinical information is supplied in the request form:

'Fever, abdominal pain, diarrhoea with blood. Two days ago was at barbeque where she ate chicken that wasn't quite cooked. One episode of vomiting. No travel, and no recent hospitalization or antibiotics. Other people at barbeque have similar symptoms.'

What test or tests would you perform on this stool samples?
A. Ova, cysts, and parasites only.
B. M, C, & S and viral PCR.
C. Viral PCR only.
D. M, C, & S only.
E. Ova, cysts, and parasites and M, C, & S.

7.10.3 Question 3

You are asked to introduce a new point of care HIV screening test for use in the A&E in order to help improve uptake of testing. You are sent sample tests to evaluate, which you do with the following results.

Provided all other elements are comparable between the tests, which test would you choose?
A. Sensitivity = 22%; Specificity = 100%.
B. Sensitivity = 50%; Specificity = 50%.
C. Sensitivity = 98%; Specificity = 22%.
D. Sensitivity = 82%; Specificity = 75%.
E. Sensitivity = 11%; Specificity = 26%.

7.11 Answers and discussion

7.11.1 Answer 1

A. Isolate the patient in a side room
Norovirus is highly infectious and is present in both stool and vomitus. It is transmitted by droplets transmitted through air to close contacts or by fomites that land on the environment and which

are then ingested by others. Most commonly it is transmitted by eating food or drinking liquids that are contaminated with norovirus, touching surfaces or objects contaminated with norovirus then putting your fingers in your mouth, or having contact with someone who is infected with norovirus. A person with norovirus is most infectious from when their symptoms start until forty-eight hours after all their symptoms have passed, although they may also be infectious for a short time before and after this.

Isolating the patient to prevent spread to others is the best practice. Barrier nursing will not stop norovirus spreading. Contacts do not need screening but should be monitored closely for symptoms, and tested and isolated if they develop any. Ideally the bay the patient was in should be closed to further admissions or patient movements until the incubation period of forty-eight hours has past to ensure the contacts do not become symptomatic. This would reduce the outbreak potential.

Answer E is not incorrect, but is not logistically feasible, as would mean a loss of bed space if a single patient is isolated in a bay, and inappropriate use of side rooms.

7.11.2 Answer 2

D. M, C & S only

Use your clinical judgement to assess the symptoms and most likely diagnosis. Based on the incubation period, possible point source, and clinical symptoms, this is most likely to be bacterial—campylobacter or salmonella. Testing all might cover all bases but is not cost effective. Development of SOPs to guide testing based on clinical information provided will help demand management and improve capacity for appropriate testing.

7.11.3 Answer 3

C. Sensitivity = 98%; Specificity = 22%

There are two measures that are commonly used to evaluate the performance of screening tests: the *sensitivity* and *specificity* of the test. The sensitivity of this test refers to the ability of the test to correctly identify those with HIV, whereas, the specificity refers to the ability of the test to correctly identify those without the virus.

Tests with a high sensitivity are used to *rule in* those with the disease, but may pick up some without; tests with high specificity are used to *rule out* those without the disease.

Selecting the optimal balance of sensitivity and specificity depends on the purpose for which the test is going to be used. A screening test should be highly sensitive and a confirmatory test should be highly specific.

The most important characteristics of any screening test depend on the implications of an error. In all cases, it is important to understand the performance characteristics of any screening test to appropriately interpret results and their implications. In this case, while a false positive will lead to great anxiety for the patient while awaiting a confirmatory test, a false negative is more serious as the diagnosis will be missed completely. The sensitivity and specificity of a screening test are characteristics of the test's performance at a given cut-off value above or below which the test is positive. In general the higher the sensitivity, the lower the specificity, and vice versa.

The *positive predictive value* (PPV) of the test reflects the probability that HIV is present when the test is positive, whereas the *negative predictive value* (NPV) reflects the probability that HIV is not present when the test is negative. The positive predictive value of a screening test will be influenced not only by the sensitivity and specificity of the test, but also by the prevalence of the disease in the population that is being screened. When the disease is more prevalent, people are

Table 7.1 Evaluation of test performance.

		Truth	
		Disease present	*Disease absent*
Test	*Positive test*	True positive	False positive
	Negative test	False negative	True negative

more frequently affected, so the probability of disease among those with positive tests will be higher (Table 7.1).

Sensitivity = True positive/(True positive + False negative)

Specificity = True negative/(True negative + False positive)

PPV = True positive/(True positive + False positive)

NPV = True negative / (True negative + False negative)

CHAPTER 8

Bacteriology diagnostic methods

Heather Dolphin, Fatima Ahmad, Gurtan Atamturk, Jennifer Henderson, Tim Linehan, Robert Serafino Wani, and Satya Das

CONTENTS

8.1 The main specimen types, containers, and tests performed

This is summarized in Table 8.1.

8.2 Methods used to process samples

a) Microscopy—A cell count is performed on sterile fluids and CSF samples using the Neubauer chamber or a similar device. The number of white blood cells (WBC) and red blood cells seen under the microscope are reported as well as the differential WBC count (i.e. the number or percentage of lymphocytes and neutrophils in the sample). A Gram stain is then done and the presence of any organism reported.

b) Culture samples are plated onto the appropriate media and streaked out for single colonies as shown (Figure 8.1). Blood agar is normally used; however, other media are used depending on the site of the specimen, e.g. chocolate agar is used if a fastidious organism is a potential pathogen such as *Haemophilus sp.*; anaerobic agar for anaerobes; selective agar such as MacConkey can be used on non-sterile specimens to differentiate between the colony types. Plates are incubated for eighteen to forty-eight hours at the correct conditions; most plates being CO_2, others at O_2 and anaerobically.

Table 8.1 Examples of specimen types, tests, containers, and storage conditions.

Specimen	Test	Container	Storage conditions/ extra information
Blood culture	Automated culture	BactAlert or Bactec Bottle	Keep at room temperature and send to lab ASAP Should be loaded onto the machine within hours
Cerebrospinal fluid (CSF)	Microscopy and culture, tests for acid fast bacilli (AFB) and Cryptococcus antigen	Sterile CSF container	Send to the lab immediately and call lab for urgent processing Store in refrigerator if needed (2–8 °C)
Body fluids and tissues	Microscopy and culture, acid fast bacillus (AFB)	Sterile container	Send to the lab immediately if urgent otherwise store in refrigerator (2–8 °C)
Swabs (throat, eye, ear, wound, genital, MRSA)	Culture	Transwab or liquid amies swab (not dry)	Refrigerate (2–8 °C)
Sputum, bronchoalveolar lavage	Culture	Sterile container	Refrigerate (2–8 °C)
Faeces	*Clostridium difficile* toxin, culture for salmonella, shigella, campylobacter, *E. coli* 0157, helicobacter antigen, parasites	Sterile container	Refrigerate (2–8 °C)
Skin, nails, hair	Mycology investigation	Sterile container	Room temperature
Urine	Microscopy and culture	Primary tube or sterile container	Refrigerate (2–8 °C)

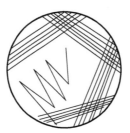

Figure 8.1 Streaking out on an agar plate to obtain a single colony.

c) Identification plates are examined for growth. Potentially significant isolates are identified either by MALDI-TOF MS, by API, or other biochemical tests.
d) Sensitivities are performed on significant organisms by manual and automated methods.

8.3 The main types of media, their use, and how they work

This is summarized in Table 8.2.

Table 8.2 Examples of media and colonial characteristics.

Type of media	Examples of media	Incubation time	Colony observation	Identification
Blood agar	Enrichment	$35 \pm 2°C$ for twenty-four to forty-eight hours at 3–10% CO_2	Different colonies observed for different organisms. Haemolysis for β-haemolytic streptococci	Growth of most bacteria, fastidious and otherwise such as *Streptococci*
Chocolate agar	Non-selective, enriched growth medium	5–10% CO_2 at 35–37°C for twenty-four to forty-eight hours	*H. Influenzae* appear as convex. Smooth, pale grey or transparent colonies	Fastidious *H. influenzae and Neisseria meningitidis*
MacConkey agar	Selective and differential	$35 \pm 2°C$ for twenty-four hours	Lactose fermenter- pink colonies Non-lactose fermenter- transparent colourless colonies	Lactose fermenter—*E. coli.* Non-lactose fermenter—*Salmonella sp. and Shigella sp*
Sorbitol MacConkey agar	Selective and differential	35–37°C for twenty-four hours	Colourless colonies	*E. coli O157*
Xylose lysine deoxycholate (XLD) agar	Selective	35–37°C for twenty-four hours	*Salmonella sp.*—Red colonies with black centre as produce H_2S *Shigella sp.*—H_2S negative, so red colonies only	*Salmonella and Shigella sp*
Chromogenic MRSA medium	Selective	37°C for eighteen to twenty-four hours	Denim-blue colonies	Presumptive MRSA
Campylobacter agar	Selective	39–42°C for ≥ forty-eight hours	Grey-coloured colonies	*Campylobacter* species
Neomycin fastidious anaerobe agar	Selective	35–37°C for twenty-four hours	Grey-coloured colonies	*Clostridium perfringens*
TCBS Agar (Thiosulfate Citrate Bile Salts Sucrose Agar)	Selective	35–37°C for twenty-four hours	*V. cholerae*—yellow colonies. *V. parahaemolyticus*—blue-green centred colonies	*V. cholerae, V. parahaemolyticus*, and other *Vibrio sp*
Columbia CNA Agar	Selective and differential	5–10% CO_2 at 35–37°C for twenty-four hours	alpha, beta, and gamma colonies	Gram-positive bacteria e.g staphylococci, haemolytic streptococci, and enterococci

8.4 When to use selective agar

Selective agar is necessary when isolating pathogens from faeces, although further confirmatory tests are needed.

8.4.1 How are salmonella and shigella confirmed?

- Black or colourless colonies on xylose lysine deoxycholate (XLD) or other chromogenic agar plates (Figure 8.2) are tested with oxidase reagent.
- Oxidase negative isolates are identified by MALDI-TOF, API and or biochemically using triple-sugar iron (TSI) tubes.
- Serology is then performed on suspicious isolates and sent to a reference laboratory for confirmation.
- Campylobacter is confirmed by testing grey flat colonies on campylobacter agar with oxidase reagent. Oxidase positive samples are Gram stained and if 'seagull'-shaped gram-negative bacteria are observed under the microscope, campylobacter is confirmed.

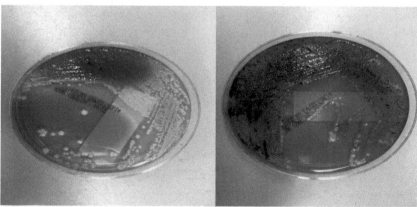

XLD agar- Negative
Proteus

XLD agar- Black colonies-*Salmonella* or
Colourless colonies-*Salmonella* or *Shigella*

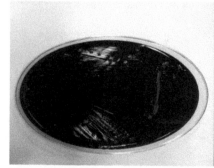

CCDA- *Campylobacter* sp.

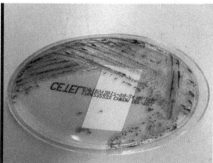

CETEL 0157 chromogenic agar: negative
(Positive (E. coli 0157) gives pink to mauve colonies)

Figure 8.2 Examples of selective plates.

8.5 Common biochemical tests to identify microbial pathogens

8.5.1 The catalase test

The catalase test is a simple biochemical test to differentiate between *Staphylococcus* species and *Streptococcus* species, with the use of hydrogen peroxide (H_2O_2). It tests for the presence of the enzyme catalase which is found in *Staphylococcus* species.

   Method: Colonies of suspect organism are introduced to slide where a drop of 3% hydrogen peroxide is added and a coverslip is placed on top.

   Result: If bubbles are observed (from the release of oxygen as catalase breaks down hydrogen peroxide into water and oxygen), the test is positive and indicates the organism is *staphylococcus species*.

8.5.2 The oxidase test

The oxidase test is used primarily to differentiate between *Pseudomonas* species from other coliforms and enteric bacteria (e.g. *E. coli*, *Klebsiella*) with the use of oxidase reagent (tetramethyl-p-phenylenediamine dihydrochloride) by testing for the presence of cytochrome c oxidase activity.

   Method: Colonies of the suspect organism can be introduced directly to swab tip with a drop of oxidase reagent on the tip, or oxidase reagent is dropped onto blotting paper and the organism is introduced to the spot.

   Result: If a colour change to dark purple occurs, this indicates the presence of *Pseudomonas* species.

8.5.3 The urease test

The urease test demonstrates urease activity by *Proteus, Providencia, Klebsiella, Morganella*, and *Clostridium sordelli*, while other enterobacteriae are negative. Other urease positive organisms include *Ureaplasma urealyticum, Helicobacter pylori, Nocardia* and *Cryptococcus* spp. Urea in the medium is broken down by organisms possessing urease into ammonia and carbon dioxide.

   Result: If a colour change from yellow to red-orange (or pink) occurs, it indicates the presence of urease.

8.6 'Rapid' biochemical tests used in the laboratory

The Analytical Profile Index (API) method relies on a series of miniaturized biochemical tests in which a single organism acts on one substrate at a time to provoke enzyme activity within a microtube (Figure 8.3).

   Method: Each microtube on the API biochemical strip is dehydrated until a bacterial suspension is added; then the biochemical strip is incubated.

   Result: After a period of incubation the panels are each scored based on a positive or negative reaction to the substrate within the panel. The scoring provides a number profile which is used to determine the identification of the organism when compared to a database, such as apiweb™.

8.7 Routine stains used in microbiology

8.7.1 Gram stain

Gram stain is the principal stain used in the demonstration and identification of bacteria. Gram-positive bacteria are purple and gram-negative bacteria are pink/red. The test uses crystal violet, Gram's iodine, acetone, and safranin or carbol fuchsin or neutral red.

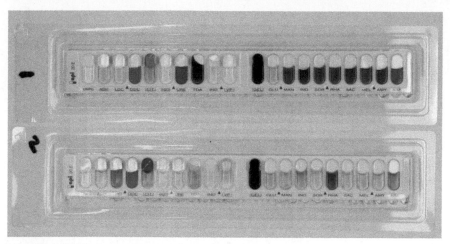

Figure 8.3 API 20E: 1- *P. mirabilis*; 2- *S. marcescens*.

8.7.2 Mycobacterial stains

Mycobacteria are detected by auramine (more sensitive, hence used for screening the slide) or Ziehl Neelsen (ZN, which is more specific) staining as they are acid fast due to the large amount of lipids in their cell wall. Auramine positive slides are usually stained with ZN to confirm the presence of mycobacteria.

8.7.2.1 Auramine

Auramine stain uses auramine-phenol solution, acid alcohol 3%, potassium permanganate 0.1%, and a UV microscope at 25x objective is used to examine the slides.

8.7.2.2 Ziehl Neelsen (ZN) stain

For the ZN stain, carbol fuchsin is heated, acid alcohol 3% is used to decolourize, and then methylene blue is used as a counterstain. The slide is examined under oil immersion (x100 objective).

8.7.3 Auramine stain for Cryptosporidium detection

Auramine O Stain uses acid alcohol to decolourize, then methylene blue as a counterstain. Slides are examined under the UV florescence microscope under low power (x25 objective).

8.8 Algorithms to identify common bacteria

The flow charts in Figure 8.4 and Figure 8.5 summarize the identification of gram-positive and gram-negative bacteria, respectively.

8.9 Commonly used manual and automated sensitivity testing in microbiology

8.9.1 Broth dilution

The Broth dilution method involves subjecting the isolate to a series of concentrations of antimicrobial agents in a broth environment which can be conveniently performed in a microtiter

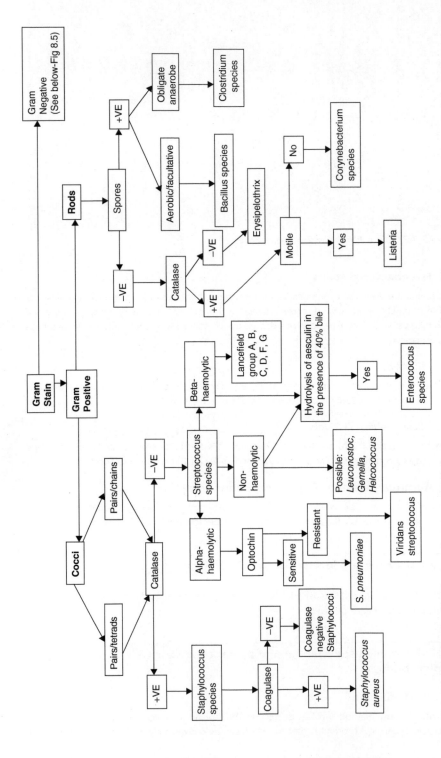

Figure 8.4 Algorithm for the identification of gram-positive bacteria.

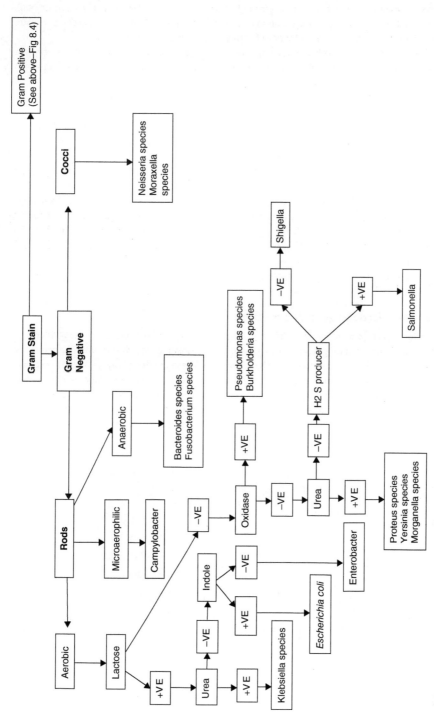

Figure 8.5 Algorithm for the identification of gram-negative bacteria.

format. The lowest concentration at which the isolate is completely inhibited (as evidenced by the absence of visible bacterial growth) is recorded as the minimal inhibitory concentration or MIC. The MIC is thus the minimum concentration of the antibiotic that will inhibit this particular isolate. Several different companies use this theory for their automated methods.

A procedure similar to broth dilution is agar dilution. Agar dilution method follows the principle of establishing the lowest concentration of the serially diluted antibiotic concentration at which bacterial growth is still inhibited.

8.9.2 Disk diffusion method

The disk diffusion susceptibility method is simple and practical and has been well-standardized. The test is performed by applying a standardized bacterial inoculum to the surface of a sensitivity agar plate, making sure that the sample is spread in more than one direction across the plate. The primary discs are applied to the plate using a disc dispenser and plates incubated overnight.

The zones of growth inhibition around each of the antibiotic disks are measured to the nearest millimetre. The diameter of the zone is related to the susceptibility of the isolate and to the diffusion rate of the drug through the agar medium. The zone diameter of each antibiotic is interpreted using the European Committee on Antimicrobial Susceptibility Testing (EUCAST) breakpoints.

The results of the disk diffusion test are 'qualitative,' and reported as either R (resistant) or S (sensitive).

8.9.3 Antimicrobial gradient method

The antimicrobial gradient diffusion method (Figure 8.6) uses the principle of establishing an antimicrobial concentration gradient in an agar medium leading to determination of susceptibility. The E-test (Figure 8.7) is a commercial version available. These are thin plastic test strips that have a dried antibiotic concentration gradient underneath and are marked on the upper surface with a concentration scale. After overnight incubation, the tests are read by viewing the strips from the top of the plate. The MIC is determined by the intersection of the lower part of the ellipse shaped growth inhibition area with the test strip and measured in μg/ml.

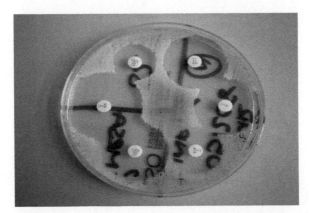

Figure 8.6 Disc sensitivities.

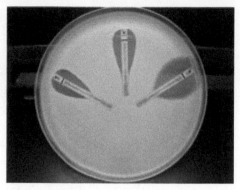

Figure 8.7 E-test sensitivities.

8.10 Using discs to detect resistance mechanisms

8.10.1 Inducible clindamycin resistance (D test)

A flattening of the zone of inhibition around the clindamycin disk proximal to the erythromycin disk (producing a zone of inhibition shaped like the letter D; see Figure 8.8) is considered a positive result and indicates that the erythromycin has induced-clindamycin resistance. Clindamycin should be reported as susceptible when the induction test is negative or as resistant when positive.

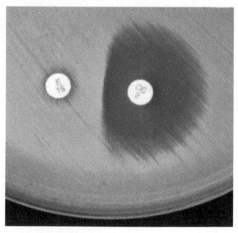

Figure 8.8 Detection of inducible clindamycin resistance.

8.10.2 Extended spectrum beta-lactamases

ESBL (extended spectrum beta-lactamase) is a bacterial enzyme which confers resistance to penicillin and cephalosporin antibiotics. The emergence of ESBL-producing organisms has become

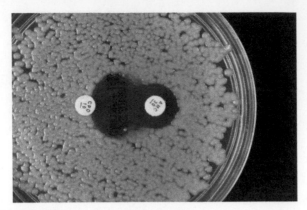

Figure 8.9 ESBLs- Extended spectrum beta-lactamases.

increasingly significant because of the limited therapeutic option available to treat infections due to these organisms and also due to their ability to spread easily between populations. The two main bacterial species that produce ESBLs are *Escherichia coli* (*E. coli*) and *Klebsiella pneumoniae*. The ESBLs that *E. coli* most often produce are called CTX-M enzymes.

The presence of an ESBL can be determined by zone-size comparison when simultaneously tested with antibiotic and with antibiotic plus inhibitor combinations (see Figure 8.9). Mutations that alter the amino acid configuration around the active site of these beta-lactamases are caused by the ESBLs.

8.11 Common pathogens found in each specimen type

This is summarized in Table 8.3.

Table 8.3 Likely pathogens isolated from different sites/specimens.

Site	Common pathogens
Blood culture	All bacteria and yeast
Body fluids and tissues including CSF	All bacteria and yeast
Swabs (throat, eye, ear, nose)	*Staphylococcus aureus, Streptococcus pneumoniae, Haemophilus influenzae,* beta haemolytic *Streptococci, Moraxella catarrhalis, Pseudomonas aeruginosa*
Wound	*Staphylococcus aureus,* beta haemolytic *Streptococci,* and coliforms if post-surgical or deep wound
Genital swab	*Neisseria gonorrhoea, Candida,* beta haemolytic *Streptococci, Trichomonas,* Bacterial vaginosis
Nasopharynx swab	*Bordetella pertussis*
Respiratory sample	*Streptococcus pneumoniae, Moraxella catarrhalis, Haemophilus influenzae, S.aureus, Mycobacteria, fungi, Legionella*
Faeces	*Salmonella, Shigella, Campylobacter, E. coli 0157,* parasites
Skin, nails, hair	Dermatophytes
Urine	*Coliforms, Staphylococcus saprophyticus, Enterococcus, Pseudomonas*

Pseudomonas, Enterococci, and Coliforms—When isolated from deep-seated wounds, abscesses, from wounds during surgery, ITU and neonatal patients can be significant.
Many other organisms can be considered significant, depending on the clinical history and specimen type.

8.12 Follow-up tests on culture-negative samples

In cases where no pathogen was isolated from standard microbial agar plate culture, it might be pertinent to order a sample for 16S PCR (polymerase chain reaction) testing.

PCR is used to detect the presence of organism from the amplification of bacterial DNA, either by using fluorescent probes/markers (i.e. 'real-time' PCR), or by more conventional means where amplification of the target DNA is determined by agarose gel electrophoresis, stained with ethidium bromide and examined under UV light. 16S PCR testing is used for the detection and identification of microorganisms from their unique 16S rRNA gene.

8.13 Further readings and useful resources

UK Standards for Microbiology Investigations
https://www.gov.uk/government/collections/standards-for-microbiology-investigations-smi

8.14 Assessment questions

8.14.1 Question 1

A neonate develops symptoms of acute meningitis a week after birth. Gram staining of the CSF shows gram-positive bacilli.

Which laboratory test is most likely to confirm the identification of this organism?
A. Catalase.
B. DNase plate.
C. Staphaurex latex agglutination.
D. Tube coagulase.
E. Tumbling motility.

8.14.2 Question 2

A gram-negative bacillus is isolated from pus drained from the wound of a nineteen-year-old farmworker's hand. It is oxidase positive and grew on blood agar but not on MacConkey agar plate.

Which is the most likely organism?
A. *Aeromonas hydrophila.*
B. *Escherichia coli.*
C. *Klebsiella pneumoniae.*
D. *Pasteurella multocida.*
E. *Pseudomonas aeruginosa.*

8.14.3 Question 3

A twenty-one-year-old student presents to his GP with headache, neck stiffness, and fever. He is given intramuscular benzylpencillin and then sent to A&E. He undergoes various investigations and the following results are obtained:

Random plasma glucose	6.1 mmol/L

Cerebrospinal fluid (CSF):

Opening pressure	350 mmH$_2$O (normal range: 120–250)
Total protein	2.90 g/L (normal range: 0.15–0.45)
Glucose	<0.5 mmol/L (normal range: 3.3–4.4)

White cell count	204/µL (normal range: ≤5)
Neutrophil count	190/µL (normal range: 0)
Microscopy	no organisms seen
CT scan of brain	no abnormality detected

Which of these investigations is most likely to identify the causative agent?
A. Blood cultures.
B. CSF culture.
C. Nasopharyngeal aspirate culture.
D. Polymerase chain reaction (PCR) on CSF sample.
E. Throat swab culture.

8.15 Answers and discussion

8.15.1 Answer 1

E. Tumbling motility.
The catalase test is used to differentiate *Streptococci* (catalase negative) from *Staphylococci* (catalase positive). Tube coagulase, Staphaurex latex agglutination, and the DNase plate are laboratory tests used to differentiate between *Staphylococcus aureus* and other staphylococcus species. *Staphylococcus aureus* gives positive results in these above tests while non-aureus Staphylococcal species give negative results. *Listeria monocytogenes* is a short gram-positive bacillus with rounded ends that causes serious infection in the elderly, neonates, pregnant women, and the immunocompromised. In adults, infection is acquired through ingestion of contaminated food whereas in neonates it is by direct contact when passing through the birth canal. Clinically, patients present with bacteraemia, meningitis, and meningo-encephalitis. *Listeria monocytogenes* is motile (by virtue of their possession of peritrichous flagella) when grown at room temperature (20–25°C) but not at 37°C, and displays characteristic 'tumbling' motility.

8.15.2 Answer 2

D. *Pasteurella multocida*.
All of the gram-negative organisms mentioned could cause wound infection. However, excepting *Pasteurella multocida*, all will grow on MacConkey agar plate, which is used in the laboratory to differentiate lactose fermentators (e.g. Enterobacteriaceae) from non-lactose fermentators (e.g. Pseudomonads). *Pasteurella multocida* is an oxidase-positive non-motile gram-negative pleomorphic organism found as a commensal in livestock and wild animals. It is associated with animal bites, scratches, or licks, but infection without epidemiological contact with animals can occur. It is usually sensitive to penicillin.

8.15.3 Answer 3

D. Polymerase chain reaction (PCR) on CSF sample.
This is a clinical presentation of bacterial meningitis. After parenteral administration of benzyl penicillin, the likelihood of isolating an organism using traditional microbiology techniques such as culture of body fluids is greatly reduced. Throat swab and nasopharyngeal aspirate may identify organisms which could be commensals of the upper respiratory tract. Finding organisms in sterile sites such as blood and CSF is diagnostic. PCR of CSF and/or blood has a better yield of identifying the causative organism. In the event that no organism is isolated this patient will usually be treated with intravenous antibiotics for up to two weeks to cover for possible pneumococcal meningitis.

CHAPTER 9

Virological diagnostic methods

Anthony R. Oliver

9.1 Questions for virologists

Every clinical virologist must step back and ask what the aim of diagnostics is, in general, i.e. the 'who/what/when/where' questions. Broadly, the clinical virologists of today must answer a limited set of questions because that is what current technology allows:

- Is this person currently infected with a virus?
- Has this person ever been infected/exposed to a virus?
- This person has a confirmed virus infection—how is it progressing with or without intervention?
- From whom was this virus infection contracted?

However, currently many questions remain remarkably difficult to answer with existing diagnostics. Increasingly the focus of diagnostics is moving from interest solely in the virus itself to how a given virus interacts with a given host pre/post infection, e.g. HIV host co-receptor testing.

Nearly all virological diagnostic methods rely on two fundamental technical principles—target and signal amplification, which both allow the visualization of virus-specific antigen/antibody or nucleic acid. Luckily, some clinical samples, e.g. stool, do not require amplification in order to detect significant virus infections, but even in these situations it is impossible to visualize the presence of viruses or their host antibodies without highly specialized equipment and chemistry. Most viruses are < 200nm in size, and therefore it is impossible to resolve virus particles even with the best optical microscopes. Nearly all of the methodologies detect surrogate markers. It is of note that viable virus numbers do not equal nucleic acid copies, which do not equal virus capsids visible by electron microscopy: these are apples and elephants when trying to compare their quantity.

9.2 Available diagnostic technology

Diagnostic technology operates in two phases or realms; detection or screening, and characterization. For example, asking if a patient has an Influenza A virus infection, followed by asking what is the haemagglutinin/neuraminidase type (e.g. H1N1). It is possible to further characterize, e.g. asking if the virus is sensitive to antiviral treatment.

Screening technologies tend to have the following characteristics:

- Relatively low cost
- High throughput/capacity
- High levels of sensitivity and specificity

Conversely, second-line technologies are:

- Higher cost
- Often low throughput/capacity
- Offering levels of sensitivity that may not be optimal for screening
- Offering considerable additional detail in terms of virus/antibody typing and character

Figure 9.1 shows the possible diagnostic approaches.

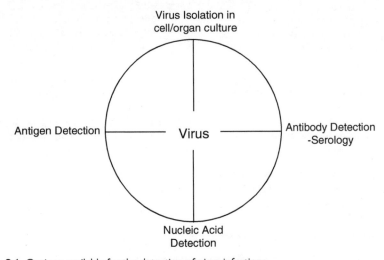

Figure 9.1 Options available for the detection of virus infections.

9.3 Achieving virus isolation/characterization

Viruses are obligate intracellular parasites. Consequently, if they are to be 'grown' or 'isolated', their substrate must be living cells. The earliest diagnostic techniques relied heavily upon animal or cell culture systems to recognize the presence of a virus. Typically, routine diagnostic laboratories used monolayer cell cultures in small test tubes or multi-well plates. While cell culture is a 'catch-all' (or at least a 'catch-many') technique, it has significant drawbacks, not least the need for cell culture infrastructure and expertise in order to produce good quality cultures with which to inoculate patient material. Secondly, different viruses and virus families have a predilection for specific cell types, so it is often necessary to maintain and inoculate two to three different cell types to give a

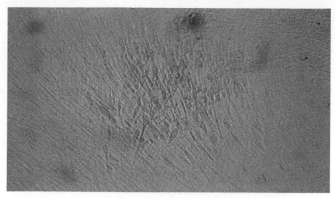

Figure 9.2 Cytomegalovirus focal CPE in human embryo lung fibroblast cell culture (D + 10).

broad coverage of different viruses. For example, human cytomegalovirus (hCMV) will only grow in human fibroblast cell lines, whereas influenza would normally only grow in monkey kidney epithelial cells. Additionally, viruses need somewhere between two and twenty-one days incubation before they are detectable by microscopic examination of their 'cytopathic' effect (CPE) (Figure 9.2). CPE alone is often insufficient to provide a definitive virus type, so subsequent physical/antibody-based pre/post inoculation methods are required to identify a virus down to its type/serotype. This methodology has been largely superseded by real-time PCR due to its scalability and speed.

9.4 Direct detection techniques

Prior to the advent of PCR in the late 1980s, two techniques more than any other contributed to the expansion of both the discovery of human viruses and to diagnostic armoury. Direct immunofluorescence (DIF) is a type of signal amplification technique. It relies on the visualization of virus-infected cells through the medium of virus-specific antibodies conjugated with a dye which fluoresces under excitation by ultraviolet light. In 1975, Köhler and Milstein discovered commercial monoclonal antibody production, which resulted in greatly enhanced specificity, the lack of which was a significant impediment to the interpretation of the first generation assays that used convalescent human or animal serum. In the 1970s and 1980s, negative staining electron microscopy (EM) led to the discovery of whole new human virus families, e.g. the 1972 discovery by Flewett and colleagues of human rotavirus , and Madeley and Cosgrove's 1975 discovery of human astrovirus. These viruses had previously been undetected due to their fastidiousness in existing cell culture systems. Both of these techniques were regarded as 'rapid' diagnostics and, in that regard, even today are almost unparalleled; it is perfectly possible to generate a single EM result in around twenty minutes! However, these diagnostic methods suffer from a lack of sensitivity and specificity compared to the molecular amplification techniques of today, and also from relatively low throughput. However, they are, and were, extremely effective and practical tools in the correct arena. Current viral infection control procedures have been based upon these tools, more than any other. It is noteworthy that for both, the relative insensitivity is not a major impediment (with the exception of norovirus) as the targets that they were used upon are present in overwhelming amounts in the majority of acute cases, e.g. respiratory syncytial virus (RSV) and rotavirus. EM has a sensitivity of around 10^5–10^6 particles per ml of sample. Indeed, an increased risk of nosocomial infection was often associated with the measureability in these direct detection methods. The use of these methodologies has waned with the rise of automated PCR; EM, in particular, suffers from the need for extremely expensive capital equipment costing several hundreds of thousands of

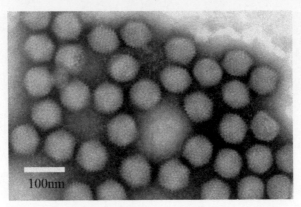

Figure 9.3 Adenovirus by negative staining EM.

pounds, coupled with a requirement for operators of the highest calibre to produce relatively low numbers of results.

Negative staining EM is a simple procedure using plastic/carbon-coated copper mesh grids and the heavy metal stain (phosphotungstic acid; Figure 9.3). An experienced operator will make a diagnosis within two to five minutes for most cases. The technique can be enhanced by the use of specific antibody at different stages. However, a major drawback is the insufficient specificity for many viruses, as identification is based normally on morphology alone (Figure 9.3). For example, it is unable to distinguish between the herpesviruses herpes simplex virus (HSV) and varicella-zoster virus (VZV), or the paramyxoviruses that cause mumps and measles.

Immunofluorescence (Figure 9.4) requires a cellular sample such as nasopharyngeal aspirate, which is washed and disaggregated to form a cell suspension. This is air-dried to a teflon (PTFE)-coated microscope slide and fixed in acetone to remove the lipid membranes, allowing a fluorescein isothiocyanate (FITC)-labelled specific antibody to be applied to one of the slide wells. Once washed to remove the unbound antibody, the slide is dried and examined under a UV microscope with an appropriate set of filters. Granular cellular apple-green fluorescence, with nuclear sparing, in 'flask'-shaped columnar ciliated epithelial cells counterstained red, is highly diagnostic of RSV with the appropriate antibody. Antibodies are available for the most significant viral pathogens.

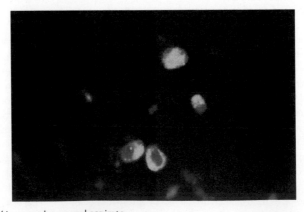

Figure 9.4 RSV in nasopharyngeal aspirate.

The modern legacy of these early detection techniques are lateral flow devices that use monoclonal antibodies affixed to a membrane solid phase and a colourimetric enzyme/substrate interaction to visualize the presence of virus-specific antigen. These are seen as 'point of care' type devices that are also used for particularly urgent cases, especially in detecting norovirus and influenza. However, they suffer from similar limitations in sensitivity and specificity.

9.5 Detecting and characterizing virus-specific antibodies

The mainstay of both small and large diagnostic virology laboratories is the serology lab. The predominant sample type analysed is serum, but other fluids such as saliva, urine, and blood spot eluates are also tested. These laboratories are typically populated with two or three different serological platforms covering the high- and low-throughput analytes, which have an appropriately broad test menu. Of these, HIV antibody, hepatitis B and C screening, and syphilis testing form the large bulk of the analyses.

Enzyme immunoassay is the predominant technology in detection and characterization. Table 9.1 shows the various approaches that can be used. A good laboratory will supply numeric data for each parameter to the authorizer, normally in the form of the signal to cutoff ratio, i.e. the value of the sample divided by the value of the cutoff used by the assay. Very often assays will have a 'grey zone' of +/- a percentage (usually 10%) around the cutoff along with a protocol for repeating or reporting values lying within. Most modern assays utilize microparticles as the 'solid phase' which is the medium that separates the isolated target and label from the excess reagents that are washed away. The detection system can be colourimetric, but fluorescence and chemi-luminescence increasingly are now used. The advantage of the latter two is that analysers can measure the rate of production of light/fluorescence rather than an endpoint colour change. This is quicker to measure and normally offers a larger dynamic range for the assay which is important for target quantitation.

9.6 Methods used for viral nucleic acid detection/ characterization

These methods are explored in Chapter 11.

9.7 Is the most sensitive method the best?

No. The assay whose sensitivity is best matched with the question asked is the one that should be used. For example, while single-copy assays exist for the detection of HIV RNA, they are not clinically useful for the routine management of HIV infection. Instead, a cutoff of fifty copies per ml of plasma is used in all clinical management algorithms.

9.8 Factors influencing the choice of diagnostics

The following parameters should be considered:

- Speed—time to first result and then subsequent rate of result production.
- Cost of reagents, including sensible quality control regime.
- Cost of capital equipment.
- Ease of use.

Table 9.1 Antibody immunoassay protocol summary.

Assay Type	Quantitative (Y/N)	Signal proportional to	Weakness	Good for specific IgM detection	Affected by input dilution
Indirect anti-globulin IgG/IgM/IgA 1.Solid phase virus specific antigen 2.Sample for detection of IgG/IgM/IgA 3.Conjugate anti-human Ig Class antibody	Y	Absolute amount of specific class Ig	Competition from other Ig classes and rheumatoid factor	N	Y
Antigen sandwich 1.Solid phase virus specific antigen 2.Sample for detection of total antibody 3.Antigen conjugate	Y	Absolute amount of virus-specific Ig all classes	Technically more difficult to conjugate antigens	Not appropriate as all classes detected	Y
Competitive 1.Solid phase virus specific antigen 2.Sample for detection of total antibody mixed with antibody conjugate	N	Inverse of the absolute amount of virus-specific Ig all classes	Enzyme poisoning if sample and conjugate mixed	Not appropriate as all classes detected	Y
μ Capture (IgM antibody Capture) 1.Solid phase anti-human IgM 2.Sample for detection of IgM 3.Virus-specific antigen 4.Virus-specific antibody conjugate	N	Amount of virus-specific Ig relative to total Ig	Not quantifiable	Y—best in class protocol for IgM detection	N

- Assay performance—sensitivity/specificity.
- Analyzer footprint.

9.9 Differences between quantitative and qualitative assays

Quantitative and qualitative assays serve different functions and are set up in different ways. For example, qualitative assays are geared to respond quickly to a small input dose (Figure 9.5). This is not the optimal response for reproducible quantitation, which works best where the signal responds in equal linear proportion to the input dose.

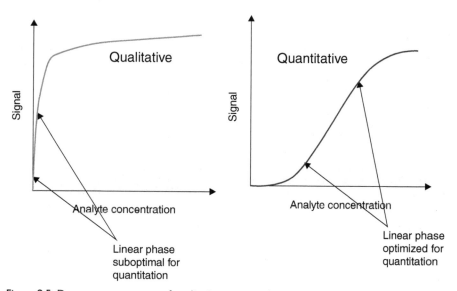

Figure 9.5 Dose-response curves of qualitative assays and quantitative assays.

9.10 Assessment questions

9.10.1 Question 1

There is an outbreak of diarrhoea and vomiting on the care of the elderly ward. A large batch of stool samples is received in the laboratory to determine the cause of the outbreak.

Which of the following techniques would you use on the stool samples?
A. Electron microscopy.
B. Immunofluorescence.
C. Rapid lateral flow device.
D. Real-time multiplex PCR.
E. Virus isolation.

9.10.2 Question 2

A previously known HIV-1 positive pregnant lady presents to the labour ward at thirty-eight weeks gestation without any record of antenatal care.

Which of the following blood tests is the most appropriate investigation?
A. A highly sensitive HIV viral load assay able to detect ten copies RNA per ml of sample with a turnaround time of seventeen days, cost £100.
B. A next-generation sequencing assay capable of producing sequence data to cover all HIV drug mutations with a turnaround time of twenty-one days, cost £300.
C. A rapid antibody typing assay with a turnaround time of two hours, cost £15.
D. An HIV viral load assay able to detect fifty copies RNA per ml of sample with a turnaround time of twenty-four hours, cost £20.
E. An HIV viral load assay able to detect 5000 copies RNA per ml of sample with a turnaround time of one hour, cost £5.

9.10.3 Question 3

The interpretation of data from enzyme immunoassays depends on the format of the assay.

Considering the type of assay used in the following options and the signal-to-cutoff ratio (S/CO) obtained, which of the following options should be reported as antibody 'NOT detected' with no further action?
A. Hepatitis A IgM, μ capture assay, S/CO = 255.4.
B. Hepatitis B core total antibody, competitive assay, S/CO = 10.5.
C. Hepatitis B core IgM, μ capture assay, S/CO = 1.40.
D. HIV 1/2 antibody, antigen sandwich assay, S/CO = 1365.9.
E. Measles IgG, indirect anti-globulin assay, S/CO = 0.99.

9.11 Answers and discussion

9.11.1 Answer 1

D. Real-time multiplex PCR
While EM might be an alternative diagnostic tool, it is not suited to the processing of large numbers of samples. Additionally, EM is not suited to the detection of norovirus as it is difficult to visualize even at the height of an acute infection. Currently, many institutions would lack the experience to use an electron microscope, even if it were available. Lateral flow devices produce quick results but always suffer from a lack of sensitivity, and often a lack of specificity as well. Virus isolation would be largely useless as it would take too long and most of the targets are fastidious. Immunofluorescence requires intact cellular material which is not readily available in stool. This leaves real-time PCR, which has the requisite sensitivity, specificity, throughput, and cost.

9.11.2 Answer 2

D. An HIV viral load assay able to detect fifty copies RNA per ml of sample with a turnaround time of twenty-four hours, cost £20.
The key here is to determine the best clinical outcome balanced against cost and turnaround time. The lady would be offered a C-section if she had a detectable viral load fifty or more copies RNA per ml. British HIV Association guidelines still use less than fifty copies RNA per ml of sample as the definition of 'undetectable'. This has been the case since the mid-1990s and is based on the output of very many clinical trials of HIV antiviral drug therapy. The time factor is determined by the late presentation relative to expected delivery date, i.e. two weeks. So option A is slightly too slow, more expensive, and un-necessarily sensitive, whereas option E is too insensitive to be of use even though it is quick and cheap. Option B provides a large amount of data but does not quantify the RNA so is, in this particular instance, clinically useless as well as being expensive and far too slow. Option C, the antibody typing assay, is of no use as we already know the virus is HIV 1. Option D provides the level of sensitivity required in a clinically useful timeframe at reasonable cost.

9.11.3 Answer 3

B. Hepatitis B core total antibody, competitive assay, S/CO = 10.5

Clearly options A, C, and D rely on methodologies where the signal is proportional to the input amount of the analyte, therefore anything ≥ 1 S/CO is positive. However, option B is a competitive or blocking assay, so the signal is inversely proportional to the input analyte amount. A positive will give rise to < 1 S/CO, giving little or no signal, whereas a negative will not compete for binding of the conjugate giving a signal, resulting in a S/CO ≥ 1. Option E merits some discussion, as on the face of it, it is a methodology giving rise to a signal proportional to the input and therefore giving a value < 1, should it not be considered as negative? In this case, the result is only 1% less than the cutoff and therefore lies within a typical 'grey-zone' for most assays. It would likely be reported as equivocal or be repeated and have an algorithm applied to the aggregate results to determine the qualitative interpretation.

CHAPTER 10

Fungal diagnostics

Shila Seaton and Rohini J. Manuel

10.1 Defining fungal diagnostics

The field of fungal diagnostics encompasses tests that are performed to help diagnose fungal disease, guide its management, and or monitor the effectiveness of its treatment. For some superficial skin and yeast infections, a clinical examination of the patient combined with microscopic examination of the sample may be sufficient to determine that fungal disease is present, even if the specific fungal pathogen is not identified.

For deep-seated and systemic infections, a combination of diagnostic tests may be required in order to obtain a definitive diagnosis. These include microscopy to detect fungal elements, culture, detection of circulating antigens and antibodies, and molecular tests.

More recently, molecular and proteomic approaches have increasingly dominated the conventional identification of pathogenic yeasts and, to some extent, filamentous fungi, since traditional methods are time consuming. More importantly, conventional methodologies have failed to identify common organisms that display uncharacteristic profiles, or fungal pathogens that are rarely encountered.

10.2 Types of fungal diagnostics

10.2.1 Conventional

The 'gold standard' for the definitive diagnosis of fungal disease is histology or culture of the fungal pathogen from a clinical specimen. A specimen will routinely be inoculated onto several different types of media (Table 10.1), and then incubated at specific conditions and temperatures for up to twenty-one days. Media plates will be examined periodically for growth, and staff will try to identify the fungus using both macroscopic and microscopic morphologies. The few biochemical tests available, e.g. the urease test, can be helpful in identification, most often for yeast species.

Microscopy of fungal isolates, histopathological examination of tissue, and fungal specific stains play fundamental roles in the diagnosis of infection for the variety of fungi that cause disease (Table 10.2).

Table 10.1 The appropriate diagnostic tests for each clinical specimen type, and the time taken to obtain a result.

Diagnostic test	Specimen type(s)	Function	Uses	Time to result(s)
Standard fungal culture media Sabouraud Dermatophyte Test medium Czapek Chromogenic Cornmeal(Tween) Dalmau Potato Dextrose Agar Malt agar	Blood, cerebrospinal fluid (CSF), body fluids,* bone marrow, catheter tips, corneal scrape, vaginal swab, skin, nail, hair	Growth of fungus on appropriate media exhibiting phenotypic features for identification	Diagnose infection by specific fungi which includes filamentous moulds and yeasts	Days to weeks
Biochemical systems	Fungal colony isolated in culture	Combination of chemical, enzymatic, and fermentation tests to provide a discriminatory profile	Identifies yeast species	24/48 hours
Microscopy GRAM Lactophenol aniline blue/fuchsin Calcofluor white India ink KOH (potassium hydroxide)	Skin, nail, hair, blood, CSF, body fluids	Identify fungal isolate with microscopic examination of fungal elements indicative of the genus, or species of the fungus	Diagnose infection by specific fungi and guide treatment	One hour
Antigen testing Mannan (ELISA) Beta-D-glucan (EIA) Galactomannan (Latex agglutination, ELISA) Cryptococcal (Latex agglutination, EIA)	Serum, CSF, bronchoalveolar lavage fluid (BAL), urine	Detects cell wall proteins associated with a specific fungus Tests available for a variety of fungi Sequential samples to monitor for disease	Diagnose infection caused by specific fungi Useful for screening and monitoring of disease using sequential samples	Days
Antibody IgG, IgM, IgE; Immunodiffusion Complement fixation ELISA/EIA	Blood, serum, CSF, body fluids	Detects immune response to a specific fungus	Diagnose current or recent infection by specific fungi. Obtain sequential samples to monitor disease and response to therapy	Days to weeks

(continued)

Table 10.1 Continued

Diagnostic test	Specimen type(s)	Function	Uses	Time to result(s)
Molecular	Fungus isolated in culture, direct detection in blood, CSF, body fluids, and tissue	Detects DNA, RNA genetic material (18rS, 28rS, ITS1, D1–D2 regions dependent on PCR) target fungi	Detects core pathogens but also atypical fungi and rare species unknown to be pathogenic**	Days to weeks
Susceptibility testing	Sample of fungus isolated in culture	Follow-up to fungal culture. When a fungus (causative agent) has been identified, susceptibility is sometimes requested to determine the most effective antifungal agent(s) to use	Guide treatment	Days to weeks after culture
Proteomics	Sample of fungus isolated in culture	Detects the cell wall proteins and identifies a wide variety of fungi	Identify causative fungal agent and guide treatment	Ten minutes for yeast isolates, filamentous fungi may take longer)

*Includes BAL, pleural, ascitic, and peritoneal fluids.
**Some methods only available in research setting.

Table 10.2 Common stains used for the diagnosis of fungal disease and for the identification of fungal isolates.

Type of stain	Specimen type	Function
Gram stain	Fungal colony, blood, sterile (e.g. cerebrospinal fluid (CSF)) and non-sterile body fluids (e.g. BAL fluid)	Yeast elements (blastospores and hyphae) stain purple. Filamentous fungi do not take up the stain, but are visible for primary identification. Stain is low/absent for *Cryptococcus* species
Fontana-Masson (MH)	Tissue section	Stains the cell wall (melanin) of *Cryptococcus neoformans*. Especially useful for differentiation of non-capsular *C. neoformans*. Cell walls stain brown/black
Giemsa	Bone marrow, peripheral blood, sputum, and BAL	Staining for *Histoplasma* and *Pneumocystis* spp
Lactophenol fuschin/aniline blue (Lactophenol: preserves fungal structures and kills the fungus. Fuschin/ aniline blue: stains the fungal elements)	Colony of fungus	Growing fungus absorbs the stain to highlight typical features* of the fungus. Fungal elements stain pink with fuschin and blue with aniline blue
KOH (potassium hydroxide) 10% w/v	Skin scrapings, nail and hair clippings	Observation of fungal elements* made visible with the softening of the matrix of the specimen
Calcofluor/bankophor white	Blood, sterile, and non-sterile body fluids	Apple green fluorescence of fungal elements*
Mayer mucicarmine	Tissue biopsies	Capsule of *Cryptococcus neoformans* stain deep rose
India Ink	CSF	Black background highlights the capsule of *Cryptococcus neoformans* budding cell
Periodic Acid Shift (PAS)	Biopsy of deep tissue (foci of infection)	Stains carbohydrates, in particular glycogen, purple-red (magenta), and epithelial mucin fungal elements* stain pink
Gomori (Grocott) methenamine silver stain (GMS)		Green/blue background highlights brown/black fungal elements*
Grindley fungus		Yellow background highlights pink/red/purple fungal elements*
Haematoxylin and Eosin (H&E)		Acidophilic cytoplasm is red, basophil nuclei are blue, erythrocytes are red Fungal elements* stain pink, red, or purple
Immunofluorescence	BAL, tissue	Green background with *Pneumocystis* cells staining black

*Spores, hyphae, and fruiting bodies.

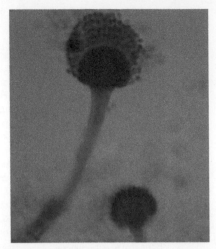

Figure 10.1 Image of *Aspergillus fumigatus* species complex fruiting bodies.
Reproduced courtesy of UK NEQAS.

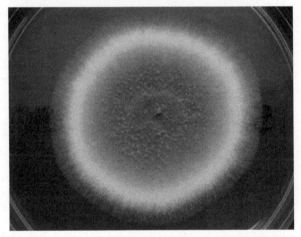

Figure 10.2 Image of *Aspergillus fumigatus* species complex colony on Sabouraud media.
Reproduced courtesy of UK NEQAS.

The most common stain for identifying fungal elements from a cultured isolate is lactophenol fuschin/aniline blue stain. Figure 10.1 depicts the fruiting body (conidiophore) of *Aspergillus fumigatus* species complex, the most prevalent fungal species responsible for invasive aspergillosis (IA) in severely immunocompromised individuals. Figure 10.2 illustrates the phenotype of a three-day old colony.

10.2.2 Serology

10.2.2.1 Antibody detection

Serological tests are beneficial when non-culture based diagnosis of fungal disease is required.

Complement fixation is predominantly used to diagnose endemic mycoses, e.g. coccidioidomycosis, blastomycosis, and histoplasmosis. These dimorphic fungi are not easily cultured, hence serological testing plays a vital role in diagnosis.

Multiple assays are available for the detection of *Aspergillus*-specific antibodies in human serum. Since raised *Aspergillus*-specific IgG, IgE, IgA, and IgM all have different interpretations in different clinical scenarios, it is important to understand which assays measure which antibody types when interpreting results. For example, IgG antibody assays are a useful aid to diagnosis in bronchopulmonary aspergillosis.

10.2.2.2 Antigen detection

Beta-D-glucan (BDG) is a polysaccharide present in the majority of fungal cell walls except for *Cryptococcus* and Mucoraceous moulds. BDG is useful for screening for suspected invasive fungal disease (IFD), but its high negative predictive value has greater impact in excluding IFD.

Mannan, a cell wall polysaccharide of yeasts, is a highly immunogenic antigen with a greater sensitivity than BDG. It can provide confirmatory results faster than a positive blood culture and is a useful indicator for the presence of yeast species, apart from *Cryptococcus*. However, a negative result does not indicate absence of IFD, as the antigen is rapidly cleared during disease.

Galactomannan (GM) is a cell wall polysaccharide of most *Aspergillus spp.*, and the detection of the antigen in serum or broncho-alveolar lavage (BAL) fluid using the Platelia *Aspergillus* enzyme immunoassay (EIA) is an important test for the early diagnosis of IA in patients with underlying risk factors, e.g. haematological malignancies and stem cell transplantation. The detection of GM in these specimens is a recommended criterion for the diagnosis of IA in the 2008 European Organisation in Research Treatment of Cancer/Mycology Study Group (EORTC/MSG) guidelines.

Several studies discuss the lack of stability of GM in serum specimens during storage prior to testing, which impacts upon the sensitivity of the antigen.

10.2.2.3 Radiological investigations

One of the most useful tools for diagnosis of IFD is high-resolution computed tomography scan (CT) of the site of infection, e.g chest. An early indicator of IA is the characteristic halo sign, which describes the ground-glass appearance around a pulmonary nodule. The other characteristic sign is the air crescent sign, which appears later in infection. Wedge-shaped pleurally based infiltrates may also be present.

10.2.2.4 Molecular detection

Molecular diagnostic tools are rapid, accurate, and quantitative, and can help in provision of a rapid diagnosis to aid patient management.

Nucleic acid hybridization probes, DNA sequencing, peptide nucleic acid fluorescence in-situ hybridization (PNA FISH) probes, and polymerase chain reaction (PCR) tests are available for the identification of fungal isolates in pure culture.

PNA FISH for direct detection of *Candida* spp. from blood cultures enables the rapid identification of the five most common species of *Candida*, with each species emitting a different fluorescence dependent on the species (*C. albicans* and *C. parapsilosis* emit bright green fluorescing cells, *C. tropicalis* yellow, *C. glabrata* and *C. krusei* bright red), which helps direct appropriate treatment. Several multicentre research studies recommend the use of a standardized PCR technique—from specimen type, DNA extraction method, and PCR technique—to allow for efficient detection of pathogenic fungi.

10.2.2.5 Proteomics

Matrix-assisted laser desorption/ionization time of flight (MALDI-ToF) mass spectrometry (MS) is increasingly available in clinical microbiology laboratories due to low operational costs, speed of detection, and specificity of analysis. Based on characteristic protein spectra obtained from intact cells, MALDI-ToF MS allows the highly discriminatory identification of yeasts and filamentous fungi such as *Aspergillus spp.* to genus and species level, with the aid of a spectral database. Direct identification of yeasts from positive blood cultures has the potential to greatly shorten turnaround times and improve the laboratory diagnosis of fungaemia.

10.3 Which diagnostic test is best?

In terms of sensitivity and specificity, there is no single test that is best for definitive diagnosis. Because of this, international guidelines recommend use of a combination of tests to optimize the management and treatment of patients.

The 2008 EORTC guidelines recommend that the combination of culture, clinical symptoms, radiographic evidence, and antigen detection will enable the diagnosis of proven IA. Hoenigl et al. (see Useful resources and further reading) showed that the combination of PCR with antigen testing provided 98% sensitivity and specificity compared to a combination of antigen and culture (89% sensitivity and specificity respectively).

Combined biomarker screening is increasingly used to diagnose IA in high-risk patients. In adults, the combination of GM and fungal DNA detection has proven to be beneficial in the diagnosis of IA.

The laboratory diagnosis of cryptococcosis is based on direct microscopy, culture and antigen detection by cryptococcal antigen testing, as false negative results from misinterpreted India ink preparations can cause misdiagnosis.

10.4 Appropriate clinical specimens

The recovery of fungi is highest from the active site of infection. Table 10.1 details the specimen type, appropriate diagnostic test(s), and the time taken to obtain a result.

10.5 Limitations of available diagnostic tests

10.5.1 Conventional methodology

One significant problem associated with traditional methods is that they can take up to four weeks to complete. They are often onerous and require highly experienced laboratory staff competent in the visual recognition of fungal morphologies.

It has been shown that traditional phenotypic and microscopic characteristics are insufficient to identify newly emerging fungal species that cause disease.

10.5.2 Histopathology

Histopathology requires a sample of the tissue section where the fungal disease is active. Biopsies are invasive, and the section of sample may not contain fungal elements.

Examination of the stained preparations requires skill and expertise to differentiate between fungal elements and various artefacts that may be present.

Standard histological stains for fungi are GMS stain and PAS (see Table 10.1). The GMS stain is more sensitive than the PAS stain, although the GMS also stains inflammatory cells and tissue reticulin alongside fungal elements.

10.5.3 Serology (antigen/antibody)

10.5.3.1 Antibody

A positive antibody test result in a single serum sample may indicate exposure to a specific fungus, but it does not indicate when the exposure occurred. Rising antibody concentrations between acute and chronic serum samples may indicate active or recent fungal disease. Antibody tests are not recommended for the classical immunocompromised population, as they are unable to mount an immune response, e.g. for the diagnosis of IA.

10.5.3.2 Antigen

BDG is ubiquitous in the environment, and false positives are a potential limitation of this test. An antigen positive test result is likely to be indicative of IFD, but a negative result cannot confirm the absence of disease.

The *Aspergillus* antigen GM is present only transiently in serum, and may not be detectable in sequential samples when utilized for screening or monitoring for disease. Issues with storage conditions have been discussed previously. The assay has also been shown to produce false positives in patients treated with piperacillin-tazabactam or co-amoxiclav.

The cryptococcal antigen test is obscured by rheumatoid interference factors if present in the test specimen or by cross-reactive organisms, e.g. *Trichosporon asahii*, leading to false positive results.

10.5.3.3 Mass spectrometry

With proteomics, identification can only be made on a cultured isolate, with final identification determined within minutes. The scope of identification is dependent on the compilation of spectra forming the database.

10.5.3.4 Molecular diagnostics/sequencing

DNA sequencing is feasible with the currently available technology, although analysis and interpretation of the data pose a significant challenge, as results are dependent on sequence quality with existing reference databases, and the skill and expertise of scientific staff.

10.6 The future of fungal diagnostics

Combinations of fungal diagnostics are enabling mycologists to significantly reduce the time taken for the detection and identification of a variety of fungi in the clinical laboratory.

Opportunities and challenges remain for the direct detection of fungi from clinical specimens; however, it is still necessary to combine the newer technologies of molecular diagnostics and proteomics with more conventional methodologies to improve patient management.

10.7 Useful resources and further reading

Borman, A., M., Szekeley, A., Johnson, E. M., 'Comparative Pathogenicity of United Kingdom Isolates of the Emerging Pathogen *Candida auris* and Other Key Pathogenic Candida Species', *American Society for Microbiology* 1(2016),

De Pauw, B., Walsh, T. J., Donnelly, J. P., Stevens, D. A., Edwards, J. E., Calandra, T., et al., 'Revised Definitions of Invasive Fungal Disease from the European Organization for Research and Treatment of Cancer/Invasive Fungal Infections Cooperative Group and the National Institute of Allergy and Infectious Diseases Mycoses Study Group (EORTC/MSG) Consensus Group', *Clinical Infectious Diseases*, 46/12 (2008), 1813–1821.

Hoenigl, M., Prattes, J., Spiess, B., Wagner, J., Prueller, F., Raggam, R. B., et al, 'Performance of Galactomannan, Beta-D-Glucan, Aspergillus Lateral-Flow Device, Conventional Culture, and PCR Tests with Bronchoalveolar Lavage Fluid for Diagnosis of Invasive Pulmonary Aspergillosis', *Journal of Clinical Microbiology*, 52/6 (2014), 2039–2045.

Leroux, S., Ulmann, A. J., 'Management and Diagnostic Guidelines for Fungal Diseases in Infectious Diseases and Clinical Microbiology: Critical Appraisal', *Clinical Microbiology and Infection*, 19/12 (2013), 1115–1121.

Posteraro, B., De Carolis, E., Vella, A., Sanguinetti, M., 'MALDI-ToF Mass Spectrometry in the Clinical Mycology Laboratory: Identification of Fungi and Beyond', *Expert Review of Proteomics*, 10/2 (2013), 151–164. doi: 10.1586/epr.13.8

Ráčil, Z, Kocmanova, I., Lengerova. M., Weinbergerova, B., Buresova, L., Toskova., M., et al., 'Difficulties in Using 1,3-Beta-D-Glucan as the Screening Test for the Early Diagnosis of Invasive Fungal Infections in Patients with Haematological Malignancies—High Frequency of False-Positive Results and their Analysis', *Journal of Medical Microbiology*, 59 (2010), 1016–1022.

Walsh, T. J., Annaissie, E. J., Denning, D. W., Herbrecht, R., Kontoyiannis, D. P., Marr, K. A., et al., 'Treatment of Aspergillosis: Clinical Practice Guidelines of Infectious Diseases Society of America', *Clinical Infectious Diseases*, 46 (2008), 327–360.

10.8 Assessment questions

10.8.1 Question 1

A bronchoalveolar lavage fluid sample from an allogeneic stem cell transplant recipient with suspected invasive aspergillosis is received in the laboratory.

Which diagnostic test is the most appropriate to help establish a diagnosis?
A. Galactomannan.
B. IgG antibody detection.
C. IgM antibody detection.
D. Mannan.
E. PCR.

10.8.2 Question 2

MALDI-ToF MS allows the highly discriminatory identification of yeasts and filamentous fungi.

What is its principle?
A. Analysis of the spectra of cell wall proteins.
B. Detection of antibodies.
C. Detection of antigens.
D. Detection of nucleic acid.
E. Mass spectrometry of DNA.

10.8.3 Question 3

You receive a serum sample from a patient with aplastic anaemia, on whom you have performed the galactomannan (GM) antigen test. What is a characteristic of the galactomannan antigen test?
A. It does not produce false positive reactions with piperacillin-tazobactam.
B. Galactomannan is present transiently in serum.
C. Galactomannan remains stable during long term storage.
D. The assay is quantitative.
E. The assay is used for the diagnosis of Pneumocystis.

10.9 Answers and discussion

10.9.1. Answer 1

A. Galactomannan

The most useful diagnostic test would be galactomannan, as an immunocompromised patient would not mount a significant immune response to determine the presence of a fungal infection. Only yeast species contain the mannan antigen.

10.9.2 Answer 2

A. Analysis of the spectra of cell wall proteins.

MALDI-ToF mass spectrometry is a process that examines the spectra obtained from the proteins of the fungal cell wall. It does not detect DNA.

10.9.3. Answer 3

B. Galactomannan is present only transiently in serum.

The galactomannan antigen test is a semi-quantitative test. Galactomannan antigen is present transiently in patients with invasive aspergillosis. The galactomannan antigen test is not used for the diagnosis of pneumonia. Recent studies have suggested that the galactomannan antigen is unstable during long-term storage. Cross-reactivity with piperacillin-tazobactam has been described in the literature.

CHAPTER 11

Molecular diagnostics

Duncan Clark and Mark Wilks

11.1 The application of molecular diagnostics in infection

Molecular diagnostics in infection generally relate to the detection and/or characterization of nucleic acid sequences of infectious agents in clinical samples which are used to provide:

- A laboratory diagnosis.
- A means of monitoring patients at risk of developing disease caused by a particular infection.
- A method to predict through genotypic analysis the susceptibility or resistance to appropriate treatments.
- A measurement of the response to therapy.

11.2 Commonly used molecular diagnostic approaches

A few key laboratory techniques underpin the majority of molecular diagnostic tests that are currently used in the field of infection, and include:

- Block-based polymerase chain reaction (PCR).
- Real-time PCR, including quantification.
- Strand displacement amplification.
- Transcription mediated amplification.
- DNA sequencing.

These can be commercially sourced, which has the advantage of CE marking, or developed in-house, sometimes referred to as laboratory developed tests (LDTs). Whatever the source, the underlying principles are often the same and rigorous evaluation and validation is required for the adoption of any molecular test in the diagnostic laboratory.

11.3 Laboratory requirements for molecular diagnostics

The majority of molecular diagnostic tests require the amplification of a specific DNA sequence and its subsequent detection by a variety of means. As such, small sequences of DNA from the infectious agent are amplified from a relatively low copy number in the clinical sample. For example, after thirty to forty cycles of PCR, a single copy of a sequence can theoretically be amplified to over a billion copies. This PCR product, commonly termed amplicon, can provide a template for any further testing with the same PCR test and therefore potentially act as a source for false positive results. Molecular diagnostic laboratories have requirements to keep the different stages of the molecular test separate and minimize the risk of amplicon contamination. Most facilities will have a 'clean PCR laboratory' that is used to store the clean reagents such as primers, probes, enzyme mastermixes, and no clinical samples, nucleic extracts, or amplification reactions are ever taken into this environment. Another laboratory is used for the nucleic acid extraction of the clinical samples and this environment is often used to set up the PCR reactions. The final requirement is a post-PCR laboratory that houses the PCR instruments for amplification and the appropriate equipment to provide any post-amplification PCR analysis. This laboratory contains the potential amplicon contamination, and it is critical that material from this laboratory does not inadvertently transit back to either the extraction laboratory or the clean PCR lab. This provides a uni-directional workflow for molecular-based amplification tests. Most diagnostic laboratories will use a degree of automation to facilitate their molecular service and there are a variety of automated extraction platforms and systems for setting up PCR reactions. Some platforms are fully automated from extraction through PCR and amplicon detection.

11.4 Preparing a sample for molecular testing

Any molecular test requires the availability of high-quality nucleic acid from the clinical sample. In microbiology and virology, common sample types that are used in molecular tests include:

- Cerebrospinal fluid (CSF);
- Blood/plasma;
- Upper and lower respiratory tract samples;
- Stool;
- Urine;
- Swabs; and
- Biopsy.

Whether done manually or using an automated nucleic acid extractor, the most common method for extracting nucleic acid from a sample relies on:

- Initial sample lysis using a buffer containing the chaotropic agent, guanidinium thiocyanate, and the protease enzyme, Proteinase K.
- Following lysis, the addition of silica (as magnetic particles or as a membrane on a spin column). Under high salt concentrations, silica binds tightly to both DNA and RNA.
- Washing steps to remove the non-nucleic acid material.
- Elution of the purified nucleic acid (DNA and RNA) from the silica matrix in the presence of a low salt buffer.

Prior to PCR, if the target to be detected has a RNA template/genome, e.g. HIV-1, influenza viruses, measles virus, hepatitis C virus, an additional step is required to convert the RNA template to complementary DNA (cDNA). This can either be carried out separately or incorporated as the first stage in the PCR test. Either way, it relies on the use of a reverse transcriptase enzyme, which is a RNA-dependent DNA polymerase, to convert single stranded RNA to cDNA. The latter is now a suitable template for PCR amplification.

11.5 Block-based PCR

PCR results in the exponential amplification of double-stranded DNA, the specificity of which is determined by the PCR primers. It is conducted through a series of thermal cycles, usually thirty to forty. The appropriate design of primers is very important and specialized software is usually used in their selection. Likewise, in designing a test to detect all the genetic variants that may exist for a particular infectious agent, targeting a conserved region of the genome is required. Although individual mismatches between a patient's infectious agent and the complementary primers used in the PCR test can be tolerated to a certain extent, the more mismatches or their positioning at the 3′ end of a primer can severely compromise the efficiency of amplification. Block-based PCR refers to a test that requires a subsequent post-amplification step such as gel analysis or hybridization to identify if the amplicon has been generated. For example, the former relies on the electrophoresis of the PCR reactions in an agarose gel, stained with a DNA binding dye such as ethidium bromide. If amplicon is present, its migration into the agarose gel is determined by the size of the DNA fragment and this is confirmed by the electrophoresis of molecular size markers in the same gel.

11.6 Real-time PCR

Real-time PCR relies on the detection of amplification as the thermal cycling proceeds. For example, in a 40-cycle PCR test, the detection of any generated amplicon is performed at the end of each thermal cycle. One of the major advantages of this approach is that it is a closed-tube system. All analysis and detection of amplicon is conducted in the reaction tube, which reduces the risk of amplicon contamination as the tube is never subsequently opened. There are different methods to measure amplification of the target amplicon, and these generally rely on the generation of fluorescence. One approach is to incorporate a dye such as SYBR Green in the PCR reaction. This molecule fluoresces over a thousandfold more when bound to double-stranded DNA. In the case of PCR amplification, where the amount of amplicon (dsDNA) can be doubling every thermal cycle, the amount of bound SYBR Green increases with amplification.

Another commonly used approach is the use of a fluorescently labelled probe in the real-time PCR. The most common format is using a hydrolysis probe (often termed Taqman probe, see Figure 11.1). In this case, apart from containing a forward and reverse primer specific for the target, there is the inclusion of a probe which is designed like a primer to be complementary to an internal sequence of the amplicon. The probe is synthesized with a fluorescent molecule at the 5′ end and a quencher molecule at the 3′ end. In this configuration, the probe does not fluoresce, and the energy emitted by the fluorophore is absorbed by the closely positioned quencher molecular and no fluorescence is detected. In a real-time PCR, which contains the target to be amplified, DNA polymerization from one of the primers progresses until it reaches the probe that is bound downstream of the primer binding site. The Taq polymerase enzyme has 5′ to 3′ exonuclease activity so will continue polymerization through the probe sitting in its path and results in the degradation of the probe. As a result, if the template is present in a PCR reaction, at each thermal cycle, greater hydrolysis probe is being degraded. In this state, the energy from the fluorophore is no longer quenched and fluorescence from the molecule can be detected.

Whether using SYBR Green or a hydrolysis probe, fluorescence is measured at each cycle and PCR amplification will result in the generation of fluorescence following a sigmoidal curve (Figure 11.2). A threshold line is plotted on the amplification plot and any fluorescence line that crosses

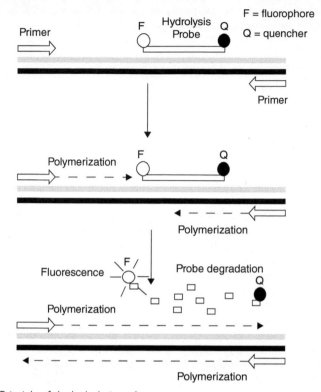

Figure 11.1 Principle of the hydrolysis probe.

this threshold is considered to be positive, i.e. a significant amount of fluorescence has been generated in that PCR reaction above the initial baseline level. When the amplification plot crosses the threshold line, this is noted at the Ct (crossing threshold), sometimes called Cq (quantification cycle).

Real-time PCR lends itself to a multiplex format. This represents multiple PCR tests in the one reaction. This can be accomplished by combining the primers and probes for different targets, i.e. three different viruses. Each probe is labelled with a different fluorophore and the real-time PCR instrument can determine which fluorescent signal is being generated from each individual probe.

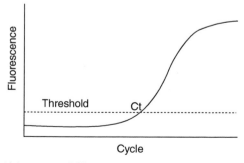

Figure 11.2 The sigmoidal curve in a PCR reaction.

Such an approach aids testing for multiple pathogens in fewer PCR reactions. Further examples of molecular multiplex testing strategies are now commercially available.

11.7 Using real-time PCR for quantification

A considerable advantage to real-time PCR is the relative ease in adapting a test to quantification. To make the test quantitative, the most common approach is to include quantitative standards in the PCR that represent a known quantity of target. These standards are amplified by the same primers and probes as the test sample. A standard curve is plotted with a line of best fit through a range of standards, and the copy number in the clinical samples can be determined from this plot. Viral loads require absolute quantification, so expression of the copy number per ml of sample. Meaningful viral load measurements require a standard sample type such as plasma, whole blood, or urine. Respiratory samples and biopsies are non-standard in composition, so applying viral load measurements is problematic. For CE marking, commercial tests require calibration to the WHO International Standards that exist for a number of viruses such as HIV-1, HCV, HBV, and CMV. Likewise, in-house or LDTs should similarly be calibrated against these international standards to provide consistency in viral load measurements by different testing laboratories. Such consistency facilitates generally applied guidelines for patient management, and this is best exemplified for HIV-1 viral load measurements in patient management. Likewise, viral load cut-offs that influence initiating therapy or measuring successful response to treatment are now established for a number of viruses, including HCV, HBV, CMV, and, to a lesser extent, BK virus and EBV. Increasingly there is the expectation that viral loads will be reported in international units (IU)/ml, which is the unitage assigned to the WHO International Standards. HIV-1 viral loads are likely to remain the exception for the time being as reporting in copies/ml is so embedded in the HIV-1 guidelines.

11.8 DNA sequencing in diagnostics

Genome analysis of infectious agents is used in a growing number of molecular diagnostic tests. In virology, there are established sequencing based approaches for HIV-1 resistance testing and tropism determination. Similarly DNA sequencing is commonly used in HCV genotyping and HBV genotyping and resistance testing. In microbiology, 16S PCR and DNA sequencing is well established as a means for bacterial identification. Most sequencing based tests within the infection field in the UK are in house developed tests, with a paucity of commercial tests available. The approach is invariably Sanger sequencing which is based on the selective incorporation of chain-terminating dideoxynucleotides by the DNA polymerase during DNA polymerization. The requirement for a genetic analyser (DNA sequencer) and the fact that tests are in house developed, means that sequencing based molecular diagnostics are less widespread than PCR testing in diagnostic laboratories, and tend to be offered by the bigger providers that have the required expertize to run such a service. Genotypic analysis frequently will make use of public access databases. For example, most laboratories will submit their HIV-1 sequences to the Stanford University HIV Drug Resistance Database for predictions on drug susceptibility or resistance based on protease, reverse transcriptase and integrase gene analysis. It is important to understand the strengths and weaknesses of any utilized database in determining a diagnostic result that may directly influence patient management.

Next generation sequencing is still in a relatively early stage of implementation in the diagnostic arena, although this is changing as the level of automation, cost and analysis pipeline become more suited to a diagnostic environment rather than a research facility. It is likely that a move to next generation sequencing will progress in the field of infection although given the additional resources required and logistical considerations in delivering a service, perhaps fewer labs will be offering this molecular approach than currently utilize Sanger sequencing methodologies.

11.9 Mass spectrometry in the detection and identification of infectious agents

The identification of bacteria and fungi has been revolutionized over the last ten years by the introduction and widespread adoption of commercially available mass spectrometry systems. Matrix-assisted laser desorption ionization time of flight mass spectrometry (MALDI-TOF MS) is used to identify bacterial or fungal proteins, and PCR combined with electrospray ionization-mass spectrometry (PCR/ESIMS), in which products of PCR are identified by electrospray ionization mass spectrometry, has been used to aid pathogen identification.

The principle is illustrated in Figure 11.3. For MALDI-TOF, laser impact causes thermal desorption of ribosomal proteins of bacteria embedded in matrix material and applied to the target plate (analytes are shown as squares or rectangles; matrix as horseshoe shapes binding to the analytes). In an electric field, ions are accelerated according to their mass and electric charge. The drift path allows further separation and leads to measurable differences in time of flight of the desorbed particles that are detected at the top of the vacuum tube. From the time of flight, the exact mass of the polypeptides can be calculated. For ESI, the DNA amplicons are dissolved in a solvent and injected though a conductive capillary and a high voltage is applied, resulting in the emission of aerosols of charged droplets of the sample. The latter are sprayed through compartments with diminishing pressure, resulting in the formation of gas-phase multiple-charged analyte ions, which then are detected by spectrometer.

MALDI-TOF MS has largely replaced biochemical methods of bacterial identification as it is much cheaper, faster, and more accurate. Typically, a bacterial colony on a plate is mixed with a small volume of a matrix such as alpha-4-cyano-4-hydroxy cinnamic acid (HCCA) which works well with Gram-positive and Gram-negative bacteria. The sample matrix mix is ionized by being irradiated by a nitrogen laser in a process called soft ionization, which largely preserves the structure of the proteins. The resultant ions are accelerated through vacuum flight tube and separation occurs depending on the mass to charge ratio. The peptide profile produced is, in fact, largely formed from ribosomal proteins, which form a major part of the growing bacterial or fungal cell. Hence, the best results with MALDI-TOF are normally obtained with rapidly growing cells. The spectra are then compared with reference spectra contained in a database and an identification normally to species level is obtained. Commercial databases are continually being updated and in the last few years have expanded to include difficult-to-identify groups of bacteria like anaerobes and mycobacteria. In addition, methods for the detection of antibiotic resistance and virulence factors are in development. Direct MALDI-TOF analysis of some clinical specimens (e.g. urine, CSF) has been reported but so far these techniques have not entered routine use. However, rapid identification of positive blood culture by MALDI-TOF has been widely reported and is in use in many laboratories. This gives typical savings in time one day over conventional methods where a positive blood culture would be sub-cultured and incubated overnight before bacterial identification was attempted.

The use of PCR/ESI-MS is a more recent development. In this case it is DNA from prior PCR amplification and not protein which is being analysed. Electrospray ionization is used to separate and identify the peaks. The main advantage of this technique over MALDI-TOF is that it allows the identification of mixed infections directly from clinical specimens such as blood. Its main disadvantages are the very high capital and running costs, and low throughput restricting its use in the diagnostic laboratory to selected specimens only.

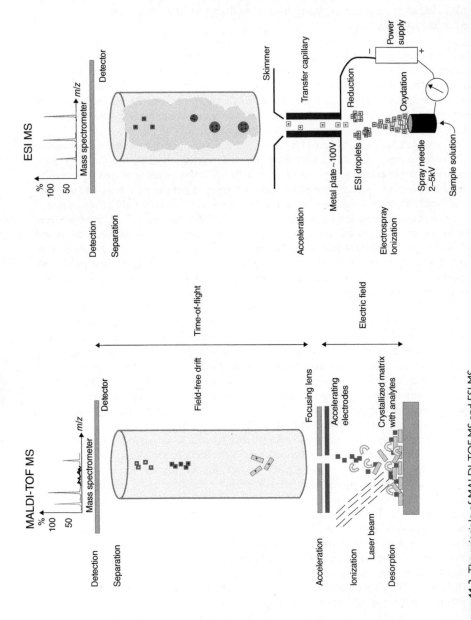

Figure 11.3 The principle of MALDI-TOF MS and ESI MS.
Reproduced with permission from S. Emonet, H. N. Shah, A. Cherkaoui, and J. Schrenzel. Application and use of various mass spectrometry methods in clinical microbiology. *Clinical Microbiology and Infection*, Nov 1, 2010.

11.10 Assessment questions

11.10.1 Question 1

Real-time PCR is now the molecular diagnostic method of choice in preference to block-based PCR.

Which of the following is not an advantage of real-time PCR over block-based PCR?
A. Real-time PCR can be used for multiple targets.
B. Real-time PCR has no problem with inhibition.
C. Real-time PCR is less susceptible to contamination.
D. Real-time PCR is more amenable to quantification.
E. Real-time PCR is quicker.

11.10.2 Question 2

Sanger sequencing is the current norm in diagnostic settings. However, next-generation sequencing (NGS) is increasingly being used.

Which of the following is not an advantage of NGS over Sanger sequencing?
A. NGS can be used for whole genome sequencing of large organisms.
B. NGS can be used to look for previously unknown pathogens.
C. NGS can detect minority species < 20% of the population.
D. NGS has a potential higher throughput.
E. NGS is less time consuming and easy to set up.

11.10.3 Question 3

A diagnostic laboratory has a choice of using an in-house developed nucleic acid amplification assay versus commercially CE marked amplification assay.

Which of the following is not an advantage of commercially CE marked assays?
A. CE marked assays are previously validated to a certain standard.
B. CE marked kits are usually user friendly.
C. CE marked tests are less prone to contamination if the manufacturers' instruction is followed.
D. The manufacturer of a CE marked assay has the responsibility to maintain the quality of the assay.
E. The manufacturer of a CE marked assay responds to genomic sequence variation of pathogens rapidly and keeps the test up to date all the time.

11.11 Answers and discussion

11.11.1 Answer 1

B. Real-time PCR has no problem with inhibition.
Real-time PCR is quicker and relies on a closed-tube system so limiting potential for contamination. Real-time PCR is generally more sensitive, can be multiplexed to detect more than one target in a reaction, and is amenable to quantification, i.e. to determine viral load. Real-time PCR is more suited to automation. PCR inhibition is a problem for both block-based PCR and real-time PCR. However, this can be controlled better in real-time PCR as an internal control can be placed in multiplex with the target PCR to detect the presence of inhibition.

11.11.2 Answer 2

E. NGS is less time consuming and easy to set up.

Sanger sequencing is the current norm in diagnostic settings, although next-generation sequencing is likely to become more widely adopted in the future. Sanger sequencing relies on the use of dideoxynucleotides in the sequencing reaction for chain termination. Sequencing tests require an appropriate genetic analyser, and as the tests are predominantly in-house developed, they therefore require an additional level of expertize compared to the use of real-time PCR in the diagnostic setting. Analysis of the DNA sequences generated relies on public access databases and it is important to understand any weaknesses with the use of these databases when generating diagnostic results. NGS has the advantages of high throughput and sensitivity. It can detect minority species that Sanger sequencing cannot detect. It can be used for whole genome sequencing for complex organisms and even in the detection of previously unknown pathogens. The future of NGS as a clinical tool is strong and is likely to replace Sanger sequencing. However, it is not easy to set up and still very time consuming to perform. These are hurdles that NGS needs to cross before it can become a routine diagnostic tool.

11.11.3 Answer 3

E. The manufacturer of a CE marked assay responds to genomic sequence variation of pathogens rapidly and keeps the test up to date all the time.

The CE marked test will have been validated by several different laboratories as well as the manufacturer, and its performance should therefore be known. The actual kit is often presented in a user-friendly form to minimize the number of manipulations required and hence contamination. The commercial test is almost always more expensive than an in-house test and may be validated for a PCR cycler to which every laboratory does not have access. Once CE marked, the manufacturer may be reluctant to change the assay even if the prevalent genomic sequence of the virus has changed. Even if change is to take place, it will take some time to pass the regulation process. In addition, the manufacturer may decide to modify the test or withdraw it altogether for commercial reasons.

CHAPTER 12

Laboratory quality control and accreditation

Anthony R. Oliver

12.1 What is accreditation?

According to the International Organization for Standardization (ISO), the 'Medical laboratories—Requirements for quality and competence (ISO 15189:2012) BS EN ISO 15189:2012' accreditation is defined as 'a procedure by which an authoritative body gives formal recognition that an organization is competent to carry out specific tasks'.

Accreditation is delivered by the 'competent authority' based on a set of defined standards and the continual internal audit of the laboratory processes and infrastructure against these standards to achieve conformance. Additionally, the 'competent authority' periodically undertakes assessments to ensure compliance with the standards. These assessments vary in frequency and nature depending upon the assessment body. In some instances (e.g. UK Accreditation Service, UKAS), the assessments are annual and based on a four-year cycle covering the whole laboratory repertoire and infrastructure.

12.2 Regulatory bodies involved in UK diagnostic pathology regulation and accreditation

12.2.1 Health and Safety Executive (HSE)

The HSE is responsible for the inspection and licencing of microbiological containment level 3 and 4 facilities.

12.2.2 Human Tissue Authority (HTA)

The HTA is responsible for legal registration of laboratories that process and store human tissue, and is mainly histology related.

12.2.3 Medicines and Healthcare Products Regulatory Authority (MHRA)

The MHRA provides guidelines on good laboratory practice, good clinical practice, good clinical laboratory practice, and good manufacturing practice, largely around clinical trial work. It is also responsible for accreditation of blood transfusion laboratories. Finally, it provides guidance on the In Vitro Diagnostic Medical Device Directive (IVDMDD, 98/79/EC) and the regulation of medical 'devices' including diagnostic devices, where a 'device' is defined as including reagent kits and analytical platforms.

12.2.4 European Federation for Immunogenetics (EFI)

EFI provides guidance and standards for transplantation and tissue typing laboratories across Europe.

12.2.5 Clinical Pathology Accreditation (CPA) to 2009

Until 2009, CPA provided accreditation for the majority of UK pathology services. CPA was acquired by the UK Accreditation Service in 2009.

12.2.6 UK Accreditation Service (UKAS)

UKAS is a government-appointed national accreditation body for the UK that is responsible for certification, testing, inspection, and calibration services, and is the competent authority for all ISO standards, not just pathology. It covers various sectors, including healthcare, food production, energy supply, climate change, and personal safety. The majority of UK pathology services will be UKAS ISO15189 accredited by 2018, including transitional 'dual' CPA standards/ISO15189 accreditation between 2015 and 2018. It also provides ISO22870:2006 accreditation that is point of care specific, as well as ISO17025:2005, which applies to calibration standards.

12.3 Standards in the context of accreditation

A standard is a statement specifying a quality attribute against which conformance can be measured. The standards that different authorities devise are often in very different styles and conformance can be measured in different ways. For example, some standards define a test or technology and are very prescriptive about how it must be performed, and by whom. ISO15189 tends to be quite an open standard—effectively an output-based specification—requiring the user to demonstrate the quality of the process, and its governance (Table 12.1). These differences notwithstanding, all standards *should* adhere to the following principles:

- The standard should be specific and worded in clear unambiguous language, and
- Conformance to the standard should be objectively measurable using evidence.

12.4 Identifying and interpreting ISO15189:2012

The following is an excerpt of standard 5.4.6:

5.4.6 Sample reception
The laboratory's procedure for sample reception shall ensure that the following conditions are met.
a) Samples are unequivocally traceable, by request and labelling, to an identified patient or site.

Table 12.1 Medical Laboratory Requirements for Quality and Competence (ISO 15189:2012) BS EN ISO 15189:2012 standards.

1	Scope	5	Technical requirements
2	Normative references	5.1	Personnel
3	Terms and definitions	5.2	Accommodation and environmental conditions
4	Management requirements	5.3	Laboratory equipment, reagents, and consumables
4.1	Organization and management responsibility	5.4	Pre-examination processes
4.2	Quality management system	5.5	Examination processes
4.3	Document control	5.6	Ensuring quality of examination results
4.4	Service agreements	5.7	Post-examination processes
4.5	Examination by referral laboratories	5.8	Reporting of results
4.6	External services and supplies	5.9	Release of results
4.7	Advisory services	5.10	Laboratory information management
4.8	Resolution of complaints		
4.9	Identification and control of nonconformities		
4.10	Corrective action		
4.11	Preventive action		
4.12	Continual improvement		
4.13	Control of records		
4.14	Evaluation and audits		
4.15	Management review		

Note that the standard does *not* establish how many patient identifiers constitute unequivocal traceability, nor that NHS number or DOB are mandatory data items. Standards are finely crafted statements and require careful reading to tease out the important information. Note here that the word 'procedure' is used. A standard of procedure (SOP) is a written document; thus, this standard implies that the laboratory must have a written document detailing sample reception. Additionally, the standard uses the word 'shall', which means it is a legal requirement. It also uses the word labelling; it could be argued that this need not be visual labelling, i.e. barcode or electronic tagging, but the test would be one of reasonableness and good practice, given the infrastructure in place. Every laboratory that is ISO15189 accredited must have a suitably competent Quality Manager; fortunately, it is their job to provide this level of interpretation with their peers across pathology.

12.5 Assessments and how they work

The ISO15189:2012 standard is structured in two main sections. Section 4 deals with the management, organization, and quality systems, whereas Section 5 focuses more on the analytical and peri-analytical processes. At an assessment visit an assessment manager, a UKAS employed general assessor, will concentrate on section 4, particularly the quality management system. (S)he will also organize the time of one or more volunteer peer assessors, who are experienced professionals and experts in the discipline/area being assessed. Typically, there is a medical peer assessor and a scientific peer assessor for each discipline visit. The assessment manager will determine the complexity of the repertoire being assessed and the resources required to do so. Visits can last variable periods of time that are determined by how the laboratory quality system is structured. Peer assessors are generally in any given area between one and three days. The laboratory, in applying for accreditation, is effectively stating its compliance with all the standards. The whole test repertoire will be reviewed over the cycle in detail for its conformity to the standards. However, assessments are sampling exercises, and are not designed to review every test against every standard on each visit.

12.6 After an assessment

Frequently, a visit will uncover things that do not conform to standards. These abberations form a major part of the report that is ultimately supplied to the laboratory as the outcome of the assessment. The laboratory management is asked to sign their agreement to the findings throughout the visit. These are reviewed within the UKAS and, if supported by peer review, the laboratory is given a period of one to three months to clear them. Clearance is accomplished via the submission of documentary evidence of compliance or by the submission of suitably governed action plans for longer-term issues. Upon clearance, as judged by the assessment manager and or peer assessor, accreditation is recommended granted by UKAS for a defined repertoire of tests.

12.7 Maintaining and improving laboratory 'quality'

ISO15189:2012 requires a laboratory to maintain a quality management system (QMS). Table 12.2 articulates the major elements of laboratory quality. The QMS is the governance framework for

Table 12.2 Major elements of laboratory quality.

ISO definition	Laboratory term	Example
Management system to direct and control an organization with regard to quality	Laboratory Quality Management System (QMS)	Governance such as document control, policies, procedures, meetings, corrective and preventative action, audit schedule
The assembly of all planned and systematic actions necessary to provide adequate confidence that a product, process, or service will satisfy given quality requirements	Quality Assurance (QA)	Internal and external quality assurance programmes (IQA/EQA). Vertical/ horizontal/observation style audits. User feedback
The operational techniques and activities that are used to satisfy quality requirements	Quality Control (QC)	Internal use of controls independent of the assay (IQCs) manufacturer, review process, analysis of positive rates

the maintenance and improvement of the laboratory output. Quality control (QC) is what is done daily to control the pre-analytical, analytical, and post-analytical processes. Quality Assurance (QA) generally has a broader scope and its activities are generally less frequent. It can be useful to view QA to confirm that QC is working.

12.8 Fitting the laboratory audit into the QMS

The audit is a critical tool in the assurance process. Audits systematically identify weaknesses. The standards are already set by the accreditation body so, within the audit cycle (Figure 12.1), audits should be designed to cover the entirety of the laboratory both by test and by standard. A typical laboratory audit schedule will cover all these over a one- to two-year period, and provides the confidence of where nonconformance gaps are and/or improvements that could be made. The output of these audits are nonconformities and it is a legal requirement to track these, from their identification through action plans, if required, to closure when the nonconformity is addressed. At re-audit, the same nonconformity should not appear, as it should have been resolved.

12.9 Managing internal quality control (IQC) in virology

'Internal' can refer to the department, the assay, or the sample. It is a generally accepted definition that an IQC is a reagent of known (positive) value that is independent of the manufacture of the assay. An IQC is normally included in addition to the positive and negative kit/run controls at a frequency dictated by the style of assay and the throughput of results. It is designed to detect assay batch-to-batch variation and long-term drift. If quantitative, it will ideally be traceable to an international standard; despite being an ISO15189 requirement, these are not currently universally available. Secondly, organism populations and antibodies are not homogenous; they are biological materials and thus have a relatively high inherent variability between samples and patients. Consequently, while useful, the rules and processes that govern much of IQC in biochemistry have

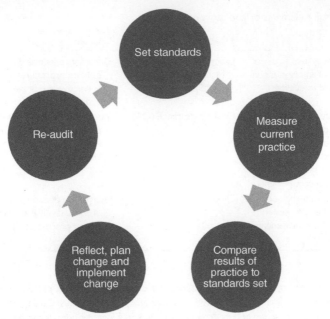

Figure 12.1 Audit cycle.

a more limited utility in microbiology, e.g. sodium is a very different analyte from HIV1. Finally, the dynamics of PCR and other target amplification techniques are very different from assays for inorganic analytes.

However, the use of one or more IQCs that represent clinically useful values in an assay does allow for control for variation in the assay over assay lots, operators, analysers, and time. In order to bring the maximum benefit to any analysis, all this information as well as the lot of the control itself should be used. Figure 12.2 shows a Shewart plot using a rolling mean/ standard deviation (SD). The use of Westgard rules is commonplace even in virology, although the selection of which to use and a knowledge of the assay is imperative. Figure 12.2 shows a realtime Adenovirus PCR assay where one value is outside +3SD, thus failing the 1_{3S} Westgard rule. In a qualitative assay that has, in real-time PCR terms, a very tight spread of values, it is questionable to reject the assay on this statistical basis alone. Therefore, a more liberal validation criterion should be chosen, given the inherent variability of the assay and the clinical relevance of the result.

12.10 Further reading and useful resources

Medical Laboratory Accreditation (ISO 15189). https://www.ukas.com/services/accreditation-services/medical-laboratory-accreditation-iso-15189/

UK Standards for Microbiology Investigations. UKAS provide quality assurance in the diagnostic virology and serology laboratory. https://www.gov.uk/government/uploads/system/uploads/attachment_data/file/482795/Q_2i7.pdf

Westgard Rules. https://www.westgard.com/westgard-rules.htm

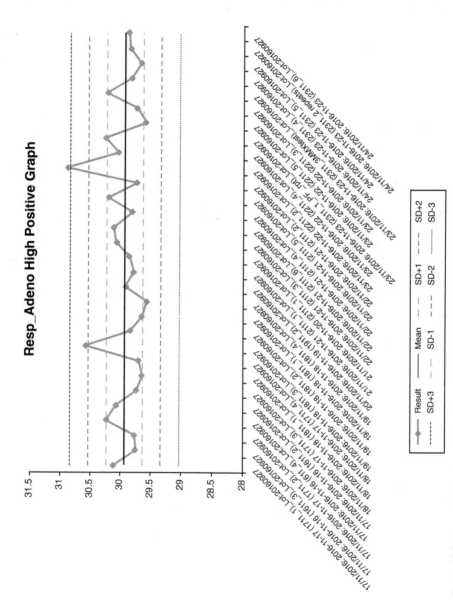

Figure 12.2 Shewart plot of a real-time adenovirus PCR assay.

12.11 Assessment questions

12.11.1. Question 1

An anti-HBs serology assay by manufacturer A with a cutoff of 10 IU/L is in use in the laboratory. The kit includes a 1000 IU/L positive control and a negative control. The laboratory also has an alternative assay made by manufacturer B.

What is the best internal quality control (IQC)?
A. A 10 IU/L kit control from the alternative kit by manufacturer B.
B. A 100 IU/L control from another source traceable to the Second International Standard for anti-hepatitis B surface antigen.
C. A 100 IU/L control from manufacturer A traceable to the Second International Standard for anti-hepatitis B surface antigen.
D. A 1000 IU/L control from another source traceable to the Second International Standard for anti-hepatitis B surface antigen.
E. A 1000 IU/L kit control from the alternative kit by manufacturer B.

12.11.2 Question 2

Westgard Rules are used in laboratories to identify systemic and random errors which can create uncertainty of measurement.

Which of the following violations of Westgard Rules would best indicate a significant trend in the results?
A. One control value exceeds the mean +3SD.
B. Three consecutive control values exceed the same mean -1SD.
C. One control value exceeds the mean ±2 SD.
D. Ten consecutive control values fall on the same side of the mean.
E. Two consecutive control values exceed the mean ±2SD.

12.12 Answers and discussion

12.12.1 Answer 1

B. A 100 IU/L control from another source traceable to the Second International Standard for anti-hepatitis B surface antigen.
Option B is preferred as it is a quantifiable standard in the clinically relevant range of 10–100 IU/L and it is independently manufactured and traceable to the latest ISO standard reference material. Options A and E are not traceable. Option C is good, but it is not verifiably independent of the kit manufacture. Finally, Option D can be used, but is a very high positive and not within the clinically relevant range.

12.12.2 Answer 2

D. Ten consecutive control values fall on the same side of the mean.
The rule described in Option D (10x rule) detects systematic error and it is violated when ten consecutive values fall on the same side of the mean. Its violation often indicates the deterioration of assay reagents and is a mandatory rejection. The other violations are warning rules and will require investigations of previous run, trigger recalibrations, or equipment maintenance. The other mandatory Westgard Rules are 1_{3SD} (one control value exceeds the mean ±3SD) and R_{4SD} (one control measurement in a group exceeds the mean +2SD and another exceeds the mean -2SD).

PART THREE

HEALTH
AND SAFETY

CHAPTER 13

Biosafety categorisations and containment levels

C. Y. William Tong

CONTENTS

13.1 Categorizing biosafety levels of micro-organisms

The Control of Substances Hazardous to Health Regulations 2002 (COSHH) classifies biological agents into four categories (Hazard Groups) according to an approved list by the Health and Safety Executive (HSE). Biological agents are bacteria, viruses, parasites, and fungi that can cause harm to human health, usually due to infection, although some are toxic or can cause an allergy. The approved list is relevant to risk assessment for work with biological agents and the application of appropriate control measures. Hazard Group 1 agents are not considered to pose a risk to human health, while Hazard Group 4 agents present the greatest risk.

The principle of the categorization is laid down by the Advisory Committee on Dangerous Pathogens (ACDP) based on the following (see also Table 13.1):

- the likelihood that it will cause disease by infection or toxicity in humans;
- how likely it is that the infection would spread to the community; and
- the availability of any prophylaxis or treatment.

The ACDP only considers the risks to human health when deciding appropriate classification. Some listed agents can also cause disease in animals (zoonoses) and have also been assigned a hazard classification under the Specified Animal Pathogens Order (SAPO). In allocating human pathogens to a hazard group, no account is taken of particular effects on those whose susceptibility to infection may be affected, for example, because of pre-existing disease, medication, compromised immunity, pregnancy, or breastfeeding.

Table 13.1 Description of the ACDP classification.

Hazard	Description
Group 1	Unlikely to cause human disease.
Group 2	Can cause human disease and may be a hazard to employees; it is unlikely to spread to the community and there is usually effective prophylaxis or treatment available.
Group 3	Can cause severe human disease and may be a serious hazard to employees; it may spread to the community, but there is usually effective prophylaxis or treatment available.
Group 4	Causes severe human disease and is a serious hazard to employees; it is likely to spread to the community and there is usually no effective prophylaxis or treatment available.

13.2 Examples of Hazard Group 3 and 4 organisms

Type 2 polio virus has been reclassified from Hazard Group 2 to Hazard Group 3 to bring the UK in line with the expectations of World Health Organization's global polio eradication programme. This reclassification also applies to attenuated type 2 polio viruses once this component is no longer used as part of the trivalent polio vaccine (Table 13.2).

Zika virus has been reclassified from Hazard Group 3 to Hazard Group 2 as there is substantial evidence that while it can cause human disease, this is generally mild. It is also unlikely to spread to the community from the laboratory.

13.3 Defining containment levels

COSHH regulations specify four containment levels for activities which involve working with biological agents. These correspond to the classification of biological agents into Hazard Groups 1 to 4, e.g. Hazard Group 2 biological agents should be handled at Containment Level 2 (CL2), and Hazard Group 3 at Containment Level 3 (CL3).

Certain Hazard Group 3 biological agents have been identified as presenting a limited risk for workers because they are not normally infectious by the airborne route (those marked with * in Table 13.2). Hence, those intending to work with such agents may not necessarily need to use all the containment measures normally required at CL3 because of the nature of the specific activity and the quantity of the agent involved. However, this does not imply that the work can be downgraded completely to CL2. For example, blood-borne viruses (BBVs) are unlikely to transmit by airborne route during diagnostic procedures not involving propagation or concentration of the virus. Providing appropriate precautions are taken, not all the stated CL3 measures may be required when testing samples containing BBVs.

13.4 Laboratory requirements at different containment levels

Basic good laboratory practice is required at all levels. Laboratory workers should use appropriate level of personal protective equipment (PPE). Basic requirements include laboratory coat or gown, disposable gloves, and eye protection when splashing is possible. The level of requirement increases with each containment level:

Table 13.2 Examples of Category 3 and 4 organisms (only some of the commoner examples are listed. Please refer to http://www.hse.gov.uk/pubns/misc208.pdf for the entire list).

	Category 3	Category 4
Bacteria	*Bacillus anthracis;* *Brucella sp.;* *Chlamydophila psittaci;* *Coxiella burnetti;* *Escherichia coli,* verocytotoxigenic strains (e.g. O157:H7 or O103);* *Francisella tularensis* (Type A); Some *Mycobacterium sp.*—including *africanum, bovis, leprae,* and *tuberculosis;* *Pseudomonas mallei;* *Rickettsia sp.;** *Salmonella typhi* and *paratyphi;** *Shigella dysenteriae* (Type 1);* *Yersinia pestis.*	None
Fungi	*Blastomyces dermatitidis;* *Coccidioides immitis;* *Histoplasma capsulatum;* *Penicillium marneffei.*	None
Helminths	*Echinococcus sp.;** *Taenia solium;**	None
Parasites	*Leishmania donovani* and *brasiliensis;** *Naegleria fowleri;* *Plasmodium falciparum;** *Trypanosoma brucei rhodesiense;** *Trypanosoma cruzi.*	None
Prions	Creutzfeldt-Jakob disease agents*—sporadic, familial, variant, iatrogenic; Bovine spongiform encephalopathy (BSE) agent and other related animal TSEs.*	None
Viruses	Lyssaviruses (including rabies*); MERS and SARS coronavirus; Poliovirus type 2; Hantavirus (sin nombre, Seoul); Rift Valley fever virus; Severe fever with thrombocytopaenia syndrome virus (SFTS); Dengue viruses types 1–4; Central European tick-borne encephalitis (TBE) virus; Japanese encephalitis virus; West Nile virus; Yellow fever virus; Hepatitis B, C, D viruses;* Monkey pox virus; HIV, SIV, HTLV.*	Herpesvirus simiae and B viruses; Ebolavirus and Marburg viruses; Hendra and Nipah viruses; Junin, Lassa and related arenaviruses causing viral haemorrhagic fevers; Crimean/Congo haemorrhagic fever (CCHF) virus; Far Eastern tick-borne encephalitis; virus (Russian spring–summer encephalitis Virus); Kyasanur Forest disease virus; Omsk haemorrhagic fever virus; Variola major and minor viruses (smallpox).

*May be used at less than the minimum containment conditions.

CL1: Applicable to secondary education and undergraduate teaching laboratories; Open laboratory benches with surfaces impervious to water and easy to clean; No mouth pipetting; No eating, drinking, or smoking; Safe handling of sharps; Avoidance of splashes/aerosols; Procedures to decontaminate work surfaces and spillages.

CL2: Applicable to all diagnostic laboratories handling pathological specimens; Greater caution is exercised compared to CL1; Controlled access; Use of appropriate biological safety cabinets (BSC); Autoclave (in building) before disposal of potentially infectious waste; Appropriate immunization of staff.

CL3: Special design and separate from main laboratory areas; Double door access (air lock); Observation window; Sealable for fumigation; Negative pressure air flow with no recirculation and ducted externally through a high-efficiency particulate air (HEPA) filter; Appropriate training of staff including the use of appropriate personal protective equipment (PPE); Strict access control; Class I BSC are generally used when handling samples; Autoclave on site.

CL4: Purpose-built facilities; High security in addition to all the requirements for CL3; High level of staff training; Class III BSC are generally used, though Class I or II BSC can be used in combination with body suit with air supply.

13.5 Biological safety cabinets (BSC)

A BSC is an enclosed, ventilated workspace in a laboratory for safe working with infectious or potentially infectious materials. The primary purpose of a BSC is to protect the laboratory worker and the surrounding environment from pathogens. Exhaust from BSC are filtered via a HEPA filter, which should remove 99.97% of particles $> 0.3\mu$m. It is important to differentiate BSC from a laminar flow clean bench, which protects the samples/products, rather than the worker. Additionally, a BSC is also different from a fume cupboard, which is a ventilated enclosure for storing and/or using harmful volatile chemicals.

There are three classes of BSC—I, II, and III. Each needs to be sited in the correct location in the laboratory and must not be affected by flow of air and personnel. Staff should be trained to use BSC correctly. They should be carefully maintained and regularly tested (e.g. smoke test) to ensure correct airflow. The cabinet should be decontaminated after each use. After each service or major contamination event, it should be fumigated using formaldehyde.

Class I BSC: provide protection for worker and environment, but not the samples/products being handled (Figure 13.1).

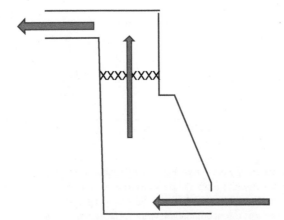

Figure 13.1 A cross-sectional diagrammatic representation of a Class I BSC showing location of HEPA filter (XXXXXXXX) and air flow (arrows).

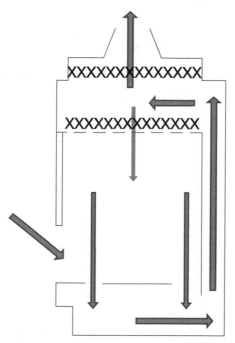

Figure 13.2 A cross-sectional diagrammatic representation of a Class II BSC showing location of HEPA filters (XXXXXXXX) and air flow (arrows).

Class II BSC – Protect both worker and environment. There are different types of Class II BSC and they are most commonly used in clinical and research laboratories. It is also used in some diagnostic CL2 laboratories for handling pathological specimens (see Figure 13.2).

Class II BSC: recirculate filtered air over the work area to reduce the risk of contamination of the work and the worker (Figure 13.2).

Class III BSC – Also known as glove box; Installed in CL4 laboratories for maximum protection; Air-tight enclosure; All materials enter and leave through a dunk tank or double-door autoclave. (see Figure 13.3).

13.6 Managing Hazard Group 4 pathogens

All Hazard Group 4 pathogens are viruses and many are causative agents of viral haemorrhagic fever (VHF), a term that encompasses severe and life-threatening viral diseases endemic in parts of Africa, South America, the Middle East, and Eastern Europe (Table 13.3). Almost all cases of VHFs in the UK are imported. They are not easy to diagnose without a high index of suspicion, very difficult to treat, and have a high case-fatality ratio. They also have a high potential of nosocomial spread. Direct contact of broken skin and mucous membrane with infected blood and body fluid is the main route of transmission. Indirect contact with contaminated environment is also believed to be important.

Any patient who has had a fever ≥ 37.5°C, or a history of fever in the previous twenty-four hours, and a travel history to a VHF-endemic area or epidemiological exposure to cases suspected of VHF within twenty-one days needs to be identified on presentation to the health care service. It is important to maintain standard precaution and good infection control procedure during initial

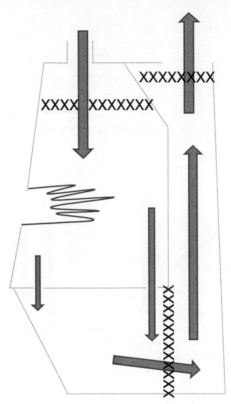

Figure 13.3 A cross-sectional diagrammatic representation of Class III BSC showing location of HEPA filters (XXXXXXXX) and air flow (arrows).

Table 13.3 ACDP Hazard Group 4 VHF viruses.

Viral families	Viruses	Geographical locations reported
Arenaviridae	Lassa	West and Central Africa
	Lujo	Southern Africa
	Chapare	Bolivia
	Guanarito	Central Venezuela
	Junin	Argentina
	Machupo	Northeastern Bolivia
	Sabia	Brazil
Flavivirdae	Kyasanur forest disease	India
	Alkhurma haemorrhagic fever**	Saudi Arabia
	Omsk haemorrhagic fever	Western Siberia
Bunyaviridae	Crimean Congo haemorrhagic fever	East and West Africa, North and Central Asia, Middle East, India and Pakistan, Balkans, West China
Filoviridae	Ebola	Western, Central, and Eastern Africa
	Marburg	Central and Eastern Africa

**Note that Alkhurma haemorrhagic fever is Hazard Group 3).

assessment. There are four possible categories. The risk category can change dependent on the available history, symptoms, and diagnostic test results.

1. **Unlikely to have VHF**: Established as not visited a VHF-endemic area within twenty-one days of becoming ill; Not become unwell within twenty-one days of exposure; Become afebrile for > 24 hours; Malaria screen is positive and responds appropriately to malaria treatment; Has a confirmed alternative diagnosis and is responding appropriately.

   ACTION: Manage according to the alternative diagnosis.

2. **Low possibility of VHF**: Fever ≥ 37.5 or history of fever in past twenty-four hours and developed symptoms within twenty-one days of leaving a VHF-endemic country, but no history of high-risk contact; No evidence of extensive bruising or active bleeding.

   ACTION: Isolate in a single room; Standard precautions include hand hygiene, gloves, and plastic apron; Additional protection for splash or aerosol generating procedures; All samples from patients in this category can be treated as standard samples; Investigations should include URGENT Malaria screen, full blood count, urea and electrolytes (U&Es), liver function tests (LFTs), glucose, C-reactive proteins (CRP), coagulation studies, urine, stool and blood cultures, and chest X-ray.

3. **High possibility of VHF**: History and symptoms as in low possibility, but also has history of close contact with body fluids from an individual or laboratory animal known or strongly suspected to have VHF within the past twenty-one days, or extensive bruising or active bleeding.

   ACTION: Isolate in a dedicated single side room immediately; Standard precaution as well as droplet precaution; Urgent discussion with Infection Consultant and Imported Fever Service regarding VHF test; Notify local Health Protection Team; Urgent malarial screen and other investigations according to CL2 condition; Analysis of specimens should not be delayed while awaiting the VHF results.

4. **Confirmed VHF**: Confirmed diagnosis of infection by a VHF agent. This is usually made by the Rare and Imported Pathogens Laboratory (RIPL).

   ACTION: Restrict staff contact; Enhance personal protection; Urgent discussion with the High Level Isolation Unit (HLIU) to arrange for immediate transfer; Notify relevant bodies and launch public health actions.

13.7 Further readings and useful resources

HSE—The Approved List of Biological Agents. http://www.hse.gov.uk/pubns/misc208.pdf

HSE—The Management, Design and Operation of Microbiological Containment Laboratories http://www.hse.gov.uk/pubns/books/microbio-cont.htm

HSE—Management of Hazard Group 4 Viral Haemorrhagic Fevers and Similar Human Infectious Diseases of High Consequence: November 2015. https://www.gov.uk/government/uploads/system/uploads/attachment_data/file/534002/Management_of_VHF_A.pdf

PHE—Imported Fever Service

https://www.gov.uk/guidance/imported-fever-service-ifs

13.8 Assessment questions

13.8.1 Question 1

Rabies virus is classified as a Hazard Group 3 pathogen by ACDP.

What is the rationale for it being classified as Hazard Group 3 and not Hazard Group 4?

A. An effective prophylaxis is available.

B. An effective treatment is available.
C. Case fatality is not 100%.
D. No human-to-human transmission has ever been reported.
E. The virus is present in nervous tissue only.

13.8.2 Question 2

Clean PCR reagents are being prepared in the laboratory.

What is the most appropriate device listed below used in the laboratory to prevent contamination of the reagents?
A. Class I biological safety cabinet.
B. Class II biological safety cabinet.
C. Class III biological safety cabinet.
D. FFP3 respirator.
E. Fume cupboard.

13.8.3 Question 3

A thirty-five-year-old man presents with a two-day history of fever after returning from military service at rural Afghanistan one week previously. He had received all the prophylaxis recommended by the army during the trip. On examination, he is very unwell and shows signs of extensive bruises and bleeding tendency.

What is the most likely diagnosis?
A. Crimean Congo haemorrhagic fever.
B. Dengue shock syndrome.
C. Ebola haemorrhagic fever.
D. Lassa haemorrhagic fever.
E. Malaria.

13.9 Answers and discussion

13.9.1 Answer 1

A. An effective prophylaxis is available.
Rabies is a deadly infection with very few known survivors once symptoms develop. An experimental treatment, the Milwaukee protocol, has reported to be successful, but the success has not been reproduced in most cases and is not recommended by most experts. Apart from transplantation, there were no known cases of human-to-human transmission. Nevertheless, the consequences of the illness made any contacts with body fluids of the patients a high risk and this includes laboratory personnel handling samples. The main reason why rabies is not Hazard Group 4 is because of the effective vaccine, which can be used as pre-exposure as well as post-exposure prophylaxis.

13.9.2 Answer 2

B. Class II biological safety cabinet.
Class II biological safety cabinets, if used appropriately, protect both the user and the environment in which the reagents are handled. A Class I BSC protects the worker but not necessarily the work environment. A Class III BSC is used only in a high-security laboratory and not generally required for routine work like preparation of reagents. A fume cupboard is for handling of volatile chemicals. FFP3 respiratory protects the worker from aerosols.

13.9.3 Answer 3

A. Crimean Congo haemorrhagic fever.

This patient is strongly suspected to have viral haemorrhagic fever. As he returned from an area known to have Crimean Congo haemorrhagic fever, this is the most likely diagnosis that needs to be excluded. Ebola and Lassa fever were not found in Afghanistan. Dengue fever is a possibility but is seldom as severe. Malaria will need to be excluded as per VHF protocol, but the geographical area he returned from and the fact that he has received standard military prophylaxis make this less likely.

PART FOUR

PRINCIPLES OF PUBLIC HEALTH IN RELATION TO COMMUNICABLE DISEASES

CHAPTER 14

Key communicable diseases of public health significance and UK legislation

Marina Basarab

CONTENTS

14.1 Reporting infections to public health

Timely reporting to public health authorities of certain infections which are transmissible between individuals and/or are likely to have been acquired from a contaminated source is essential to prompt immediate action to reduce further spread. In England, Health Protection Teams (HPTs) effect health protection actions at local level. They act as the 'proper officer' carrying out the function of receiving notifications in relation to the statutory regulations for both attending registered medical practitioners and diagnostic laboratories (see Section 14.6 and Section 14.7). Notification to public health authorities is a legal requirement. It is critical to the control and prevention of outbreaks of communicable diseases and is an integral part of wider local and national infection surveillance.

Clinical recognition is the first step and public health authorities should be notified on clinical suspicion before obtaining laboratory test results to look for causative pathogens. As soon as a notification has been made, public health risk assessment and appropriate measures can be initiated. These may include preventing others being exposed to cases or a possible source of contamination, offering chemoprophylaxis, vaccination, education, and closing down of premises. The intervention will depend on the clinical syndrome, the confirmed or presumed infectious agent involved, and any further supporting or refuting diagnostic laboratory results. Time is of the essence; there should be no delay in notifications (see Table 14.1 and Table 14.2).

Table 14.1 Notifiable infectious diseases in Schedule 1 of Health Protection (Notification) Regulations 2010.

Notifiable diseases	Urgent or routine notification required
Acute encephalitis	Routine
Acute meningitis	Urgent if suspected bacterial infection
Acute poliomyelitis	Urgent
Acute infectious hepatitis (A,B,C,E)	Urgent
Anthrax	Urgent
Botulism	Urgent
Brucellosis	Routine; urgent if possibly UK acquired
Cholera	Urgent
Diphtheria	Urgent
Enteric fever (typhoid/paratyphoid)	Urgent
Food poisoning	Routine; urgent if possible cluster
Haemolytic uraemic syndrome	Urgent
Infectious bloody diarrhoea	Urgent
Invasive group A streptococcal disease	Urgent
Scarlet fever	Routine
Legionnaire's disease	Urgent
Leprosy	Routine
Malaria	Routine; urgent if possibly UK acquired
Measles	Urgent
Meningococcal septicaemia	Urgent
Mumps	Routine
Plague	Urgent
Rabies	Urgent
Rubella	Routine
SARS	Urgent
Smallpox	Urgent
Tetanus	Routine; urgent if associated with injecting drug abuse
Tuberculosis	Routine; urgent if healthcare worker or multidrug resistant
Typhus	Routine
Viral haemorrhagic fever	Urgent
Whooping cough	Urgent if diagnosed in acute phase, routine if in later phase
Yellow fever	Routine; urgent if possibly UK acquired

14.2 Notification responsibilities

Health protection legislation is set out in the Health Protection (Notification) Regulations 2010. It requires both registered medical practitioners (RMPs) and laboratories to notify cases of infection or contamination that could present a significant risk to human health, on the basis of clinical suspicion or laboratory confirmation.

Table 14.2 Notifiable organisms (causative agents) in Schedule 2 of Health Protection (Notification) Regulations 2010.

Causative organism	Urgent or routine notification required
Bacillus anthracis	Urgent
Bacillus cereus (only if associated with food poisoning)	Routine; urgent if part of a known cluster
Bordetella pertussis	Urgent if diagnosed during acute phase
Borrelia spp.	Routine
Brucella spp.	Routine; urgent if possibly UK acquired
Burkholderia mallei	Urgent
Burkholderia pseudomallei	Urgent
Campylobacter spp.	Routine; urgent if part of a known cluster
Chikungunya virus	Routine; urgent if possibly UK acquired
Chlamydophila psittaci	Urgent if diagnosed in acute phase or part of a known cluster
Clostridium botulinum	Urgent
Clostridium perfringens (only if associated with food poisoning)	Routine; urgent if part of a known cluster
Clostridium tetani	Routine; urgent if associated with injecting drug abuse
Corynebacterium diphtheriae	Urgent, prior to results of toxigenicity being available
Corynebacterium ulcerans	Urgent, prior to results of toxigenicity being available
Coxiella burnetii	Urgent if diagnosed in acute phase or part of a known cluster
Crimean-Congo haemorrhagic fever virus	Urgent
Cryptosporidium spp.	Routine; urgent if part of a known cluster, known food handler, or evidence of increase above expected numbers
Dengue virus	Routine; urgent if possibly UK acquired
Ebola virus	Urgent
Entamoeba histolytica	Routine; urgent if part of a known cluster or known food handler
Francisella tularensis	Urgent
Giardia lamblia	Routine; urgent if part of a known cluster, known food handler, or evidence of increase above expected numbers
Guanarito virus	Urgent
Haemophilus influenzae (invasive)	Urgent
Hanta virus	Routine; urgent if possibly UK acquired
Hepatitis A, B, C, delta, and E viruses	Urgent for all acute cases and also for chronic cases who might represent a high risk to others, i.e. healthcare workers who perform exposure prone procedures
Influenza virus	Routine; urgent if known to be a new subtype or associated with known cluster or closed communities e.g. care home
Junin virus	Urgent
Kyasanur Forest disease virus	Urgent

(Continued)

Table 14.2 Continued

Causative organism	Urgent or routine notification required
Lassa virus	Urgent
Legionella spp.	Urgent
Leptospira spp.	Routine
Listeria monocytogenes	Urgent
Machupo virus	Urgent
Marburg virus	Urgent
Measles virus	Urgent
Mumps virus	Routine
Mycobacterium tuberculosis complex	Routine; urgent if healthcare worker or suspected cluster or multidrug resistant
Neisseria meningitides (excluding throat carriage)	Urgent
Omsk haemorrhagic fever virus	Urgent
Plasmodium falciparum, vivax, ovale, malariae, knowlesi	Routine; urgent if possibly UK acquired
Polio virus (wild or vaccine types)	Urgent
Rabies virus (classical rabies and rabies-related)	Urgent
Rickettsia spp.	Routine; urgent if possibly UK acquired
Rift Valley fever virus	Urgent
Rubella virus	Routine
Sabia virus	Urgent
Salmonella spp non-typhi and paratyphi	Routine; urgent if associated with an outbreak, food handler or closed community e.g. care home
Salmonella typhi/paratyphi	Urgent
SARS coronavirus	Urgent
Shigella bodyii, flexneri, dysenteriae	Urgent
Shigella sonnei	Routine; urgent if associated with an outbreak, food handler or closed community e.g. care home
Streptococcus pneumoniae (invasive)	Routine, unless part of a known cluster
Streptococcus pyogenes (invasive)	Urgent
Varicella zoster virus	Routine, urgent if primary VZV in a healthcare worker
Variola virus	Urgent
Verocytotoxigenic Escherichia coli (including E. coli O157)	Urgent
Vibrio cholerae	Urgent
West Nile Virus	Routine; urgent if possibly UK acquired
Yellow fever virus	Routine; urgent if possibly UK acquired
Yersinia pestis	Urgent

14.3 Notification duties of registered medical practitioners

The medical doctor (and no other healthcare professional) attending the patient with possible or probable or confirmed infection is responsible for notification to the public health authorities. The first doctor who forms a clinical suspicion, without waiting for laboratory results, should notify the public health authorities of the case to avoid delay in commencing prevention and control actions. Notification is required if there are 'reasonable grounds' for suspecting a patient:

- has a notifiable disease that is listed in Table 14.1; or
- has an infection that is not listed in Table 14.1 but which, in the doctor's opinion presents, or may present, significant harm to human health; or
- has died with, but not necessarily of, a notifiable disease or other infection not listed in Table 14.1 that presents or may present significant harm to human health in life or in death.

Importantly, prior notification of the causative agent by a diagnostic laboratory does not remove the doctor's responsibility for notification. If laboratory test results refute the clinical diagnosis later, the clinician is not required to denotify the case.

All cases of acute infectious hepatitis should be notified; there are separate mechanisms for reporting HIV, sexually transmitted infections, healthcare-associated infections, and Creutzfeldt-Jakob disease (CJD).

The regulations allow for identification and action in cases of emerging or novel infections in the requirement for doctors to notify on suspicion of an infection which may present significant harm to human health as a result of, for example, potential high transmissibility, number of people affected, significant morbidity or mortality. This notification should be undertaken even before the syndrome is fully characterized or case definitions have been developed.

The statutory Notification Regulations apply to individual cases only. However, it is important, although not a legal requirement, for doctors to report suspected outbreaks or clusters of infection to public health for further investigation and management, regardless of whether or not the disease is notifiable, e.g. a parvovirus outbreak on a haematology ward.

There is also a requirement for notification if a patient is suspected to be contaminated with chemicals, radioactive material, or other radiation that the doctor believes presents or could present significant harm to human health. Such situations would not usually involve an infection specialist.

14.4 Notification duties of diagnostic laboratories

Diagnostic laboratories also have a legal duty to notify public health authorities when they identify evidence of infection, in life or death, with a causative agent listed in Table 14.2. The person responsible for notification is the director of the laboratory (e.g. the clinical microbiologist, other registered medical practitioner, or other person in charge) or anyone else working in the laboratory to whom the director has delegated this function. Evidence of infection caused by a notifiable organism includes:

- direct identification of organisms by microscopy, culture, detection of nucleic acids, or antigens; or
- antibody response to the agent or histological findings that are considered diagnostic of a specific agent.

It is important to note that prior notification of the notifiable disease by a medical doctor attending the individual case does not remove the laboratory's responsibility for notification. The diagnostic laboratory must always notify a case if they identify any evidence of infection by a notifiable causative agent. Confirming (or refuting) a clinical diagnosis may have an important impact on implementation of public health actions, such as excluding someone from work and recommending prophylactic antibiotics for contacts.

14.5 How and when to notify

There are clear time frames for notification by attending medical doctors and diagnostic laboratories of suspected or confirmed infections to HPTs; these are indicated in the second column of Table 14.1 and Table 14.2. The level of urgency is guided by consideration of factors, including:

- the nature of the disease, e.g. significant morbidity, mortality, a rare/re-emerging disease;
- the transmissibility and route of spread of the infection, e.g. highly infectious with respiratory transmission;
- the potential interventions for control and prevention interventions, e.g. the opportunity to use vaccination early to prevent spread;
- individual case circumstances, e.g. a healthcare worker, exposure to pregnant women; and
- identification of a cluster of cases, e.g. food poisoning.

14.6 Attending doctors: how and when to notify

The attending doctor should notify the local HPT (http://www.gov.uk/health-protection-team). If the case requires urgent notification, this should be done by telephone as soon as possible and always within twenty-four hours. It is good practice to document notification in the patient's case notes. If non-urgent, notification can be made within three days of the initial clinical suspicion, either by telephone or by completion of a notification form (https://www.gov.uk/government/publications/notifiable-diseases-form-for-registered-medical-practitioners) which may be sent to the HPT by secure email, fax, or post.

14.7 Diagnostic laboratories: how and when to notify

Diagnostic laboratories must report causative organisms which require urgent notification (see Table 14.2) as soon as possible by telephone and always within twenty-four hours. Routine notification should be undertaken either electronically or on paper within seven days.

The majority of NHS laboratories already undertake voluntary reporting to public health authorities of laboratory diagnoses of a wider range of causative agents than those listed in Table 14.2, via the electronic CoSurv system. While some notification requirements can be met by the CoSurv system of electronic extraction of data, there is still a requirement to separately notify urgent cases by telephone.

14.8 Further reading and useful resources

Health Protection Legislation (England) Guidance 2010: http://webarchive.nationalarchives.gov.uk/20130107105354/http:/www.dh.gov.uk/prod_consum_dh/groups/dh_digitalassets/@dh/@en/@ps/documents/digitalasset/dh_114589.pdf

Laboratory reporting to Public Health England: https://www.gov.uk/government/uploads/system/uploads/attachment_data/file/545183/PHE_Laboratory_Reporting_Guidelines.pdf

The Health Protection (Notification) Regulations 2010: http://www.legislation.gov.uk/uksi/2010/659/contents/made

14.9 Assessment questions

14.9.1 Question 1

A blood culture flags positive and gram-positive cocci in chains are seen on microscopy. The medical registrar tells you it is from a thirty-five-year-old woman admitted with fever and rapidly progressing severe cellulitis extending from the hand to shoulder and anterior chest wall, with muscle tenderness. Urgent imaging with a view to operate is being undertaken.

Which is the most appropriate course of action with respect to notification to public health?

A. Agree with the registrar that you will speak again when the imaging results and operation findings are available and make a decision as to how to approach public health notification.

B. Ask the registrar to phone the local HPT as a case of clinically suspected invasive group A streptococcus and follow up the blood culture the following day.

C. Telephone the local HPT as soon as possible and inform them that this is a case of probable necrotizing fasciitis clinically, with a positive blood culture consistent with streptococcal species, being followed up urgently in the laboratory.

D. The case must be notified by telephone to the local HPT as an invasive group A streptococcus as soon as possible.

E. Wait until identification of the blood culture isolate is complete and, if it is a group A streptococcus, phone public health as soon as possible.

14.9.2 Question 2

A paediatric registrar telephones asking to send away urgently a blood for PCR for meningococcus in a fourteen-year-old patient with a fever, purpuric rash, and vomiting. Ceftriaxone was commenced before the blood culture was taken.

From the public health perspective, what is the most appropriate course of action?

A. Arrange to speak with the registrar again as soon as possible when the full history and admission blood tests are available, to agree between you the likelihood of this being meningococcal disease and then contact the local HPT urgently if necessary.

B. Ask the registrar to take a vaccine history for the child and a list of all close contacts and that when this has been done, they should telephone the local HPT as soon as possible.

C. Ask the registrar to take blood cultures now anyway and that you will contact them urgently with the result of the PCR.

D. Inform the registrar that they must telephone the local HPT as soon as possible and that you will arrange for the blood to be sent for PCR urgently.

E. Tell the registrar that you will liaise with the local HPT as soon as possible by telephone, to advise them that you are sending off a meningococcal PCR on a patient.

14.9.3 Question 3

A twenty-four-year-old Ukrainian man is sent home from A&E with a discharge summary indicating only that the patient had a sore throat, evidence of mild pharyngitis, and cervical lymphadenopathy, but was otherwise well. His throat swab has grown a *Corynebacterium diphtheriae*, which the laboratory scientist informs you was being sent to the reference laboratory for toxigenicity testing.

What is the best course of action in the first instance?

A. Advise A&E that they must inform the local HPT as soon as possible that this is suspected case of diphtheria.

B. Arrange for the isolate to be sent away urgently and let A&E staff know that it has been sent.

C. Ask A&E to check if there are any further clinical details documented that are suggestive of diphtheria and to phone you back when they have done this so that you can assess whether this is a possible or probable case.

D. Ask A&E to review the patient urgently while you phone the local HPT as soon as possible and advise them of the isolate identification and that it is being sent away for toxigenicity testing.

E. The reference laboratory will report the result directly to the local HPT if it confirmed as a toxigenic strain, and public health action can be taken.

14.10 Answers and discussion

14.10.1 Answer 1

C. Telephone the local health protection team as soon as possible and inform them that this is a case of probable necrotizing fasciitis clinically, with a positive blood culture consistent with streptococcal species, being followed up urgently in the laboratory.

Invasive group A streptococcal disease should be notified urgently to public health by the medical doctor who has made the clinical diagnosis, prior to microbiological confirmation. In this scenario, as the infection registrar in receipt of the blood culture result *combined with* clinical information consistent with necrotizing fasciitis, you have a clear basis on which to notify public health urgently, without incurring further delay waiting for radiology reporting and surgical intervention. The local health protection team will contact the clinical team—who also have a responsibility to notify—risk assess the case, and, as deemed necessary, identify and inform close contacts, advising them of symptoms and the need to seek health care if indicated. In the meantime, the infection registrar should expedite laboratory identification and ensure sending away of invasive group A isolates to the reference laboratory for typing.

See Interim UK guidelines for management of close community contacts of invasive group A streptococcal disease https://www.gov.uk/government/uploads/system/uploads/attachment_data/file/344610/Interim_guidelines_for_management_of_close_contacts_of_iGAS.pdf

14.10.2 Answer 2

D. Inform the registrar that they must telephone the local health protection team as soon as possible and that you will arrange for the blood to be sent for PCR urgently.

Meningococcal septicaemia is the most likely diagnosis based on the information the paediatrician has given. In this situation, and in all cases where meningococcal disease is considered to be likely, prior to microbiology results, it is the responsibility of the paediatrician, as the medical doctor attending the patient, to contact the local health protection unit at the earliest opportunity. Health protection practitioners will undertake a risk assessment of the case and categorize it as 'probable' or 'possible' meningococcal disease and, as necessary, they will lead in identifying close contacts who require prophylaxis. The role of the infection registrar in this scenario is to facilitate the meningococcal PCR test being done as soon as possible, which may confirm the diagnosis and potentially direct public health action further in vaccination options for prolonged close contacts according to the serogroup identified.

See guidance for public health management of meningococcal disease in the UK https://www.gov.uk/government/uploads/system/uploads/attachment_data/file/322008/Guidance_for_management_of_meningococcal_disease_pdf.pdf

14.10.3 Answer 3

D. Ask A&E to review the patient urgently, while you phone the local health protection team as soon as possible and advise them of the isolate identification and that it is being sent for toxigenicity testing.

Corynebacterium diphtheriae is a notifiable organism, even before results of toxigenicity are known. In all such cases, the local diagnostic laboratory must notify the local health protection team at the point they have confirmed the organism identification and are planning to send it to the reference laboratory, so that the HPT can undertake a risk assessment. In many cases, public health action will then be delayed until toxigenicity results become available. However, in situations where there are factors that increase the likelihood that the isolate is toxigenic, or where the risk to public health is potentially high (e.g. possible disease in a healthcare worker), reporting to the local the HPT may prompt preliminary interventions, and particularly if there is going to be delay in reference laboratory testing. In this scenario, the patient comes from a high-risk area where vaccination coverage is low—a significant epidemiological risk factor that may warrant earlier public health action. The local HPT will liaise with the A&E doctors when the patient is reviewed clinically to refine their risk assessment to inform actions such as antibiotics treatment/prophylaxis for the patient/contacts.

Diphtheria: Public Health Control and Management in England and Wales https://www.gov.uk/government/uploads/system/uploads/attachment_data/file/416108/Diphtheria_Guidelines_Final.pdf

CHAPTER 15

Vaccine-preventable diseases

C. Y. William Tong

15.1 Defining vaccine-preventable diseases

These are diseases in which an effective preventive vaccine exists. A death that could have been prevented by vaccination is a vaccine-preventable death. The World Health Organization (WHO) has identified twenty-five diseases as vaccine preventable (Table 15.1). This list may expand as new vaccines are being developed.

15.2 The Expanded Programme on Immunization (EPI)

The Expanded Programme on Immunization, or EPI, is vaccination programme introduced in 1974 by the WHO to all nations. The EPI initially targeted diphtheria, whooping cough, tetanus, measles, poliomyelitis, and tuberculosis. The aim was to provide universal immunization for all children by 1990 and to achieve health for all by 2000.

In 2010, about 85% of children under one year of age in the world had received at least three doses of DTP vaccine (diphtheria, tetanus, and polio). Additional vaccines have now been added to the original six targets. Most countries have now added Hepatitis B (not in UK) and Haemophilus influenzae type b (Hib) to their routine infant immunization schedules, and an increasing number are in the process of adding pneumococcal conjugate vaccine and rotavirus vaccines to their schedules.

15.3 Can vaccination eradicate diseases?

Immunization is a proven tool for controlling and even eradicating infectious diseases. The immunization campaign against smallpox between 1967 and 1977 resulted in the eradication of smallpox. Apart from smallpox, the only other viral infection that was declared eradicated through vaccination campaign was rinderpest in cattle (2011), a close relative of measles virus in humans.

Table 15.1 Vaccine-preventable diseases recognized by the WHO.

Bacterial infections	Viral infections
Anthrax	Hepatitis A
Cholera	Hepatitis B
Diphtheria	Hepatitis E
Haemophilus influenzae type b	Human papilloma virus
Meningococcal disease	Influenza
Pertussis	Japanese encephalitis
Pneumococcal disease	Measles
Tetanus	Mumps
Tuberculosis	Poliomyelitis
Typhoid fever	Rabies
	Rotavirus gastroenteritis
	Rubella
	Tick-borne encephalitis
	Varicella and herpes zoster
	Yellow fever

Another major infection target for global eradication is against poliomyelitis—the global polio eradication initiative (GPEI). When the programme began in 1988, polio threatened 60% of the world's population. Eradication of poliomyelitis is now within reach: infections have fallen by 99%; wild type polio type 2 was last detected in 1999 and declared eradicated in 2015; wild-type poliovirus type 3 has not been detected in the world since 2012. Poliovirus type 1 is the only wild-type virus in circulation and endemic transmission is only reported in Afghanistan and Pakistan. Currently, the old trivalent oral poliovirus vaccine is replaced by the more potent bivalent poliovirus type 1 and 3 vaccine. Many western countries have switched from oral vaccine to the injected inactivated vaccine to avoid the problem of vaccine-induced paralysis, which could be associated with the oral live attenuated vaccine.

Other infections in which elimination programmes through vaccination are being undertaken are measles and congenital rubella.

15.4 Factors that make smallpox relatively easy to eradicate

The success of smallpox eradication is due to a combination of factors:

- Availability of an effective vaccine:
  - Immunogenic and high efficacy;
  - Stable and easy to transport;
  - Simple to administer;
  - Effective in single dose.
- Easy to diagnose and perform surveillance:
  - Patients had a characteristic rash;
  - Infected patients can be spotted with little training.
- Easy to contain once diagnosed:
  - Transmission through droplets spread by face-to-face contact;
  - Simple isolation can result in successful containment.
- No asymptomatic carriers:
  - Permanent immunity after disease;

- No carrier state;
- No animal reservoir.

In order to be considered eradicable, the following three factors need to be present:

- Humans must be critical to maintaining circulation of the organism;
- Sensitive and specific diagnostic tools must be available; and
- An effective intervention must be available.

15.5 Why is measles still prevalent when the vaccine is effective?

Measles is highly contagious and a high level of immunity in the population (herd immunity) is required to prevent transmission in the community. The herd immunity threshold in western countries is at least 93–95% in the entire population. This is even higher in developed countries, particularly in urban areas, as the average age at infection may be lower and can occur before the age when vaccination is recommended. On the whole, a vaccination coverage required to prevent measles outbreaks is 96–99%. Using the vaccine at a younger age, e.g. nine months rather than one year, protects the younger infants, but the vaccine efficacy is lower when given at a younger age due to the presence of passive maternal antibodies. Hence, additional doses are required to maintain population immunity.

There is an added problem of the population not accepting the vaccine. This 'anti-vax' campaign is due to scare stories of the MMR vaccination being associated with diseases such as autism. This association has widely been discredited, but its continued circulation has significantly affected the vaccine acceptance rate in some communities.

15.6 New vaccines in the pipeline

There are many new vaccines on the pipeline. Two notable ones which have been implemented in a small scale are vaccines for dengue and malaria.

The first dengue vaccine, Dengvaxia (CYD-TDV) was licensed in Mexico, Brazil, El Salvador, and the Philippines. It is a live recombinant tetravalent vaccine based on the yellow fever 17d backbone and is given on a 0/6/12-month schedule. The WHO recommended its use in countries with prevalence > 50%. Several other dengue vaccine candidates are in clinical or pre-clinical development.

RTS,S/AS01 (RTS,S) is a malaria vaccine developed against *Plasmodium falciparum*. It is given in a four-dose regimen at 0/1/2/18 month schedule. In infants aged five to seventeen months, vaccine efficacy against clinical malaria was 39%. With a four-dose schedule, the overall efficacy against severe malaria among children in this age group was 31.5%, with reductions in severe anaemia, malaria hospitalizations, and all-cause hospitalizations. Based on these data, the WHO recommended pilot implementation studies to be conducted for further evaluation.

15.7 Where are the vaccines for HIV and hepatitis C?

Infections targeted for vaccine development are those with a high global prevalence. Hence, significant work has been done on developing a vaccine against HIV and hepatitis C. The presence of multiple genotypes, evolution of quasispecies, and development of immune escape mechanism are some of the major challenges. Additionally, for hepatitis C, there is a lack of in-vitro culture systems and lack of suitable animal models. Some vaccine developments are now directed to modify diseases rather than as an agent to prevent disease.

15.8 Further reading and useful resources

WHO. *Immunization, Vaccines, and Biologicals.* http://www.who.int/immunization/monitoring_surveillance/en/

European Centre for Disease Prevention and Control. *Vaccine-preventable diseases.* http://ecdc.europa.eu/en/healthtopics/vaccine-preventable-diseases/Pages/vaccine-preventable-diseases.aspx

Public Health England. *Immunisation Against Infectious Disease.* https://www.gov.uk/government/collections/immunisation-against-infectious-disease-the-green-book

15.9 Assessment questions

15.9.1 Question 1

The polio eradication programme has met with more challenges than smallpox.

Which common factor is shared by smallpox and polio making them targets for eradication?
A. Easy case finding.
B. Isolation is an effective strategy.
C. No animal reservoir.
D. No asymptomatic infections.
E. Single dose of immunization effective.

15.9.2 Question 2

Dengue is a global health problem. Scientists have been trying to develop a vaccine against dengue for many years.

What pathogenetic factor makes vaccine development in dengue particularly challenging?
A. Ability to establish latency.
B. Absence of neutralizing antibody response.
C. Antibody dependent enhancement between serotypes.
D. Cross reaction with other flaviviruses.
E. Presence of asymptomatic infection.

15.9.3 Question 3

The basic reproductive number (R0) of measles is said to be twelve to eighteen. Vaccination coverage of 96–99% is required to bring down the effective reproductive number.

What level of effective reproductive number is required in order to prevent transmissions in community?
A. A negative value.
B. Half of the basic reproductive number.
C. Less than one.
D. One.
E. Zero.

15.10 Answers and discussion

15.10.1 Answer 1

C. No animal reservoir.

Unlike smallpox, most polio infections are asymptomatic (95–99%). Case finding is therefore difficult. Smallpox is transmitted through direct contact whereas polio is transmitted faecal-orally. Hence, isolation strategy is effective in preventing further transmission of smallpox but not possible in polio. Immunization with vaccinia is effective after a single dose, but multiple doses are required in polio. The only common feature that are shared by smallpox and polio that favour eradication is the lack of an animal reservoir with humans being the only source of infection.

15.10.2 Answer 2

C. Antibody-mediated enhancement between serotypes.

The problem with development of a successful dengue vaccine is the presence of four serotypes and the phenomenon of antibody-dependent enhancement of pathogenesis. Antibodies generated during a primary infection with one serotype of dengue virus will not be of sufficient concentration or avidity to neutralize a secondary infection with dengue virus of a different serotype. However, they might opsonize the secondary virus and target it for Fc-receptor-mediated endocytosis into the replicative target myeloid cells, such as monocytes and macrophages, resulting in higher viral loads, increase in viral activity, and virulence. Therefore, any vaccine development not only needs to address the serotype variations but also to ensure that the immune response across the serotypes is balanced.

15.10.3 Answer 3

C. Less than one

The basic reproductive number (R0) is the average number of individuals who are directly infected by a single infectious individual in a totally susceptible population. The role of vaccination is to reduce the proportion of susceptible individuals in the population, i.e. to increase the herd immunity. This will bring down the effective reproductive number. As long as the effective reproductive number is greater than one, continuous transmission will occur. The higher the R0, the greater the coverage is required. In the case of measles, a coverage of 96–99% is required to bring the effective reproductive number to less than one when the outbreak cannot be sustained.

PART FIVE

INFECTION PREVENTION AND CONTROL

CHAPTER 16

Common organisms responsible for healthcare-associated infection (HCAI)

George Jacob and Martina N. Cummins

CONTENTS

16.1 Meticillin-resistant *Staphylococcus aureus* (MRSA)

MRSA are *S. aureus* which become methicillin resistant by the acquisition of the *mec* A gene which is on a mobile chromosomal determinant called staphylococcal cassette chromosome *mec* (SCC *mec*). The *mec* A gene encodes for a penicillin-binding protein (PBP2a) which has a low affinity for isoxazolyl-penicillins (MICs to oxacillin/meticillin $\geq 4\mu g/ml$) and is resistant to all classes of beta-lactam antibiotics.

16.2 Screening for MRSA

Current Department of Health (DOH) guidance (2014) recommends that mandatory MRSA screening be streamlined to include only:

- All patient admissions to high-risk units;
- Healthcare workers; and

- All patients previously identified as colonized or infected with MRSA.

The guidance also advises Trusts to follow *local risk assessment* policies to identify other potential high-risk units or units with a history of high endemicity of MRSA; and The guidance also recommends regular auditing of compliance with MRSA screening policy.

16.3 Healthcare setting infection control and prevention measures for MRSA

The 2006 guideline for the control and prevention of MRSA in healthcare facilities recommends the following four measures.

- Isolation

MRSA-positive patients should be nursed in a single room or if none is available, cohorting into a bay after risk assessment. Patient movement, and the number of staff and visitors looking after the patient, should be minimized.

- Hand hygiene and use of personal protective equipment (PPE)

All staff and visitors should decontaminate their hands with soap and water/or an alcohol rub before and after contact with the patient or their immediate surroundings. Single-use disposable gloves and aprons/non-permeable gowns should be used by staff and visitors if there is a risk of contamination with body fluids.

- Disposal of waste and laundry

All waste from colonized/infected patients should be placed in the infectious waste stream. All linen and bedding from patients colonized/infected with MRSA should be considered as contaminated and processed as infected linen.

- Cleaning and decontamination

The patient's room should be cleaned/disinfected daily with an appropriate detergent/disinfectant as per local policy. On discharge of the patient, the room needs to be terminally cleaned before it is reused. All patient equipment should either be single-patient use or be cleaned, disinfected, and sterilized.

In addition to following the 2006 guidelines, information leaflets and education about MRSA should be provided to the patient and visitors. Instituting antimicrobial stewardship programmes helps in raising awareness of the risks of resistance and encourages prescriber compliance.

16.4 Treatment options available for a patient colonized/infected with MRSA

Thirty per cent of healthy individuals carry *Staphylococcus aureus* in their nose, groin, and axillae, and around 30% are occasional carriers. The 2006 guidelines for the control and prevention of MRSA in healthcare facilities recommends the following patient decolonization protocols help eradicate skin and nasal caarriage.

16.4.1 Nasal carriage

Use of 2% mupirocin (*Bactroban Nasal®*) ointment thrice daily for five days Mupirocin can still be used for low-level resistance (MIC = 8-256 mg/L)[1]. For high-level resistance (MIC > 512 mg/L),

Naseptin® (0.5% neomycin and 0.1% chlorhexidine) nasal ointment should be used four times daily for ten days, but Naseptin® is contra-indicated in patients with a peanut allergy.

16.4.2 Throat carriage

Antiseptic gargles or sprays (Chlorhexidine gluconate) can be used although their efficacy is unknown. Systemic treatment should only be used on the advice of a microbiologist.

16.4.3 Skin/body carriage

Four per cent chlorhexidine, 2% triclosan, or Octenisan® body wash and shampoo once daily for five days. Octenisan® is the only product licensed to be used on neonates. In patients with eczema or other skin conditions, the advice of a dermatologist should be sought.

16.4.4 Treatment

All MRSA infections should be treated based on advice from a microbiologist. Antibiotics commonly used as empirical treatment include vancomycin or teicoplanin, as well as newer agents like oxazolidinones (linezolid) or lipopetides (Daptomycin). Treatment should be based on the antibiotic susceptibility of individual strains and the area where the infection occurs.

MRSA infections must be treated before surgery. A glycopeptide should be given as surgical prophylaxis and patients should be operated on at the end of a list.

16.5 Glycopeptide-resistant enterococci (GRE)

Enterococci are gram-positive cocci that colonize the human bowel; *E. faecalis* is the predominant species. Glycopeptides inhibit cell wall synthesis by binding to the D-alanyl-D-alanine terminal sequences of the muramyl pentapeptide of the elongating peptidoglycan polymer. There are several *van* resistance genes which confer glycopeptide resistance in Enterococci. The most important resistance mechanism is by the acquisition of the *vanA* gene encoded on a transposon located on a transferable plasmid, which results in high-level, inducible resistance to both vancomycin and teicoplanin. It is commonly seen in *E. faecalis* and *E. faecium*. It results in the replacement of D-alanyl-D-alanine terminal sequences with D-alanyl-D-lactate or D-alanyl-D-serine, resulting in a peptidoglycan polymer with a reduced affinity to glycopeptides.

16.6 Screening for GRE

The 2006 guidelines for the control of GRE in hospitals recommend screening of patients in the event of 'suspected GRE outbreaks and in response to important incidents defined by risk assessment' by taking stool samples or rectal swabs which should then be cultured on a selective media for GRE. Additional sites of colonization include wounds, urine, vagina, perineum, and vascular catheter sites.

16.7 Infection control and prevention measures for GRE in hospitals

It is important to control the spread of GRE in hospitals as there are limited treatment options and there is the potential for transference of this resistance to more pathogenic bacteria like *S.aureus*.
Control measures must be influenced by a risk assessment which must include:

- Extent of GRE colonization.
- Faecal incontinence.
- Resistance to other antibiotics.
- Patient susceptibility.
- Prevalence of GRE colonization/infection.

The control and prevention measures as recommended by the 2006 GRE guidelines are as follows:

- Hand hygiene and the use of personal protective equipment

The 1995 Hospital Infection Control Advisory Committee (HICPAC) guidelines recommend the use of an antiseptic soap or a waterless antiseptic agent like an alcohol rub by healthcare workers to disinfect their hands before and after patient contact.

Single use disposable gloves and apron /non-permeable gowns should be used by staff and visitors as per MRSA guidelines.

- Isolation

The decision to isolate is based on clinical risk assessment as described above. . Ideally, patients should be isolated in single rooms but can be cohorted in bays or open wards.

- Cleaning and waste disposal (as per MRSA)
- Antibiotic stewardship

All hospitals should have antibiotic policies to restrict the use of broad-spectrum agents especially cephalosporins and glycopeptide use to reduce the incidence of GRE

16.8 Treatment options available for GRE

Enterococci are low grade pathogens which commonly cause colonization rather than infection. The oxazolidinone, linezolid, is often used for empiric treatment. Other antimicrobials can be used based on the organsim's susceptibility profile.

16.9 *Clostridium difficile*

Clostridium difficile is an anaerobic gram-positive, spore-forming bacteria. *C. difficile* asymptomatically colonizes 67% of infants and 3% of healthy adults. Colonization increases with age, especially above the age of 65 years.

16.10 *Clostridium difficile* risk factors, pathogenesis, and clinical features

The risk factors for developing *Clostridium difficile* infection (CDI) are:

- Use of broad spectrum antibiotics, especially quinolones, co-amoxiclav, clindamycin, and cephalosporins;
- Use of gastric acid suppressants, for example-proton-pump inhibitors (PPIs);
- Age > 65 years;
- Prolonged hospital admission; and
- Enteral tube feeding.

The spores of C. *difficile* survive in the environment for prolonged periods of time. Antibiotics disrupt the gut, and spores, the transmissible form, germinate in the disrupted gut. C. *difficile* produces two toxins—A and B—which cause diarrhoea, pseudomembrane formation, and colitis. The attack rate is variable.

Clinical features range from mild diarrhoea to fever with severe colitis called pseudomembranous colitis and dehydration. Pancolitis, toxic megacolon, perforation, and septic shock can occur.

16.11 Diagnosing CDI in the laboratory

The 2012 DOH updated guidance on the diagnosis and reporting of C. *difficile* recommends:

- Testing of stool samples for CDI from all hospital patients aged two years or older, and all patients from the community sixty-five years or older with diarrhoea not attributable to an underlying condition or treatment.
- The two-stage testing method consists of a screening test: Glutamate Dehydrogenase Enzyme Immunoassay (GDH EIA), a Nucleic Acid Amplification Test (NAAT), or PCR test, followed by a sensitive toxin EIA test (or cytotoxin assay). If the screening test is negative, the second test is not required.

GDH is a protein produced by both toxigenic and non-toxigenic C. *difficile* strains, but it is not specific to C. *difficile*.

Interpretation of results:

- GDH-EIA (or NAAT) positive, toxin EIA positive: CDI is likely to be present.
- GDH-EIA (or NAAT) positive, toxin EIA negative: CDI could be present, so may have transmission potential. The patient could be a potential CDI excretor. An optional third test like PCR can be added to clarify the results of samples from potential excretors.
- GDH-EIA (or NAAT) negative, toxin EIA negative: CDI is very unlikely to be present.

16.12 Infection prevention and control measures for CDI

The 2008 DOH guidance (see Further readings and useful resources) for *Clostridium difficile* infection recommends that:

- All Trusts should follow the SIGHT protocol:
    - S: Suspect that the case may be infective if there is no clear alternative explanation.
    - I: Isolate within two hours. Suspected cases should be nursed in isolation in a side room with an *en suite* toilet. Cohorting patients in a bay or in a dedicated C. *difficile* ward can be considered. The patient should remain isolated until forty-eight hours post passing formed stool. Patient movement must be minimized.
    - G: Gloves and apron should be used when in contact with patient and their surroundings.
    - H: Hand washing with soap and water before and after contact with patient and their surroundings. Alcohol hand gel *must not* be used as an alternative to soap and water as it has no effect on eliminating spores.
    - T: Test stool sample for C. *difficile* infection.
- Environmental cleaning and disinfection

See Chapter 20 on cleaning and disinfection

- Education and antibiotic stewardship

Unnecessary overuse/misuse of broad-spectrum antibiotics must be avoided.

16.13 Available CDI treatment options

The 2013 DOH/PHE updated guidance on CDI (see Further readings and useful resources) recommends:

- Clinical assessment and regular review of patients by a dedicated multi-disciplinary team;
- Supportive therapy;
- Review/stop broad-spectrum antibiotics and acid-suppressing medication like PPIs. Avoid antimotility agents in acute infections;
- Follow SIGHT protocol; and
- Base any treatment on CDI severity.

Markers of severity include:

- WCC > 15 × 10^9/L;
- Rising blood creatinine (> 50% increase above baseline);
- Temperature > 38.5°C;
- Evidence of severe colitis (clinical or radiological).

Mild disease: Not associated with raised WCC and fewer than three stools of type 5–7/day on the Bristol Stool Chart.

Moderate disease: Raised WCC but < 15 × 10^9/L and three to five stools of type 5–7/day.

For mild and moderate CDI, oral metronidazole 400 mg three times daily for ten to fourteen days. The latest evidence suggests oral vancomycin or oral fidaxomicin are superior to oral metronidazole.

Severe disease: Oral vancomycin 125mg four times daily for ten to fourteen days. If no response, start fidaxomicin 200mg twice daily for ten to fourteen days (if there are risk factors for disease recurrence, or elderly) or high-dose oral vancomycin 500mg four times daily +/- IV metronidazole 500mg three times daily. Oral rifampicin 300mg twice daily or IV immunoglobulin 400mg/kg may also be considered as additional treatment

Life-threatening disease:

Vancomycin 500mg four times daily for ten to fourteen days via nasogastric tube/rectal instillation plus IV metronidazole 500mg three times daily. These patients need monitoring in high-dependency units with specialist surgical input.

Recurrent CDI: Recurrent disease occurs in up to 20% of patients treated with oral metronidazole or vancomycin. There are two mechanisms for recurrence:

- Relapse: Usually occurs within two weeks of stopping therapy;
- Reinfection with a different strain.

Oral fidaxomicin 200mg twice daily is the treatment of choice, but oral vancomycin 125mg four times daily can also be used. In an outbreak setting, all isolates must be ribotyped, and public health authorities must be notified.

16.14 Carbapenem-resistant organisms (CRO)

CROs are bacteria which are not susceptible to carbapenems. Resistance can be intrinsic or acquired. Intrinsic resistance, e.g. *Stenotrophomonas maltophilia*, are naturally resistant to carbapenems.

Acquired resistance may involve the following:

- Carbapenemase production: The important acquired carbapenemases in the UK are:
  - KPCs: Hydrolyze all carbapenems and are partially inhibited by clavulanic acid. KPCs are plasmid-encoded.
  - Metallo-beta-lactamases (MBLs): They require zinc ions for activity. They are inactivated by metal ion chelators, such as EDTA. MBLs seen in the UK include NDM, VIM, and IMP types.
  - Members of the OXA family of beta-lactamases: OXA-23, -40, -51, and -58 seen mainly in *Acinetobacter* species and OXA-48 in Enterobacteriaceae.
- ESBL or AmpC enzyme production with porin loss: Enterobacteriaceae that produce ESBL or Amp C enzymes have reduced uptake of carbapenems when they lose their outer membrane proteins. This mechanism is commonly seen in *Enterobacter* and *Klebsiella* spp. Ertapenem is the carbapenem most affected by this.
- OprD porin loss: The most common mode of carbapenem resistance in *Pseudomonas aeruginosa*, which confers resistance to imipenem.
- Porin loss plus efflux pump: Up-regulated MexAB-OprM efflux pump with OprD porin loss confers resistance to meropenem. This mechanism is seen in *P. aeruginosa*.
- Acquired carbapenemases are the most important mechanism from an infection control and public health perspective, especially when present in Enterobacteriaceae (CPE), given the potential for spread between strains, species, and genera as it is plasmid-mediated.

16.15 Who should be screened for Carbapenemase-Producing Enterobacteriaceae (CPE)

The 2013 Acute Trust Toolkit (see Further readings and useful resources) for the early detection, management, and control of CPE advises that all patients meeting the following criteria should be screened for CPE on admission:

- Inpatient in a hospital abroad (see guidance for list of countries) in last twelve months;
- Inpatient in a hospital within the UK known to have problems with CPE in the last twelve months;
- Previously colonized/infected with CPE; or
- Previously had close contact with a patient colonized/infected with CPE.

16.16 Managing a 'suspected or confirmed case of CPE' in an acute trust

The 2013 Acute Trust Toolkit (see Further readings and useful resources) for the early detection, management, and control of CPE makes the following recommendations:

- All trusts must have a CPE management plan;
- Early identification of patients who may be colonized/infected;
- Early isolation of suspected and confirmed cases;
- Admit patient into a single room with en-suite toilet facilities;
- Early diagnosis of suspected cases and contacts and screening:
  - Screening of patient contacts of a confirmed positive case should be done. For suspected cases, if initial screening result is negative, two more samples should be taken forty-eight hours apart. If all three are negative, the patient can come out of isolation.

- Treatment of confirmed cases of infection:
  - All cases *must* be discussed with a microbiologist. Combination therapy is preferred over monotherapy. Treatment should be guided by the isolate's susceptibility profile (MICs): consider combining a polymyxin (e.g. colistin) with either tigecycline or an aminoglycoside;
  - Decolonization with antibiotics is not recommended.

Antibiotic stewardship: Ensure programmes are in place to minimize the overuse/misuse of carbapenems:

- Strict adherence to infection control and prevention measures;
- Environmental cleaning and decontamination:
  - Terminal cleaning and decontamination of the patient's room after discharge or transfer is essential;
- Early communication on transfer or discharge of patient:
  - Good communication including advice and education about condition is key with the patient, carers, and other healthcare colleagues.

16.17 Further readings and useful resources

Damani, N., Manual of Infection Prevention and Control (Oxford, 2011).

Coia, J. E., Duckworth, G. J., Edwards, D. I., Farrington, M., Fry, C., Humphreys, H., et al., 'Guidelines for the Control and Prevention of Meticillin-resistant *Staphylococcus aureus* (MRSA) in Healthcare Facilities', *Journal of Hospital Infection*, 63S (2006), S1–S44, https://www.his.org.uk/files/7113/7338/2934/MRSA_Guidelines_PDF.pdf

Wilcox, M., Cowling, P., Duerden, B., Fry, C., Hopkins, S., Jenks, P., et al. *Implementation of Modified Admission MRSA Screening Guidance for NHS (2014).* (London, 2014). https://www.gov.uk/government/uploads/system/uploads/attachment_data/file/345144/Implementation_of_modified_admission_MRSA_screening_guidance_for_NHS.pdf

Cookson, B. D., Macrae, M. B., Barrett, S. P., Brown, D. F. J., Chadwick, C., French, G. L., et al., 'Guidelines for the Control of Glycopepetide-Resistant Enterococci in Hospitals', *Journal of Hospital Infection*, 62 (2006), 6–21, https://www.his.org.uk/files/4113/7338/2928/GRE_guidelines.pdf

Centers for Disease Control and Prevention. *Recommendations for Preventing the Spread of Vancomycin Resistance. Recommendations of the Hospital Infection Control Practices Advisory Committee (HICPAC)* (Washington, DC, 1995). https://www.cdc.gov/mmwr/preview/mmwrhtml/00039349.htm

Public Health England. *The Characteristics, Diagnosis, Management, Surveillance and Epidemiology of Clostridium difficile (C. difficile).* https://www.gov.uk/government/collections/clostridium-difficile-guidance-data-and-analysis

Department of Health. Clostridium difficile *Infection: How to Deal with the Problem.* (London, 2008), https://www.gov.uk/government/uploads/system/uploads/attachment_data/file/340851/Clostridium_difficile_infection_how_to_deal_with_the_problem.pdf

Department of Health. *Updated Guidance on the Diagnosis and Reporting of Clostridium difficile.* (London, 2012), https://www.gov.uk/government/uploads/system/uploads/attachment_data/file/215135/dh_133016.pdf

Wilcox, M. H., *Updated Guidance on the Management and Treatment of Clostridium difficile Infection.* (London, 2013), https://www.gov.uk/government/uploads/system/uploads/attachment_data/file/321891/Clostridium_difficile_management_and_treatment.pdf

Public Health England. Screening and Detection of Bacteria with Carbapenem-Hydrolysing β-Lactamases (Carbapenemases). (London, 2015), https://assets.publishing.service.gov.

uk/government/uploads/system/uploads/attachment_data/file/552945/B_60i1_RUC_September_2016.pdf

Stokle, L., *Acute Trust Toolkit for the Early Detection, Management and Control of Carbapenemase-producing Enterobactericeae.* (London, 2013), https://www.gov.uk/government/uploads/system/uploads/attachment_data/file/329227/Acute_trust_toolkit_for_the_early_detection.pdf

16.18 Assessment questions

16.18.1 Question 1

An elderly patient with continual diarrhoea (Bristol stool chart type 6 stool) twice a day tests positive for *C. difficile* toxin. She was afebrile with blood pressure of 120/70. Her abdomen is soft, not distended, and non-tender to palpation. Her white cell count is 4.1×10^9 /L, and creatinine 66μmol/L. She can tolerate oral medications.

What is the most appropriate antibiotic treatment advice?
A. No treatment is necessary as the infection is self-limiting.
B. Intravenous metronidazole 500mg thrice daily and review after ten to fourteen days.
C. Oral vancomycin 125mg four times daily and review after ten to fourteen days.
D. Oral fidaxomicin 200mg twice daily and review after ten to fourteen days.
E. Oral metronidazole 400mg thrice daily and review after ten to fourteen days.

16.18.2 Question 2

On examining the blood agar plate which was incubated aerobically, large, flat colonies with a sweet caramel odour and serrated edges are observed. Pale yellow colonies are seen on the MacConkey agar. The isolate is oxidase positive, and identification from MALDI-TOF is awaited (Table 16.1).

What is the most appropriate advice concerning further supplementary testing?
A. No further testing is required.
B. Plate isolate on CPE selective chromogenic agar.
C. Send isolate away to the reference laboratory for further testing.
D. Send isolate for inhibitor-based testing.
E. Send isolate for molecular testing.

Table 16.1 A gram-negative isolate had the following zone diameters and MICs (EUCAST):

Antibiotic	MIC (mg/L)	Disk content (μg)	Zone diameter (mm)
Piperacillin	14	30	22
Piperacillin-tazobactam	12	30–6	24
Ceftazidime	6	10	20
Doripenem	0.5	10	30
Imipenem	10	10	12
Meropenem	0.5	10	30
Ciprofloxacin	0.2	5	28
Amikacin	4	30	22
Gentamicin	2	10	20
Tobramycin	2	10	20
Colistin	2	–	–

16.18.3 Question 3

A patient who has been repatriated from an ICU in India is admitted to the ICU for sepsis secondary to a laparotomy wound infection. He had an emergency laparotomy in India for peritonitis from a ruptured appendix secondary to appendicitis four weeks ago. The patient received linezolid, meropenem, and colistin when he was an in-patient in India. A swab taken on admission is negative for CPE/CRO.

What follow-up screening approach is the most appropriate in this scenario before declaring the patient CPE/CRO free?

A. No further CPE/CRO screening is required.
B. One further negative CPE/CRO screening swabs taken forty-eight hours later.
C. Two further negative CPE/CRO screening swabs taken twenty-four hours apart.
D. Two further negative CPE/CRO screening swabs taken forty-eight hours apart.
E. Two further negative CPE/CRO screening swabs taken seventy-two hours apart.

16.19 Answers and discussion

16.19.1 Answer 1

E. Oral metronidazole 400mg thrice daily and review after ten to fourteen days.
This patient has a mild *C. difficile* infection as per clinical risk assessment for severity: afebrile, normal WCC and creatinine, and no clinical signs of colitis. Oral metronidazole 400mg thrice daily is the recommended drug of choice to treat mild-to-moderate *C. difficile* infection. The clinical risk assessment for any signs of severity must be performed on a daily basis and treatment modified as per assessment.

16.19.2 Answer 2

A. No further testing is required.
It is important to identify the isolate first to elucidate the resistance mechanism. The isolate is *Pseudomonas aeruginosa* from the colonial morphology: large, flat colonies with serrated edges with a sweet caramel odour. They are non-lactose fermenters, hence the pale yellow colonies on the MacConkey agar. These organisms are oxidase positive.

The isolate is sensitive by MIC and zone diameter to all classes of antibiotics except for imipenem (see the EUCAST Clinical Breakpoints Table for *Pseudomonas* spp. for MIC and zone diameter values). The most common mechanism of resistance to imipenem in *P. aeruginosa* is OprD (D2) porin loss. Such isolates must be sent to the reference laboratory or sent for further testing if there is resistance to different classes of antibiotics like carbapenems (except for ertapenem-intrinsically resistant), tazobactam-piperacillin, and ceftazidime.

16.19.3 Answer 3

D. Two further negative CPE/CRO screening swabs taken forty-eight hours apart.
This patient is high risk for the presence of CPE/CRO for the following reasons:

1. Treatment in an intensive care unit from a hospital in a high-risk country for CPE/CRO.
2. Prior broad-spectrum antibiotic exposure contributing to increased selection pressure. As per national guidance for CRO/CPE, this patient would need to be screened for carbapenemase-producing organisms: stool, rectal, and wound swabs, and also swabs from any in-dwelling medical devices must be included in the CRO/CPE screen. If the first set of swabs are negative, two more screening swabs taken forty-eight hours apart must be sent before the patient is declared to be CPE/CRO free.

CHAPTER 17

The concept of chain of infection and infection control principles

George Jacob and Martina N. Cummins

CONTENTS

17.1 The concept of the chain of infection

For an infectious agent to spread to cause disease, certain conditions must be present. This process is called the chain of infection, which consists of six links:

- Causative agent;
- Infectious reservoir;
- Path of exit;
- Mode of transmission;
- Path of entry; and
- Susceptible host.

Infection can occur when all six links are intact. By breaking this chain, the spread of infection can be stopped.

17.2 The six links in the chain of infection

- Causative agent

A micro-organism capable of causing infection is called a causative agent. Most commonly they are bacteria, viruses, fungi, and parasites.

- Infectious reservoir

A reservoir of infection is the source from which infection can spread by allowing the pathogen to survive and possibly multiply. Humans, animals, and even inanimate environmental objects can serve as reservoirs of infection.

There are many sources of infection in a healthcare setting. These include patients, healthcare workers, visitors, inanimate objects like medical equipment, and even the hospital environment.

A human reservoir can be either an infected case, or a carrier, i.e. the person is colonized by a particular pathogen and does not present with any symptoms or signs of acute infection. Adherence to standard infection control practices is important as these asymptomatic carriers present a risk of cross infection, especially in healthcare surroundings.

- Path of exit

The path of exit is how a pathogen leaves its reservoir. It normally refers to the site where the micro-organism grows. Common sites of exit associated with human reservoirs include the skin, mucous membranes, and the respiratory, gastrointestinal, and genitourinary tracts.

- Mode of transmission

The mode of transmission is the route by which an infection spreads. Certain pathogens may use more than one route of transmission from reservoir to host. There are three common modes of transmission.

17.2.1 Contact transmission

This is the most common mode of infection transmission in a healthcare setting. It can occur either through direct contact when there is direct physical contact with the patient or indirect contact when the pathogen is transmitted from a contaminated intermediate object.

17.2.2 Airborne transmission

Infection spreads through the airborne route when the susceptible person inhales infected particles in droplet nuclei of less than 5 μm. These particles can remain airborne for long periods of time and can be dispersed over one metre from the source of infection especially when the infected person coughs or sneezes. Due to their small size, they can bypass the host's respiratory defence mechanisms and reach the alveoli, causing infection. Some of the common diseases which spread via this route are chickenpox, measles, and tuberculosis.

17.2.3 Droplet transmission

Infection spreads via the droplet transmission route when infected particles in droplet nuclei of more than 5 μm come into contact with the mucous membranes of the susceptible person's eyes, nose, and mouth. These heavier particles do not remain airborne for long periods of time but settle into the surrounding environment, causing contamination of the surfaces (especially when the infected person coughs or sneezes). It can be considered a form of contact transmission. Some of the common pathogens which spread via this route are Neisseria meningitides, Bordetella pertussis, and influenza viruses.

- Path of entry

It is the path used by the pathogen to invade a susceptible host. The path of entry is usually the same site as the path of exit.

- Susceptible host

A competent immune system fights off micro-organisms seeking to cause disease. If the immune system is compromised in any way, i.e. the host is susceptible to infection, the invading pathogen can cause disease. Patients in healthcare settings are usually very young, elderly, or suffer from certain chronic illnesses (chronic renal, hepatic, or lung diseases, uncontrolled/poorly controlled diabetes mellitus, or malignancy) which result in an ineffective immune system making them vulnerable to acquiring infection after exposure. Also, certain treatments like chemotherapy and steroid use also weaken the immune system and increase the risk of acquiring the infection. Adherence to standard and specific transmission-related infection control practices minimizes the spread of infection in these patients.

17.3 The aim of a hospital infection control and prevention programme

The aim of infection control is to prevent or reduce the risk of healthcare-associated infection. A hospital infection control programme should have the following main components:

- Surveillance;
- Outbreak management;
- Prevention of infection—standard and isolation precautions;
- Education about infection prevention and development of infection control policies; and
- Environmental cleaning, disinfection, and sterilization of equipment and safe disposal of infectious waste.

17.4 Surveillance in infection control

Surveillance is defined as the systematic collection, validation, analysis, and interpretation of data on specific events and infections, followed by the timely dissemination of information to those who can influence practice, implement change, and provide the financial and managerial support necessary to improve outcomes.

17.5 The main aims of surveillance in infection control

The main aims of surveillance in infection control are:

- To obtain the baseline rate of infections;
- To compare healthcare-associated infections within and between healthcare facilities after the data is risk adjusted;
- To ensure that best practice is adhered to by all hospital clinical teams;
- To reduce the rates of healthcare-associated infections by introducing evidence-based and cost-effective interventions;
- To identify and manage outbreaks;
- To measure the success of infection control interventions; and
- To prioritize local infection control issues so as to allocate resources accordingly.

17.6 What is targeted surveillance?

Surveillance is labour intensive and expensive. Ideally, surveillance must be directed or targeted towards preventable HCAIs either in high-risk areas like intensive care units and neonatal units, or towards infections such as surgical site infections or procedure-related infections, e.g. central line or urinary catheter-related infections, to make it cost-effective and practical.

17.7 The surveillance method commonly used by the hospital infection control and prevention team (ICPT)

A laboratory-based ward liaison surveillance method is commonly used on a daily basis by the ICPT. It involves daily ward visits by the ICPT for the purpose of collecting information about patients suspected of having an infection that may require specific infection control and prevention measures. Every hospital will have a list of these alert organisms or diseases based on the local epidemiology, which will require specific infection control and prevention measures. The ICPT should be notified of all such cases by the ward teams. This method also requires follow-up of any positive result generated by the microbiology laboratory for these patients to confirm the initial suspected diagnosis by the ICPT. Patients confirmed as cases, as well as their contacts, are followed up with further ward reviews by the ICPT.

17.8 Process surveillance

A process is defined as a succession of steps that lead to the desired outcome. Process surveillance involves the monitoring of compliance with evidence-based steps considered to be best practice. Monitoring compliance with the various steps in the care bundle to reduce catheter-associated urinary tract infections is an example of process surveillance. These steps also need to be performed effectively to guarantee the desired outcome, which is to minimize or prevent the risk of HCAIs.

17.9 Outbreak of infection

An outbreak is defined as:

- Two or more cases linked in time or place;
- A single case of a rare disease caused by a significant pathogen (polio, viral haemorrhagic fever, rabies, diphtheria);
- A greater than expected rate of infection when compared with the usual background rate within a specific geographical area and over a defined time frame.

17.10 Steps in managing an outbreak

- Recognize the presence of an outbreak:
  - Initial investigations to ascertain the nature of the outbreak has to start within twenty-four hours;
  - Perform an immediate risk assessment following receipt of initial information and institute immediate control measures.
- Declaration of an outbreak;
- Convene an outbreak control team (OCT) ideally within three days of outbreak declaration:
  - Members of the team should include all agencies/disciplines involved in the management and control of the outbreak. An OCT is normally comprised of a

director of public health (or nominated deputy), consultant microbiologist, consultant in communicable disease control, infection control nurse specialist, senior member of the clinical team: ward manager or consultant, senior member of the Trusts management: health and safety executive, communications officer, and administrative support;

- Roles and responsibilities should be delegated at the meeting and a lead organization selected to lead the outbreak response.

- Outbreak response (investigations and control measures):
  - Agree and record the case definition;
  - Control measures to be reviewed with agreement on the timescale for implementation and responsibility;
  - Descriptive epidemiology which should include number of cases as per case definition, epidemic curve, and description of key characteristics like gender, geographical spread, risk factors, severity;
  - Generate hypothesis;
  - Review risk assessment as per evidence obtained;
  - Consider analytical study and prepare an investigation protocol if study is undertaken.

- Communications strategy:
  - To be agreed at first OCT meeting and should be reviewed in subsequent meetings;
  - There should be absolute clarity concerning who is leading the outbreak with appropriate handovers;
  - Communications officer should be responsible for liaising with the media.

- End of outbreak:
  - Prepare final outbreak report within twelve weeks of outbreak closure;
  - Recommendations made and lessons learnt should be reviewed within twelve months of outbreak closure.

17.11 Standard precautions

Standard precautions are advised whenever care is given to any hospitalized patient. They reduce the risk of transmission of infection even if the infection is unknown or not apparent. As per the 2007 Centers for Disease Control (CDC)/Hospital Infection Control Advisory Committee (HICPAC) guidelines, these include:

- Hand hygiene before and after patient contact. It means handwashing with either soap and water or the use of alcohol-based gels or foams. The World Health Organization (WHO) 'SAVE LIVES: Clean Your Hands initiative' includes 'My Five Moments for Hand Hygiene', which recommends hand hygiene:
  - Before touching patients;
  - Before aseptic procedures;
  - After body fluid exposure;
  - After touching patients; and
  - After touching patient surroundings.

Handwashing with soap and water is recommended when looking after infectious patients with spore forming bacteria like *Clostridium difficile* as alcohol-based hand disinfectants have no effect against such infections. Also, its effectiveness is variable on diarrhoeal viruses, particularly the non-enveloped viruses.

- Use of personal protective equipment (PPE) like gloves, gowns, and eye protection if exposure to blood and body fluids is possible;
- Safe disposal of sharps in designated sharps containers; and
- Disposal of soiled linen in appropriate laundry bags and clinical waste in designated yellow bags as per local policy.

17.12 Different types of transmission-related precautions

The infection control precautions followed will depend on upon the mode of transmission.

- *Contact transmission*: Use of standard precautions, cohorting of cases or isolation in a single room, environmental cleaning, disinfection, and sterilization of equipment used helps to minimize the risk of infection through contact transmission.
- *Droplet transmission*: In addition to the above precautions, use of surgical masks while within one metre of patient contact will help minimize the risk of infection through droplet transmission.
- *Airborne transmission*: Use of standard precautions and isolation of patients in negative-pressure ventilation rooms with a minimum of six to twelve air changes per hour helps to dilute the infective particles. Doors to these rooms must remain closed. All healthcare workers must wear particulate respirators (FFP2 or FFP3) as part of their PPE. Environmental cleaning, disinfection and sterilization of equipment used also helps to minimize transmission via this route.

17.13 Special precautions required for neutropenic patients

In addition to standard precautions, neutropenic patients need to be nursed in special protective environments. They should be nursed in isolation in positive pressure rooms relative to corridors with a minimum of twelve air changes per hour with directed room HEPA filtered air flow. Strict adherence to effective environmental cleaning, disinfection, and sterilization of equipment and consideration of single use/dedicated equipment should be considered for each patient if possible

17.14 Further readings and useful resources

Anderson, D. J., 'Infection prevention: Precautions for preventing transmission of infection'. UpToDate. https://www.uptodate.com/contents/infection-prevention-precautions-for-preventing-transmission-of-infection

Damani, N. N., *Manual of Infection Prevention and Control* (Oxford, 2012).

MacAuslane, H., Morgan, D., CIDSC. *Communicable Disease Outbreak Management: Operational Guidance* (2nd ed., London, 2014). https://www.gov.uk/government/uploads/system/uploads/attachment_data/file/343723/12_8_2014_CD_Outbreak_Guidance_REandCT_2__2_.pdf

17.15 Assessment questions

17.15.1 Question 1

A twenty-year old man presents with an acute onset of fever, headache, photophobia, neck stiffness, and a purpuric non-blanching rash over his body.

What is the most appropriate infection control and prevention advice?
A. No special infection control and prevention measures needed.
B. Standard precautions only, admit patient to an open bay.
C. Standard precautions and isolate patient in a positive-pressure ventilated room with HEPA-filtered room directed air flow
D. Standard precautions, isolate patient in a negative-pressure ventilated room, all healthcare workers should wear a particulate respirator while nursing the patient.
E. Standard precautions, isolate patient in a single room, all healthcare workers should wear a surgical mask while nursing the patient.

17.15.2 Question 2

A twenty-six-year-old man from India presents with a history of fever, productive cough, haemoptysis, and significant weight loss.

What is the most appropriate infection control and prevention advice?
A. No special infection control or prevention measures needed.
B. Standard precautions only, admit patient to an open bay.
C. Standard precautions and isolate patient in a positive-pressure ventilated room with HEPA-filtered room directed air flow.
D. Standard precautions, isolate patient in a negative-pressure ventilated room, all healthcare workers should wear a particulate respirator while nursing the patient.
E. Standard precautions, isolate patient in a single room, all healthcare workers should wear a surgical mask while nursing the patient.

17.15.3 Question 3

A fifty-year-old woman presents to the oncology day unit with fever and cellulitis over her left leg. She has a background of breast cancer and has just completed her last cycle of chemotherapy one week ago. She is admitted for intravenous antibiotics and GCSF injections.

What is the most appropriate infection control and prevention advice?
A. No special infection control or prevention measures needed.
B. Standard precautions only, admit patient to an open bay.
C. Standard precautions and isolate patient in a positive-pressure ventilated room with HEPA-filtered room directed air flow.
D. Standard precautions, isolate patient in a negative-pressure ventilated room, all healthcare workers should wear a particulate respirator while nursing the patient.
E. Standard precautions, isolate patient in a single room, all healthcare workers should wear a surgical mask while nursing the patient.

17.16 Answers and discussion

17.16.1 Answer 1

E. Standard precautions, isolate patient in a single room, all healthcare workers should wear a surgical mask while nursing the patient.

This patient is likely to have Neisseria meningitides meningitis given the symptoms of fever, headache, photophobia, and a non-blanching purpuric rash. It is transmitted by droplet transmission. These infectious particles are heavier and tend to settle down quickly contaminating hospital environments, especially surfaces. Isolating the patient in a single room, good compliance to standard precautions (especially hand hygiene), and wearing a surgical mask if within one metre of the patient will help prevent transmission of any infection by the droplet route.

17.16.2 Answer 2

D. Standard precautions, isolate patient in a negative-pressure ventilated room, all healthcare workers should wear a particulate respirator while nursing the patient.

This patient is likely to have pulmonary tuberculosis with the symptoms of fever, productive cough, haemoptysis, and significant weight loss. It is transmitted by airborne transmission. All healthcare workers must strictly adhere to standard precautions, wear personal protective equipment, which must consist of a particulate respirator (FFP2 or FFP3 mask) capable of filtering small particles (1–5 μm) which remain airborne for longer periods of time. The masks must fit close to form a tight seal. All healthcare workers must be 'fit tested' before using particulate respirators like FFP3. Patients with pulmonary tuberculosis must also be nursed in negative-pressure ventilated rooms (airflow directed towards the patient). Negative-pressure ventilation helps in 'containing' infections spread by the airborne route and protects other patients, healthcare workers, and visitors.

17.16.3 Answer 3

C. Standard precautions and isolate patient in a positive-pressure ventilated room with HEPA-filtered room directed air flow.

This patient is likely to have neutropenic sepsis given that she is post chemotherapy and about to be started on GCSF (Granulocyte Colony Stimulating Factor). All neutropenic patients must be nursed in positive-pressure ventilated rooms (airflow directed away from the patient) as the aim of ventilation is to protect the vulnerable patient from infections originating from the hospital environment. Strict adherence to standard precautions and HEPA-filtered air both help reduce the incidence of infection in such immunocompromised patients.

CHAPTER 18

Antimicrobial stewardship

Sarfaraz Ameen and Caoimhe NicFhogartaigh

18.1 What is antimicrobial stewardship?

Antimicrobial stewardship (AMS) is a healthcare-system-wide approach to promoting and monitoring the judicious use of antimicrobials (including antibiotics) to preserve their future effectiveness and optimize outcomes for patients. Put simply, it is using the right antibiotic, at the right dose, via the right route, at the right time, for the right duration (Centres for Disease Control, 2010).

18.2 The scale of the problem and why AMS is important

Antimicrobial resistance (AMR) is a serious and growing global public health concern. Antibiotics are a unique class of drug as their use in individual patients may have an impact on others through the spread of resistant organisms. Antibiotics are essential for saving lives in conditions such as sepsis, and without effective antibiotics even minor operations could be life-threatening due to the risk of resistant infections. Across Europe approximately 25,000 people die each year as a result of hospital infections caused by resistant bacteria, and others have more prolonged and complicated illness. By 2050, AMR is predicted to be one of the major causes of death worldwide.

Protecting the use of currently available antibiotics is crucial as discovery of new antimicrobials has stalled. Studies consistently demonstrate that 30–50% of antimicrobial prescriptions are unnecessary or inappropriate. Figure 18.1 shows some of the reasons behind this. As well as driving increasing resistance, unnecessary prescribing leads to unwanted adverse effects, including avoidable drug reactions and interactions, *Clostridium difficile*-associated diarrhoea, and healthcare-associated infections with resistant micro-organisms, all of which are associated with adverse clinical outcomes, including increased length of hospital stay and mortality, with increased cost to

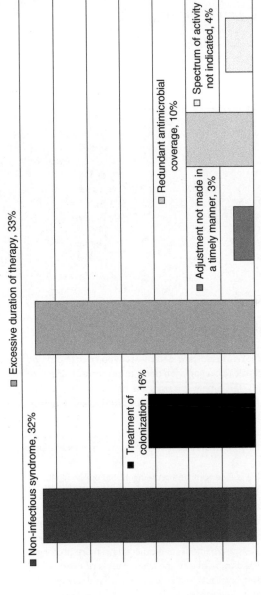

Figure 18.1 Scale of inappropriate antimicrobial usage and their reasons.

Source: data from Hecker, M. T. et al. Unnecessary use of antimicrobials in hospitalised patients. *Archives of Internal Medicine*, 163(8), 972–978. © 2003 JAMA.

healthcare systems. Prudent use of antibiotics improves patient care and clinical outcomes, reduces the spread of antimicrobial resistance, and saves money.

18.3 The gold standards of AMS

There are a number of global and national guidelines outlining what a robust AMS programme should consist of (see Further reading and useful resources), including:

- Infectious Diseases Society of America (IDSA): *Guidelines for Developing an Institutional Programme to Enhance Antimicrobial Stewardship.*
- National Institute for Health and Care Excellence (NICE): *Antimicrobial Stewardship: Systems and Processes for Effective Antimicrobial Medicine Use* [NG15].
- Department of Health (DoH): *Start Smart Then Focus*, updated 2015.
- DoH: *UK 5-Year Antimicrobial Resistance Strategy 2013 to 2018.*

There are a number of models used to illustrate good AMS standards. The *DoH Start Smart Then Focus* summarizes prudent antimicrobial treatment (Figure 18.2).

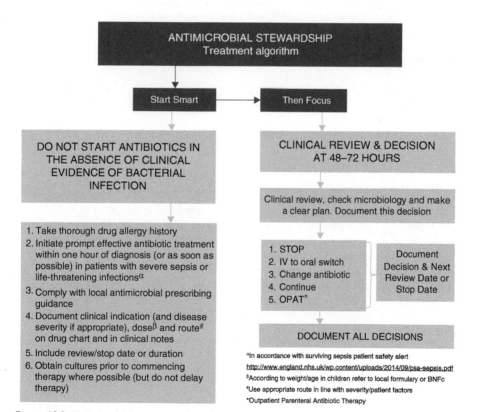

Figure 18.2 Antimicrobial treatment algorithm.
Reproduced with permission from Public Health England. Start Smart - Then Focus: Antimicrobial Stewardship Toolkit for English Hospitals, 2015. London, UK: Public Health England. Copyright © 2015 Public Health England. Available at: https://www.gov.uk/government/publications/antimicrobial-stewardship-start-smart-then-focus

18.4 Key elements of a successful AMS programme

Key elements of AMS include:

- The establishment of an AMS team to lead the local agenda on AMR and AMS;
- Development and implementation of antimicrobial guidelines with built-in decision support systems to aid prescribers;
- Education and training in antimicrobial prescribing and stewardship;
- AMS ward rounds focusing on targeting and rationalizing inappropriate antimicrobial prescribing;
- Formulary restriction (see Different types of AMS strategies);
- Monitoring and feedback to individual prescribers on:
  - Antimicrobial consumption;
  - Compliance with antimicrobial guidelines;
  - Adverse incidents related to antimicrobial use; and
  - Trends in AMR.
- Quality microbiology diagnostics and reporting; and
- Patient education and communication.

Key elements will vary in importance depending on the healthcare setting (primary care, secondary care, or long-term care facility) and the existing infrastructure and resources available. Commitment from local leaders and managers is essential to ensure that human and financial resources, as well as information technology support systems, are available to deliver sustainable stewardship activities.

18.5 The core members of an AMS team

NICE recommends that an AMS committee should be a multi-disciplinary team made up of the following core membership:

- A microbiologist / infection specialist and
- An antimicrobial pharmacist.

IDSA also recommend representation from infection control, physician, and surgical champions, the microbiology laboratory, and emphasize the importance of support from information technology, a data analyst/epidemiologist, the clinical effectiveness/quality and safety team (to monitor patient outcomes), and administration. The AMS team should have clear terms of reference with clear objectives. It is essential that there is engagement from clinical staff within the organization to understand local challenges to delivery of AMS goals, and to incorporate quality assurance processes into the AMS framework. There should be clear lines of accountability to a single leader responsible for programme outcomes. Figure 18.3 shows a proposed framework for an AMS team.

18.6 Different types of AMS strategies

AMS programmes should incorporate a variety of strategies and interventions appropriate to the healthcare setting and co-ordinated by the AMS committee. The core strategies can be divided into 'restrictive' or 'persuasive'.

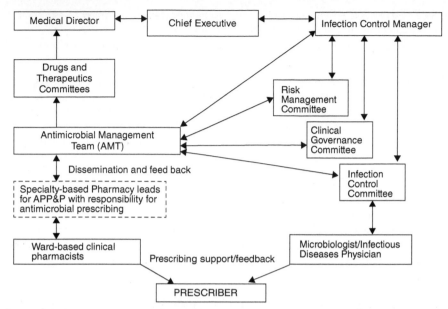

Figure 18.3 Proposed structure of AMS team.
Reproduced with permission from Nathwani, D, et al. Antimicrobial prescribing policy and practice in Scotland: recommendations for good antimicrobial practice in acute hospitals. Journal of Antimicrobial Chemotherapy, 57(6), 1189–1196. Copyright © 2006 Oxford University Press.

Restrictive strategies involve a change to the antibiotic formulary or policy implemented through an organizational change that restricts the freedom of prescribers to select some antimicrobials (usually broad-spectrum antibiotics and expensive antifungals). Examples include:

- *Formulary restriction*, whereby only a limited selection of antimicrobials is available on formulary to limit the use of particularly expensive or broad-spectrum agents;
- *Removal of restricted antibiotics from ward*;
- *Compulsory order forms*, where it is necessary to provide clinical information to justify use of the restricted antimicrobial;
- *Expert approval*, whereby approval is required from a microbiologist, ID specialist, or antimicrobial pharmacist before the drug can be used. This authorization may be required at time of initiation of the antimicrobial, or a limited prescription of forty-eight hours may be permitted before approval to continue is required; and
- *Automatic stop orders*, whereby an antibiotic is automatically discontinued after a number of days.

Restrictive strategies may only apply to certain patient groups, for example, use of cephalosporins may be restricted in elderly patients, but permitted to treat urinary tract infection in pregnancy. Restrictions may also be removed for certain indications, for example, the use of piperacillin-tazobactam permitted in empirical treatment of neutropenic sepsis.

Persuasive strategies provide physicians with guidance and feedback on antimicrobial prescribing. Examples include:

- *Education and training* on antimicrobial prescribing and local guidelines;
- *Prospective audit and feedback*;

- *AMS ward rounds* to review antimicrobials and recommend changes, e.g. timely de-escalation of antibiotics and intravenous (IV) to oral switch; and
- *Reminders/prompts* to review antibiotic prescriptions documented on the drug chart or in patient notes.

Restrictive and persuasive strategies each have advantages and disadvantages. Both have been shown to lead to a reduction in antimicrobial consumption without adverse clinical outcomes. Restriction leads to immediate reduction in consumption and has a more rapid effect on reversing antimicrobial resistance, but such measures are often unpopular with prescribers and their impact is not sustained once the restrictions are removed. If not carefully managed they may lead to delays in antibiotic administration. Persuasive strategies are usually more labour intensive, and slower to show an impact on antimicrobial prescribing and resistance but have a more sustained effect which may be due to the great opportunity for education with this type of intervention and wider acceptance by prescribers. A 2013 systematic review by Davey and colleagues provides more detailed information on the impact of AMS strategies.

The choice of strategy will depend on priorities, for example, in the setting of an outbreak of resistant organisms; a restrictive policy should lead to more rapid control. In practice, restrictive and persuasive strategies are usually combined into bundles for a greater overall effect.

18.7 How antimicrobial guidelines can help with AMS

Guidelines defining the optimal first- and second-line antibiotics for specific infections ensure the correct spectrum of antimicrobial cover for the most likely pathogens, while limiting collateral damage in terms of adverse effects, resistance, and unnecessary cost. Antimicrobial guidelines for pneumonia have been shown to significantly reduce mortality. Guidance may also include advice on microbiological tests to optimize pathogen-specific diagnosis and subsequent rationalization of therapy, and include appropriate durations to reduce unnecessary prolonged courses. Utilization of diverse classes of antimicrobials in the guidance helps to prevent resistance to a single, commonly used antibiotic class, but 'cycling' of different antibiotics over time is not currently recommended due to lack of good quality evidence.

Antimicrobial treatment guidelines should be written in accordance with national evidence-based guidance where available, but must take into consideration local patient demographics and resistance patterns and be adapted accordingly. Relevant prescribing stake-holders should be involved in guideline development as this will enhance implementation and adherence.

18.8 Measuring the impact of AMS interventions

The surveillance of antimicrobial consumption, antibiotic resistance, adverse effects, and compliance with guidelines is crucial to monitor the impact of AMS interventions and ensure ongoing quality improvement and targeted activity in areas of greatest need. Expenditure on antimicrobials should also be monitored to ensure the cost effectiveness of AMS resources, although the additional savings made by reductions in *C. difficile* and resistant organisms are difficult to measure.

18.9 The microbiology laboratory role in AMS

Quality diagnostics for rapid identification and susceptibility-testing of isolates with timely reporting facilitates the optimization and de-escalation of antibiotic therapy in individual patients. Advances in molecular diagnostics for pathogen (and resistance mechanism) detection should further facilitate timely, targeted therapy.

Selective reporting of susceptibility results in line with local antibiotic guidelines can enhance adherence to guidelines by supressing results for restricted antibiotics. Suppressing all susceptibility results for isolates which are of doubtful clinical significance, e.g. catheter urine specimens, can also help to reduce unnecessary antibiotics.

Further work is required to establish the role of biomarkers, e.g. procalcitonin as AMS tools; however, when used in an algorithm to aid antibiotic prescribing decisions in respiratory tract infection, procalcitonin significantly reduced antibiotic prescribing in primary care, emergency, and intensive care settings with no adverse outcomes reported.

18.10 Potential barriers to establishing an AMS programme

Implementation of a robust AMS programme requires a number of barriers to be successfully addressed:

- *Changing attitudes and behaviours and breaking cultural barriers*: there may be a tendency or pressure to treat the patient with antibiotics 'just in case' due to perceived safety or concern about litigation, without considering the bigger picture of AMR, side effects, and costs. Clinical engagement and awareness from all healthcare staff within the health organization regarding the challenges of AMR and the vital role all healthcare staff play in AMS is crucial. This must be driven from senior management within healthcare organizations.
- *Resource and time constraints*: organizations must invest to ensure the AMS team consists of the appropriate experts with dedicated time for stewardship activities, education and training sessions, and resources for surveillance of antibiotic consumption and resistance.
- *Inadequate education and training*: education must target medical, nursing, pharmacy, and allied healthcare professionals, including at undergraduate level.
- *Patient expectation*: there is an expectation from patients to receive a course of antibiotics to treat coughs, colds, and 'flu, which may be overcome with improved verbal and written communication to enhance patient education.

18.11 Further reading and useful resources

Department of Health; UK 5 Year Antimicrobial Resistance Strategy 2013 to 2018. https://www.gov.uk/government/publications/uk-5-year-antimicrobial-resistance-strategy-2013-to-2018

Zarb, P., Amadeo, B., Muller, A., Drapier, N., Vankerckhoven, V., Davey, P., et al., 'Identification of Targets for Quality Improvement in Antimicrobial Prescribing: The Web-Based ESAC Point Prevalence Survey 2009', *Journal of Antimicrobial Chemotherapy*, 66 (2011), 443–449.

Hecker, M. T., Aron, D. C., Patel, N. P., Lehmann, M. K., Donskey, C. J., 'Unnecessary Use of Antimicrobials in Hospitalised Patients', *Archives of Internal Medicine*, 162 (2003), 972–978.

de Kraker, M. E., Wolkewitz, M., Davey, P. G., Koller, W., Berger, J., Nagler, J., et al., 'Burden of Antimicrobial Resistance in European Hospitals: Excess Mortality and Length of Hospital Stay Associated with Bloodstream Infections Due to *Escherichia coli*-Resistant to Third-Generation Cephalosporins', *Journal of Antimicrobial Chemotherapy*, 66/2 (2011), 398–407.

Department of Health; Start smart then focus, 2015. https://www.gov.uk/government/publications/antimicrobial-stewardship-start-smart-then-focus

Nathwani, D., Scottish Medicines Consortium (SMC) Short Life Working Group; Scottish Executive Health Department Healthcare Associated Infection Task Force, 'Antimicrobial Prescribing Policy and Practice in Scotland: Recommendations for Good Antimicrobial Practice in Acute Hospitals', *Journal of Antimicrobial Chemotherapy*, 57 (2006), 1189–1196.

Davey, P., Brown, E., Charani, E., Fenelon, L., Gould, I. M., Holmes, A., et al., 'Interventions to improve antibiotic prescribing practices for hospital inpatients', *Cochrane Database of Systematic Reviews*, 4 (2013), CD003543. doi: 10.1002/14651858.CD003543.pub3

Schuetz, P., Chiappa, V., Briel, M., Greenwald, J. L., 'Procalcitonin Algorithms for Antibiotic Therapy Decisions: A Systematic Review of Randomized Controlled Trials and Recommendations for Clinical Algorithms', *Archives of Internal Medicine*, 171/15 (2011), 1322–1331.

National Institute for Health and Care Excellence (NICE). *Antimicrobial Stewardship: Systems and Processes for Effective Antimicrobial Medicine Use* [NG15] (2015). https://www.nice.org.uk/guidance/ng15?UNLID=32944887020166410438

Dellit, T. H., Owens, R. C., McGowan, J. E., Jr., Gerding, D. N., Weinstein, R. A., Burke, J. P., et al., 'Infectious Diseases Society of America and the Society for Healthcare Epidemiology of America Guidelines for Developing an Institutional Program to Enhance Antimicrobial Stewardship', *Clinical Infectious Diseases*, 44 (2007), 159–177.

TARGET antibiotics toolkit. http://www.rcgp.org.uk/clinical-and-research/toolkits/target-antibiotics-toolkit.aspx

18.12 Assessment questions

18.12.1 Question 1

Rates of piperacillin-tazobactam usage are increasing on one of the surgical wards.

Which of the following educational tools is likely to be most effective in optimizing antibiotic prescribing?
A. Academic detailing ('one-to-one' teaching opportunity).
B. Interactive workshop.
C. Lecture format departmental teaching session.
D. Posters in key areas.
E. Printed guidelines.

18.12.2 Question 2

The vast majority (80%) of antibiotics are prescribed in the community.

Which of the following is *not* useful in reducing antibiotic prescribing in the primary care setting?
A. Delayed prescribing strategies.
B. Enhanced doctor-patient communication.
C. Financial incentives.
D. Patient information leaflets.
E. Restricting duration of appointment.

18.12.3 Question 3

Due to an outbreak of carbapenemase-producing enterobacteriaceae you are co-ordinating a strict carbapenem restriction programme.

Which of the following is a persuasive stewardship strategy?
A. Antimicrobial stewardship ward rounds.
B. Automatic stop orders.
C. Compulsory order forms.
D. Expert approval.
E. Formulary restrictions.

18.13 Answers and discussion

18.13.1 Answer 1

A. Academic detailing ('one-to-one' teaching opportunity).

Poor antimicrobial prescribing has been linked with inadequate training in antimicrobial pharmacotherapy at undergraduate and postgraduate levels. Educational approaches which involve active participation of the prescriber have been shown to be more effective in changing prescribing behaviour than passive dissemination of information. Academic detailing is a 'one-to-one' educational session between an educator (physician or pharmacist) and the clinician prescriber. These face-to-face educational approaches have greater and more sustained effects on prescribing behaviour than printed material or group interactions alone.

18.13.2. Answer 2

E. Restricting duration of appointment.

Providing patients with verbal and written communication on the rationale for not prescribing antibiotics, or adopting a delayed prescribing approach (whereby the patient can collect a prescription at a later date should symptoms not improve), has reduced antibiotic prescribing for minor conditions (sore throat and cough) without adverse outcomes or reduced patient satisfaction. The NHS England Quality Premium scheme financially rewards clinical commissioning groups for quality improvements, and has recently included targets to reduce antibiotic prescribing, in particular, broad-spectrum agents, with successful outcomes. TARGET (Treat Antibiotics Responsibly: Guidance, Education, Tools) is a multi-faceted toolkit developed by Public Health England in collaboration with Royal College of GPs and various other groups aiming to influence prescriber and patient attitudes and overcome barriers to optimal antibiotic prescribing.

18.13.3 Answer 3

A. Antimicrobial stewardship ward rounds.

AMS ward rounds are a persuasive intervention as they provide prescribers with guidance and feedback on antimicrobial prescribing, rather than restricting prescribers' selection of antibiotics.

CHAPTER 19

Tools in infection prevention and control

Stephanie J. Smith and Martina Cummins

CONTENTS

19.1 Legal responsibilities placed on healthcare organizations to ensure quality infection prevention and control (IPC)

The Health Act (2008) Code of Practice on the Prevention and Control of Infections and Related Guidance provides a legal statutory requirement to which all hospital trusts in England should abide to ensure the safety of patients and healthcare workers. There are similar laws in both Scotland and Wales. Prevention and control of healthcare-associated infections (HCAI) remains integral to provide safe, quality patient care and requires an effective management team to implement the Act.

In July 2015, a revised Code of Practice was introduced for the prevention and control of HCAI. The Code of Practice is also referred to as the 'Hygiene Code' and is regulated by the Care Quality Commission (CQC). A requirement of this Act is that the board of directors receive an annual report from the Director of Infection Prevention & Control (DIPC), with acknowledgement of the report and approval of a proposed programme of delivery prior to public release and implementation.

All trusts must register with the CQC, whose role is to regulate and inspect care services in the public, private, and voluntary sectors in England. Part of the CQC assessment against the Act includes Outcome 8: Cleanliness and Infection Control. Under this outcome the trust is required to demonstrate compliance (Table 19.1).

The DIPC within an organization will assume responsibility to provide assurances that criteria are met by ensuring regular committee meetings to discuss compliance with standards, monitoring of trends, and provide strategies to reduce HCAI. The trust has to be made accountable for any infection control issues for their staff and patients and have evidence of a clear framework to provide assurances that safety has been met.

Table 19.1 The areas of compliance in The Health and Social Care Act (2008, reviewed 2015).

Compliance criterion	What the registered provider will need to demonstrate
1	Systems to manage and monitor the prevention and control of infection. These systems use risk assessments and consider the susceptibility of service users and any risks that their environment and other users may pose to them
2	Provide and maintain a clean and appropriate environment in managed premises that facilitates the prevention and control of infections
3	Ensure appropriate antimicrobial use to optimize patient outcomes and to reduce the risk of adverse events and antimicrobial resistance
4	Provide suitable accurate information on infections to service users, their visitors, and any person concerned with providing further support or nursing/medical care in a timely fashion
5	Ensure prompt identification of people who have, or are at risk of developing, an infection so that they receive timely and appropriate treatment to reduce the risk of transmitting infection to other people
6	Systems to ensure that all care workers (including contractors and volunteers) are aware of and discharge their responsibilities in the process of preventing and controlling infection
7	Provide or secure adequate isolation facilities
8	Secure adequate access to laboratory support as appropriate
9	Have and adhere to policies designed for the individual's care and provider organizations that will help to prevent and control infections
10	Providers have a system in place to manage the occupational health needs and obligations of staff in relation to infection

The IPC Team will implement a plan across their trust that requires quarterly and annual reports to ensure implementation and remedial actions listed and acted on as appropriate.

19.2 What care bundles provide in the provision of IPC

A care bundle is a set of evidence-based interventions that are grouped together to ensure that patients receive optimal management consistently. Ideally, each part of the bundle should be based on evidence from at least one systematic review composed of multiple randomized control trials. Care bundles have been implemented in England since June 2005. They have been shown to improve patient outcomes and remain a useful strategy to reduce infections in the healthcare environment. Development of a bundle must be supported by education to the team delivering the care, such as healthcare workers. A regular audit process must occur to ensure that the bundle is followed appropriately, that there is 100% compliance and that continuous improvement in care is provided by regular evidence review.

Care bundles can be implemented in the following examples:

- Prevention of ventilator-associated pneumonia;
- Prevention of intravascular line infections;
- Urinary catheter care;
- Surgical site infections.

Most care bundles are composed of three to five practice recommendations that are highlighted as vital in reducing risk of infections. These recommendations may be called *high impact interventions*

Table 19.2 Example of a care bundle approach to peripheral cannula insertion and care.

1. Hand hygiene and personal protective equipment (PPE)	- Hand hygiene in line with World Health Organization (WHO) 'Five Moments for Hand Hygiene' - Use of disposable gloves, and apron if necessary, to be disposed of post procedure
2. Insertion and skin preparation	- Use of aseptic non-touch technique (ANTT) - Appropriate topical antiseptic agent (such as 2% chlorhexidine gluconate) placed on skin, allowing it to dry for a minimum thirty seconds
3. Skin dressing	- Use of a sterile, semi-permeable transparent dressing to allow for viewing the cannula insertion site for signs of infection
4. Documentation	- Clear documentation of date of insertion, staff member who performed the task, and reason
5. Care of the cannula	- Site inspection daily with documentation of any signs of infection (Visual Infusion Phlebitis score, VIP). If VIP score is ≥ 2, the cannulae will need to be removed and antibiotic treatment for infection may be required - Cannula to be re-sited before seventy-two hours or if becoming infected prior to this time

(HII). The Department of Health issued the Saving Lives guidelines (2010) that advocate utilizing HII and care bundles in prevention of HCAI (Table 19.2).

19.3 IPC surveillance required in a healthcare organization

Mandatory and voluntary surveillance of infections make a healthcare organization accountable for their rates and also allows comparisons to be made with other institutions.

Public Health England maintains mandatory surveillance for the following:

- Meticillin-resistant *Staphylococcus aureus* (MRSA) since 2005;
- *Clostridium difficile* toxin positive cases (and other cases that meet pre-determined case definitions) since 2007;
- Meticillin-susceptible *Staphylococcus aureus* (MSSA) since 2011;
- *Escherichia coli* bloodstream infections since 2011; and
- Surgical site infections—orthopaedic cases (all NHS Trusts must carry out three months' surveillance in each financial year in at least one of four categories such as hip prosthesis, knee prosthesis, repair of neck of femur, or reduction of long bone fracture).

Examples of voluntary surveillance includes:

- Carbapenemase-producing *Enterobacteriaceae* (CPE);
- Glycopeptide-resistant enterococci (GRE); and
- Surgical site infections (cardiothoracic, abdominal hysterectomy, etc.)

19.4 A serious untoward incident (SUI) in IPC and how it is investigated

An example of a serious untoward incident (SUI) in IPC would be a bloodstream infection with Meticillin-resistant *Staphylococcus aureus* (MRSA) resulting in the death of a patient.

With any SUI, a root cause analysis (RCA) of the incident should be performed, the purpose of which is to produce a formal record of the SUI and also to discuss what can be learned to prevent the incident occurring again. The SUI investigation is led, most commonly, by the DIPC or clinical lead from the area affected. The team involved should include doctors involved in the patient's care, nursing staff, IPC practitioners, allied health professionals, and a representative from the Clinical Commissioning Groups (CCG). The SUI meeting addresses the following points:

- *what* happened (i.e. chronology of events);
- *who* it happened to;
- *when* it happened;
- *where* it happened;
- *how* it happened (i.e. what went wrong); and
- *why* it happened (i.e. what underlying, contributory, or deep-rooted factors caused things to go wrong).

A series of outcomes would be established, which may include areas of immediate improvement or educational/training issues to prevent another SUI occurring.

In line with the Health and Social Care Act (2008, 2015) and the Francis Report (2010), it is expected that healthcare professionals provide *duty of candour*, with the patient and their relatives being informed of the MRSA bacteremia, receive an apology, and be given an open and transparent review of what happened and measures that will be implemented to prevent it happening again. An action plan is developed to address issues identified as deviation from best practice or learning needs.

19.5 Key performance indicators in relation to IPC

These objectives are often monitored through *key performance indicators* (KPI).

KPI are reviewed at the end of the financial year, thus allowing for production of the annual IPC report, with appropriate changes. Such areas, and methods of their measurement, include:

- IPC training;
- IPC audits with appropriate review and action planning;
- Compliance with antimicrobial guidelines; and
- Compliance with hand hygiene guidance (observational audits/usage figures for alcohol gel).

19.6 Defining a period of increased incidence and investigating a norovirus outbreak in a hospital ward

Hospital trusts should have active surveillance methods in place to ensure that any outbreaks are identified rapidly, to ensure that they do not disrupt patient care, and to reduce any associated morbidity and mortality.

Large hospital infection outbreaks can cause professional embarrassment and can be costly both financially and personally. Therefore, it is important for healthcare organizations to be prepared for outbreaks with a clear action plan to be initiated if required.

Periods of increased incidence (PII) are when the incidence of infection is increased above acceptable/expected levels, which should prompt the IPC team to investigate the reasons why. If the increase in infections is particularly high or uncontrolled, then an official outbreak declaration should occur.

Table 19.3 Norovirus Outbreak Control Measures (based on Health Protection Scotland guidelines).

Ward
• Close affected bay(s) to admissions and transfers
• Keep doors to single-occupancy room(s) and bay(s) closed
• Place signage on the door(s) informing all visitors of the closed status and restricting visits to essential staff and essential social visitors only
• Place patients within the ward for the optimal safety of all patients
• Prepare for reopening by planning the earliest date for a terminal clean

Healthcare Workers (HCWs)
• Ensure all staff are aware of the norovirus situation and how norovirus is transmitted
• Ensure all staff are aware of the work exclusion policy and the need to go off duty at first symptoms

Patient and Relative Information
• Provide all affected patients and visitors with information on the outbreak and the control measures they should adopt

Continuous Monitoring and Communications
• Maintain an up-to-date record of all patients and staff with symptoms
• Monitor all affected patients for signs of dehydration and correct as necessary
• Maintain a regular briefing to the organizational management, public health organizations, and media office

Personal Protective Equipment (PPE)
• Use gloves and apron to prevent personal contamination with faeces or vomitus

Hand Hygiene
• Use liquid soap and warm water as per WHO 'Five Moments'
• Encourage and assist patients with hand hygiene

Environment
• Remove exposed foods, e.g. fruit bowls, and prohibit eating and drinking by staff within clinical areas.
• Intensify cleaning ensuring affected areas are cleaned and disinfected. Toilets used by affected patients must be included
• Decontaminate frequently touched surfaces with detergent and disinfectant containing 1000 ppm available chlorine

Equipment
• Use single-patient use equipment wherever possible
• Decontaminate all other equipment immediately after use

An outbreak declaration should trigger the creation of an outbreak investigation team. The members of this group most often include the DIPC, IPC practitioners, clinicians of the affected ward(s), laboratory scientists, and may involve a public health epidemiologist to assist with the investigation.

Norovirus outbreak control measures (see Table 19.3) should be initiated.

Declaring the end of a norovirus outbreak is usually defined as forty-eight hours after resolution of vomiting and/or diarrhoea in the last known case and at least seventy-two hours after the initial onset of the last new case. This endpoint should also coincide with terminal cleaning of the wards/bays affected.

19.7 Further readings and useful resources

Guidelines for the Management of Norovirus Outbreaks in Acute and Community Health and Social Care Settings. Norovirus Working Party. https://www.gov.uk/government/uploads/system/uploads/attachment_data/file/322943/Guidance_for_managing_norovirus_outbreaks_in_healthcare_settings.pdf

Department of Health, The Health and Social Care Act 2008 Code of Practice on the Prevention and Control of Infections and Related Guidance https://www.gov.uk/government/uploads/system/uploads/attachment_data/file/449049/Code_of_practice_280715_acc.pdf

Guidance on the Reporting and Monitoring Arrangements and Post-Infection Review Process for MRSA Bloodstream Infections from April 2014. NHS England. https://www.england.nhs.uk/patientsafety/wp-content/uploads/sites/32/2014/02/post-inf-guidance2.pdf

Health Technical Memorandum 04-01: Safe Water in Healthcare Premises. Part B: Operational Management. Department of Health. https://www.gov.uk/government/uploads/system/uploads/attachment_data/file/524882/DH_HTM_0401_PART_B_acc.pdf

Legionnaires' Disease Part 2: The Control of Legionella Bacteria in Hot and Cold Water Systems. HSG274 Health and Safety Executive (HSE). http://www.hse.gov.uk/pUbns/priced/hsg274part2.pdf

Root Cause Analysis Investigation. National Patient Safety Agency (NPSA) http://www.nrls.npsa.nhs.uk/resources/collections/root-cause-analysis/

19.8 Assessment questions

19.8.1 Question 1

A sixty-year-old man on an oncology ward develops clinical signs of pneumonia fourteen days post admission. Bilateral pulmonary infiltrates are seen on his chest X-ray and a rapid urinary antigen test is positive for *Legionella pneumophila* serogroup 1. The patient is started on levofloxacin and the Public Health Team (PHT) is informed.

What is the most appropriate further action?
A. Close the oncology ward to new admissions.
B. Investigate his contacts to exclude cross-infection.
C. Investigate his home environment for potential sources of legionella.
D. Investigate potential sources of legionella in the hospital environment.
E. Monitor the patient for clinical improvements.

19.8.2 Question 2

A patient on the Care of the Elderly Unit develops diarrhoea on Friday evening and there are no available siderooms on the nightingale style ward. Subsequently, over the weekend, five further patients develop acute vomiting and diarrhoea.

What is the most appropriate immediate management over the weekend?
A. Call an emergency outbreak meeting.
B. Close the ward to any new admissions.
C. Cohort all the symptomatic patients next to each other.
D. Keep the ward functioning as normal.
E. Move the symptomatic patients to available siderooms on other wards.

19.8.3 Question 3

A patient with a MRSA bacteraemia has unfortunately passed away. The cause of her death is likely related to her infection. An SUI is declared and an RCA is performed.

What is the most important function of the RCA?
A. Identify the cause of death.
B. Complete the Datix form.
C. Correct documentation on the death certificate.

D. Learn lessons to prevent the occurrence from happening again.

E. Satisfy Care Quality Commission (CQC) requirement.

19.9 Answers and discussion

19.9.1 Answer 1

D. Investigate potential sources of legionella in the hospital environment.

Legionnaires' disease is an uncommon cause of pneumonia caused by *Legionella pneumophila* and other *legionella* species. This case would be classified as a nosocomial in light of the confirmation by a validated urinary antigen test (which only identifies serogroup 1, which causes around 70–90% infections in immunocompetent patients) and as the patient was in hospital for at least ten days prior to the onset of symptoms. Legionella is not spread from person to person, although recent literature suggests some very rare cases of probable transmission between close contacts. A nosocomial case related to a healthcare setting must be immediately investigated, including review of water outlets and the hospital water safety plan, prevention of water stagnation by removal of dead ends, and prevention of biofilms with disinfection methods. Regular flushing regimes of low-use outlets and review of ventilation systems in conjunction with the hospital Estates Team should also be performed. An incident control team should always be convened in this situation. This is a notifiable disease and Public Health must be informed.

19.9.2 Answer 2

B. Close the ward to any new admissions.

This appears to be a gastroenteritis outbreak, most likely due to norovirus. If multiple patients have symptoms of suspected/confirmed gastrointestinal infection in a nightingale ward, it is imperative that the ward be closed to further admissions to reduce the risk of spread. Confirmed norovirus patients should be isolated in a side room or cases may be cohorted in a bay. There must be no transfer of patients to other departments or hospitals from this affected area unless there is an urgent clinical need. Dedicated nursing staff should be allocated to nurse symptomatic and exposed patients. Visiting should be restricted, including the reduction in any unnecessary clinical staff or excess visitors entering the ward. Hospital Senior Management and the Health Protection Team need to be informed of the outbreak. It is important to provide updates to other wards/departments to manage access to the ward, and the Trust Communications Department, in case of external interest.

19.9.3 Answer 3

D. Learn lessons to prevent occurrence again.

Root cause analysis (RCA) can be used to investigate patient safety incidents, such as MRSA contributing to a patient's death. The investigation encompasses a variety of tools and techniques to analyse areas to prevent future cases or gaps in clinical practice. This includes the post infection review (PIR) tool to investigate MRSA bacteraemias. The priority in this patient's case is to establish whether there are any areas of her care that may have lapsed and where lessons can be learned to prevent the situation happening again. The safety of both current and future patients is the main reason an RCA should be initiated, although it does satisfy CQC requirements by doing so.

CHAPTER 20

Sterilization and decontamination

Sylvia Chegra and Martina Cummins

20.1 Cleaning, sterilization, disinfection, and decontamination

Decontamination is the combination of processes (including cleaning, disinfection, and sterilization) used to make a re-usable item safe for medical use. It is important to have an understanding of the meaning of each of these terms as well as their application.

Cleaning: a process to remove infectious agents and organic matter. The effectiveness of reducing microbial contamination will vary dependent upon the efficacy of the cleaning process and the initial bio-burden. It is important to note that this process does not necessarily destroy infectious agents and is a pre-requisite to disinfection and/or sterilization.

Disinfection: a process to reduce the number of viable infectious agents and which is commonly achieved either chemically or thermally. For some infectious agents (such as certain viruses and bacterial spores) it is not an effective method for inactivation and will not achieve the same level of reduction as is achieved through terminal sterilization.

Sterilization: a process which renders an object free from viable infectious agents, including viruses and bacterial spores. Sterilization is achieved most commonly using a prescribed ratio of time, temperature, and steam or chemicals such as hydrogen peroxide, gas plasma, or ethylene oxide.

The effective decontamination of re-usable medical devices is essential in reducing the risk of transmission of infectious agents with the chosen method of decontamination being detailed in the manufacturer's decontamination guidance or instructions for use (IFU), supplied when a medical device is purchased. The guidance will reflect the validation that was carried out prior to the release of the product by accredited laboratories to ensure that the cleaning guidance is both effective and will not adversely affect the device.

20.2 The aim of medical device decontamination

The aim of the decontamination process is to:

1. Reduce or completely remove microbial contamination to such a level that it is both safe to handle for staff and safe for further use on patients.
2. Ensure that there is no toxic chemical residue on the surface of the device that could cause adverse reactions when used on a patient.
3. Ensure that the decontamination process is compatible with the device and that it does not damage the device through the use of chemicals that can have an adverse effect on the device or by exposing it to either heat or water, which may cause damage.

To ensure that a medical device is compatible with the decontamination process it is essential to ensure that the manufacturer's decontamination guidance or IFU are followed. These detail the required process for not only how to disassemble (if appropriate) and clean the device but also the validated cleaning agents against which the medical device manufacturer has validated the equipment. By following these instructions, we can ensure that no damage occurs to the device during the decontamination process and that the device itself, through inappropriate cleaning, does not cause harm to either patients or staff.

20.3 Why cleaning the hospital environment is important

Cleaning and decontamination of the patient's room and equipment are crucial in minimizing the spread of micro-organisms. The patient's room has to be cleaned/disinfected daily with an appropriate detergent/disinfectant as per local policy.

Cleaning and decontamination of the environment is an essential component of infection prevention in the healthcare setting. It aims to minimize dust and remove fomites from patient contact areas. Contaminated surfaces may harbour pathogens for prolonged periods of time, which in turn may cause cross-infection, thus appropriate cleaning of surfaces and near patient equipment is essential to reduce exposure and opportunity, e.g. *Clostridium difficile*, meticillin-resistant *Staphylococcus aureus* (MRSA), norovirus, etc.

All patient equipment should either be single-patient use or be cleaned and disinfected/sterilized as per local policy or the manufacturer's instruction.

Disinfectants may be used in conjunction with physical cleaning when a known infection is identified, i.e. when there is a patient with a known transmissible infection or in an outbreak situation.

There are a variety of disinfectants used in healthcare settings; the most common ones are sodium hypochlorite and quaternary ammonium compounds. The efficiency of these agents depends on cleaning technique, their antimicrobial activity, and how they are used, including correct strength and contact time.

Areas to consider when setting up cleaning contracts:

- Governance of cleanliness services;
- Assessment of the risk of a lack of cleanliness (for infection and damage to patient, public, or staff confidence);
- Providing cleaning tasks/schedules/roles/responsibilities;

- Measuring cleanliness on the basis of visual inspection; additional technology is available to support this process, including ultraviolet light and/or adenosine triphosphate (ATP) monitoring system to evaluate the cleanliness of environmental surfaces;
- Implementing corrective action;
- Conducting performance analysis and implementing improvement actions.

20.4 Classifying medical devices

The classification system first proposed by E. H. Spaulding divides medical devices into categories based on the risk of infection involved with their use. This classification system is widely accepted and is used to help determine the degree of disinfection or sterilization required for medical devices. Three categories of medical devices and their associated level of disinfection are recognized.

- **Critical**

A device that enters normally sterile tissue or the vascular system or through which blood flows should be sterile. Such devices should be sterilized, which is defined as the destruction of all microbial life (e.g. Critical—surgical instruments).

- **Semi-critical**

A device that comes into contact with intact mucous membranes and does not ordinarily penetrate sterile tissue. These devices should receive at least high-level disinfection, which is defined as the destruction of all vegetative micro-organisms, mycobacterium, small or non-lipid viruses, medium or lipid viruses, fungal spores, and some bacterial spores (e.g. Semi-critical—Rectal Probe).

- **Non-critical**

Devices that do not ordinarily touch the patient or touch only intact skin. These devices should be cleaned by low-level disinfection (e.g. Non-Critical—stethoscope).

For flexible endoscopes the classification is based on the following criteria:

- **High Risk**: endoscopes that enter sterile body tissues. eg. arthroscope

Manual cleaning, automated cleaning, and disinfection; rinse-water with limited bacterial contamination, followed by sterilization.

- **Medium to High Risk**: endoscopes that enter sterile body cavities via contaminated body cavities. eg. flexible cystoscope

Manual cleaning, automated cleaning, and disinfection; rinse-water with very low bacterial contamination.

- **Medium to Low Risk**: endoscopes that enter contaminated body cavities. eg. flexible sigmoidoscope

Manual cleaning, automated cleaning, and disinfection; rinse-water with limited bacterial contamination.

- **Low Risk**: endoscopes without lumens. eg. nasoendoscope

Manual cleaning and manual disinfection is an essential requirement, and use of manual cleaning followed by an automated endoscope washer-disinfector (EWD) is considered best practice.

20.5 Classifying cleaning risks and audit time

British Standards Institution (BSI) in 2014, published a version of the standard for planning and measuring hospital cleanliness (PAS 5748). In line with the PAS guidance, areas to be cleaned are broken down into functional areas; maintaining the required standard of cleanliness is more important in some functional areas than in others, which are assessed and characterized by an associated risk.

Very High Risk: consistently high levels of cleanliness must be maintained. Very high-risk areas include operating theatres, critical care areas, special care baby units, accident and emergency departments, and other departments where invasive procedures are performed. Over a period of a week all rooms within these areas should be audited at least once.

High Risk: outcomes should be maintained by regular and frequent cleaning with 'spot' cleaning in between. High-risk areas include general wards, sterile supplies, public thoroughfares, and public toilets. Over a period of one month all rooms within these areas should be audited at least once.

Significant Risk: in these areas high levels of cleanliness are required for both hygiene and aesthetic reasons. Outcomes should be maintained by regular and frequent cleaning with 'spot' cleaning in between. Significant risk areas include out-patient departments, laboratories, and mortuaries. Over a period of three months all rooms within these areas should be audited at least once.

Low Risk: in these areas high levels of cleanliness are required for aesthetic and, to a lesser extent, hygienic reasons. Outcomes should be maintained by regular and frequent cleaning with 'spot' cleaning in between. Low-risk areas include administrative areas, non-sterile supply areas, record storage, and archives. Over a period of twelve months all rooms within these areas should be audited at least twice.

One approach to managing the risk category is through a clear cleaning programme that details the following:

- the outcome required;
- the equipment required;
- the process to be applied;
- the cleaning frequencies required.

Auditing the operational processes linked with environmental cleaning services, and providing in-depth training to domestic staff are important in preventing cross-infection. Confusion may arise when adhering to the new system of risk area stratification and identifying different risks within a ward or unit.

Planning is an important part of providing an effective cleaning service. Consideration must be given to human factors and logistical concerns that interrelate with environmental cleaning procedures, including recruitment, workflow, staffing, staff training, team work, technology, supervision, collaboration between support services and clinical staff, institutional leadership, and patient preferences.

20.6 The stages of decontamination

There are three stages of decontamination. All or some of these stages may be employed in decontaminating a medical device.

1. **Physical cleaning**: removal of visible contamination plus some micro-organisms is achieved using detergent, and is either a manual or automated process.
2. **Disinfection**: reduces micro-organisms to a level that is unlikely to cause infection, i.e. destroying or inactivating pathogenic micro-organisms but not spores. Disinfection is achieved either thermally (using an automated process, typically in a washer-disinfector) or chemically (using a manual process to clean a device with a specific disinfectant in compliance with the manufacturers decontamination guidance/flexible endoscope washer disinfector).
3. **Sterilization**: this is an absolute term denoting destruction of all micro-organisms including spores. Sterilization is achieved through a time/temperature ratio required to achieve a specific log reduction using either steam or chemicals like hydrogen peroxide or ethylene oxide in autoclaves (commonly referred to as sterilizers).

20.7 Carrying out the process of decontamination

To comply with current statutory requirements healthcare providers are required to ensure that decontamination takes place in a suitable environment preferably via an automated process.

To comply with these requirements, options are available dependent upon the device and the setting.

1. **Sterile Services Department**: a centralized facility that uses washer-disinfectors to wash and disinfect devices (using water, detergent, and temperature) and autoclaves (either steam or chemical) to sterilize them.
2. **Endoscope Decontamination Unit**: a unit that processes flexible endoscopes through endoscope washer-disinfectors, which use water, detergent, and chemical disinfectant to clean and disinfect.
3. **Dedicated Local Areas**: some devices are not compatible with standard automated reprocessing, for example: ultrasound or transoesophageal echocardiogram (TOE) probes, or, in the case of non-lumened flexible endoscopes, naso-endoscopes. For these types of devices manual decontamination is permitted as a minimum. While new developments in the field of decontamination of these devices includes alternative methods such as hydrogen peroxide or ultraviolet light, a validated manual disinfection system is still acceptable.

It is worth remembering that whether the process is manual or automated the regulations relating to compliance are still the same:

- Decontamination is to be carried out by trained, competent staff;
- Traceability is required between device and process;
- There must be a validation of process;
- Procedures must comply with manufacturers guidance/IFUs;
- Decontamination process must take place in a suitable environment;
- Written protocols detailing the required process (often referred to as Standard Operating Procedures) must be followed.

20.8 The legislative requirements for decontamination

Decontamination is provided in accordance with a number of documents. Currently the decontamination process follows International (ISO), European (EN), and British (BS) standards and guidance documents. While there are over 100 regulatory documents specifically referred to in relation to the provision of decontamination, there currently exist a number of key documents, including:

1) Health Technical Memorandum (HTM)

    HTM 01-01—Decontamination in an Acute Setting

    HTM 01-06—Endoscope Decontamination https://www.gov.uk/government/collections/
        health-technical-memorandum-disinfection-and-sterilization

2) Health Technical Memorandum 01-05—Dental in the Community Setting

    https://www.gov.uk/government/collections/
        health-technical-memorandum-disinfection-and-sterilization

3) Health and Social Care Act 2008 (updated 2015)—Code of Practice on the Prevention and Control of Infections and Related Guidance

    https://www.gov.uk/government/uploads/system/uploads/attachment_data/file/449049/
        Code_of_practice_280715_acc.pdf

4) Prevention of CJD and vCJD by Advisory Committee on Dangerous Pathogens Transmissible Spongiform Encephalopathy (ACDP TSE) Subgroup—including Annex A1 to M guidance

    https://www.gov.uk/government/publications/
        guidance-from-the-acdp-tse-risk-management-subgroup-formerly-tse-working-group

5) EN 16442—Controlled Environment Storage Cabinet for Processed Thermolabile Endoscopes

6) EN 285—Steam Sterilization

7) EN 15883 Part 1-6—Management of Washer-Disinfectors (including Endoscope Washer Disinfectors and Bed Pan Washers)

8) PAS 5748:2014 Specification for the Planning, Application, Measurement, and Review of Cleanliness Services in Hospitals

    http://qna.files.parliament.uk/qna-attachments/175888%5Coriginal%5CPAS5748%20
        Specification%20for%20the%20planning,%20application,%20measurement%20and%20
        review%20of%20cleanliness%20services%20in%20hospitals.pdf

9) National specifications for cleanliness in the NHS 2007—NPSA http://www.nrls.npsa.nhs.
    uk/resources/?EntryId45=59818

10) The Revised Healthcare Cleaning Manual 2009—NPSA

    http://www.nrls.npsa.nhs.uk/EasySiteWeb/getresource.axd?AssetID=61814

20.9 Assessment questions

20.9.1 Question 1

Testing rinse water is an important part of the controls within the Endoscopy Unit. The quarterly water testing of the final rinse water cultured 12 CFUs of mycobacterium species.

What is the most appropriate action to take?

A. Change filters and decontaminate the outlet.

B. Change filters and retest next quarter.

C. Nothing.

D. Wait for the next quarterly results before acting.

E. Take the machine out of service, sanitise pipework and retest.

20.9.2 Question 2

A patient colonised with a Carbapenemase-producing enterobacteriaceae (CPE) was discharged from a side room.

What type of clean would you recommend?

A. Deep clean.

B. Deep clean with additional technology (steam/UV light/HPV).

C. Discharge clean.

D. Increase frequency clean.

E. Routine clean.

20.9.3 Question 3

One of the surgical team contacts you to say that they have found rust on four surgical instruments that are required for an operation this afternoon. They have no other sets available.

What is the most appropriate advice?

A. Cancel the operation.

B. Continue with the procedure.

C. Look for loan equipment.

D. Return the complete set to Sterile Services for reprocessing and use a new set .

E. Wipe the rust off with a disinfectant wipe and use.

20.10 Answers and discussion

20.10.1 Answer 1

E. Take the machine out of service, sanitise pipework and retest.

Environmental non-pathogenic mycobacteria present a particular problem when they occur in the final rinse-water of instruments used for diagnosis of mycobacterial infection. The presence of environmental mycobacteria in a sample taken with this instrument may lead to misdiagnosis. Mycobacteria that occur in water, for example, *Mycobacterium kansasii* and *M. chelonae*, are opportunistic pathogens and may cause disease in susceptible individuals. Tests of the final rinse water of the washer disinfector should be conducted quarterly with no mycobacteria identified in a 100 ml sample. If any mycobacteria are detected in the sample, the machine should be taken out of service, cleaned, and retested.

20.10.2 Answer 2

B. Deep clean with additional technology (steam/UV light/HPV).

Once a patient with CPE is discharged, a deep clean with additional technology is undertaken prior to another patient being admitted to the area. This clean includes steam and hypochlorite as a minimum. All disposable equipment in the room must be disposed of including unused dressings, gloves, etc. Nursing equipment must be cleaned with hypochlorite solution or a sporicidal product. Other equipment, including curtains, must be removed from the room, cleaned, or disposed of appropriately. The pillows and mattress need to be assessed as safe before they can be used by another patient. Hired specialist mattresses will be returned to the company for cleaning and decontamination.

20.10.3 Answer 3

D. Return the complete set to Sterile Services for reprocessing and use a new set.

Surgical instruments are made from high-grade stainless steel that has been given a coating during the manufacturing process to protect the instruments from the aggressive nature of the decontamination process. Over time this layer, known as the passivation layer, builds up and forms a protective layer on the instrument and prevents the steel from rusting. If at any time rust is found on the surface of an instrument it indicates that either the passivation layer is compromised or there is a weakness in the metal from which the instrument is made. When rusty instruments are found the items need to be taken out of service so as not to compromise patient care. Loan equipment or alternative instruments need to be provided as a replacement.

PART SIX

IMPORTANT CLINICAL SYNDROMES

CHAPTER 21

Sepsis—recognition, diagnosis, and management in adult patients

Mark Melzer

CONTENTS

21.1 Defining sepsis

Sepsis is defined as life-threatening organ dysfunction caused by a detrimental host response to infection. Septic shock is a subset of sepsis in which underlying circulatory and cellular abnormalities are profound enough to substantially increase mortality. Septic shock is characterized by:

- The need for vasopressors to maintain mean arterial pressure (MAP) > 65mmHg despite adequate volume resuscitation.
- A serum lactate > 2mmol/L

In lay terms, it is hypoperfusion with evidence of metabolic derangement. The mortality for both criteria is ~40%, compared to 20–30% for a single item.

Please also refer to:

https://www.nice.org.uk/guidance/indevelopment/gid-cgwave0686

21.2 Why were definitions of sepsis changed in 2016?

The old definitions of sepsis described a heterogeneous group of patients and did not discriminate between infectious and non-infectious causes such as pancreatitis and trauma. The new definitions also allow easier recognition, based on a combination of symptoms and signs. Key parameters include: decreased level of consciousness, rigors, severe myalgia, high or low temperature, pulse > 130/min, systolic blood pressure < 90mmHg, respiratory rate (RR) > 25/min, creatinine > 170μmol/L, platelets < 100 x 10^9/l and bilirubin > 33μmol/L. The Clinical Quality Commission recommend that NHS trusts use the national early warning score (NEWS), and a score > 5 is an indication to consider moving a patient to critical care.

21.3 Is Systemic Inflammatory Response Syndrome (SIRS) still part of the definition?

SIRS is defined as any of the two following criteria: acutely altered mental state, temperature < 36°C or > 38°C, pulse > 90/min, RR > 20/min, WCC > 12 or < 4 x 10^9/L and hyperglycaemia in the absence of diabetes mellitus. In the former definitions (1991 and 2001), sepsis was defined as infection plus SIRS. SIRS, however, was not good at separating infected patients who died from those who recovered from infection. SIRS was often an appropriate reaction to infection and many hospitalized patients meet the SIRS criteria. Also, as many as one in eight patients admitted to critical care units with infection and new organ failure did not have two SIRS criteria required to fulfil the sepsis definition. SIRS is no longer part of the new definitions.

21.4 Identifying organ dysfunction

Organ dysfunction is defined as an increase of two points or more in the Sequential Organ Failure Assessment (SOFA) score. This group have a mortality of 10%. The baseline SOFA score can be assumed to be zero in patients not known to have pre-existing organ dysfunction. For calculation of a cumulative total, the key parameters are the Glasgow Coma Score, O$_2$ requirements (with or without respiratory support), mean arterial pressure (with or without inotropic support), serum creatinine and urine output, bilirubin, and platelets. A screening test for sepsis, the quick SOFA criteria (qSOFA) is defined as at least two of the following: altered mental state, systolic BP < 100mmHg and RR > 22/min. Estimated mortality associated with each is 0–2% (score 0–1), 8% (score 2) and 20% (score 3).

21.5 Limitations to the new definitions

The new definitions were developed from a cohort of adult patients, aged > 18, where body fluids were taken for culture, antibiotics administered, and patients admitted to hospital. All the data were derived from patients in high-income countries, e.g. US.

21.6 Managing sepsis

Immediate implementation of the 'sepsis 6 care bundle' has been shown to increase the chances of survival. The following actions comprise the sepsis 6 care bundle:

- Administer O_2.
- Take blood cultures. Consider sites of infection and source control.
- Based upon likely site of infection, give most appropriate intravenous antibiotics within one hour.
- Start fluid resuscitation.
- Measure serum lactate.
- Monitor fluid balance. Aim for urine output > 0.5ml/kg/hour.

21.7 Microbiological samples (other than blood cultures) to be taken before commencing antibiotics

For acute infections, the ability to take other samples before antibiotic treatment will depend upon the stability of the patient. Examples include mid-stream urine, cerebrospinal fluid (CSF), stool, line tips, and pus. For chronic infections, empirical treatment can often be delayed. Examples include deep tissue samples or pus. Superficial swabs are rarely useful.

21.8 Further useful samples from a patient already on antibiotics

If a patient is already on antibiotic treatment, consider Polymerase chain reaction (PCR) testing. Examples include meningococcal PCR on whole blood for suspected meningococcal sepsis and 16S PCR on multiple deep-tissue samples when cultures are negative, e.g. prosthetic joint infections.

21.9 Considerations before starting empirical antibiotics

All NHS trusts will have an empirical antimicrobial policy which should be consulted. Policies differ depending upon the local prevalence of antimicrobial resistance to key surveillance organisms. To prescribe appropriately, the likeliest site of infection must be determined based upon clinical assessment and radiology. Previous microbiology results, e.g. previous infection/colonization with extended spectrum betalactamase (ESBL)-producing Enterobacteriaceae, may help to determine appropriate choices of antimicrobials, e.g. whether or not to prescribe a carbapenem. Consider also:

- Route of administration;
- Frequency of dosing;
- Duration of treatment;
- Monitoring for potential toxicity and, where appropriate, drug levels;
- Dose adjustment in renal/hepatic failure;
- Need for adjuvant therapy (e.g. rifampicin or fusidic acid for severe *S. aureus* infection); and
- Alternative antibiotics for severe or non-severe penicillin allergy.

21.10 When to use targeted antimicrobial therapy

A key component of good antimicrobial stewardship (the right antibiotic for the right condition, given at the right dose, for the right time) is switching to a narrow-spectrum agent when culture results are available. This reduces the risk of *Clostridium difficile* infection and colonization with multi-drug-resistant (MDR) organisms and is therefore safer for patients and more cost effective. For uncomplicated infections, e.g. pneumonia or pyelonephritis, treatment can normally be switched from IV to oral after two to three days if the patient is clinically stable and showing signs of improvement.

21.11 The commonest sites of infection requiring source control

Biomedical devices are commonly associated with infection. Source control necessitates the removal of infected intravascular catheters and urinary catheters, particularly if they are blocked. Obstructed biliary and urinary tract systems are common causes of severe sepsis and, under these circumstances, ERCP and placement of a common bile duct stent, or placement of a urinary catheter or nephrostomy tube may be required. Intra-abdominal collections require drainage, as do empyema and paraspinal collections. If a native peripheral joint is infected an arthroscopic washout is required and an infected prosthetic joint may require debridement and explantation of the prosthesis. Valvectomy is increasingly used to optimize management of infective endocarditis, particularly for acute infections caused by *S. aureus*. Surgical debridement of infected tissue is required for optimal management of necrotizing fasciitis or Fournier's gangrene.

21.12 When patients can complete treatment outside hospital

Most patients will complete antibiotic treatment in the community. For uncomplicated infections such as pneumonia or urinary tract infection (UTI), antibiotics can be stepped down to oral and patients sent home to complete treatment in the community. Where outpatient parenteral antimicrobial treatment (OPAT) services exist, IV treatment can be continued in the community, typically for lower limb cellulitis and MDR UTIs.

21.13 Infection control or public health implications in managing a septic patient

It is important to consider the need for isolation, but not if this is detrimental to patient management. Infections acquired in the community, e.g. meningococcal disease, should be notified immediately to Health protection team, and to prevent further transmission administration of rifampicin or ciprofloxacin chemoprophylaxis to household and kissing contacts should be provided. Another community-aquired infection is invasive Group A streptococcal disease, where early notification and antibiotic prophylaxis may also prevent further community-acquired cases. In terms of severe hospital-acquired infections, which are often medical devices and procedure related, implementation of care bundles should prevent these infections.

21.14 Further follow-up after hospital discharge

Follow-up is normally required to ensure treatment has been successful and to offer advice on prevention of some types of infection. Depending upon the site of infection, and whether it is complicated, the patient may be seen by either a GP or an infection specialist. The patient may need to be seen by other specialists, for example, an orthopaedic surgeon for joint infections.

21.15 Assessment questions

21.15.1 Question 1

A twenty-six-year-old man presents to hospital with a two-day history of altered mental state and severe myalgia.

On examination, the patient is:

- Apyrexial;
- Confused;
- Exhibits a non-blanching purpuric rash;
- Has a BP 90/60.

A diagnosis of meningococcal septicaemia was suspected by the GP, who administered intramuscular benzylpenicillin.

What is the most appropriate investigation?
A. Blood culture.
B. CSF examination.
C. EDTA blood for meningococcal PCR.
D. Throat swab for M/C&S.
E. Wound swab for M/C&S from a disrupted purpuric lesion.

21.15.2 Question 2

A forty-two-year-old man presents with difficulty weight bearing on his right foot. He has poorly controlled insulin dependent diabetes mellitus.

On examination you find:
- A deep infected looking ulcer under the head of the first metatarsal joint;
- The patient is alert and orientated;
- Apyrexial;
- Pulse 82/min;
- BP 130/82.

What is the next most appropriate investigation?
A. Blood culture and start empirical treatment.
B. Deep tissue sampling for M/C&S and withhold empirical treatment.
C. MRSA screen and withhold empirical treatment until screen result obtained.
D. Rectal screen for carbapenemase-resistant enterobacteriaceae (CRE) and start empirical treatment.
E. Wound swab for M/C&S and withhold empirical treatment.

21.15.3 Question 3

A twenty-eight-year-old accountant presents with a six-day history of generalized lethargy and nausea. He returned from a holiday in New Delhi four weeks previously.

On examination the patient is:
- Alert and orientated;
- T 37.8°C;
- Icteric sclera;
- Mild hepatomegaly;
- Blood results shown in Table 21.1

Table 21.1 Investigations

Blood Results	
ALT	395 U/l
Bilirubin	102 μmol/L
ALP	106 U/l
Hepatitis A IgM	Detected

What is the most appropriate public health response?

A. Advise need for hepatitis A immunization in the event of future overseas travel.
B. Delay notification until reference lab confirmation of hepatitis A received.
C. Delay notification unless food handler.
D. Immediately inform the health protection team.
E. Reassure patient that with good hand hygiene secondary transmission is unlikely.

21.16 Answers and discussion

21.16.1 Answer 1

C: EDTA blood for meningococcal PCR.

The patient's confusion and hypotension are key indicators of severe sepsis. In these circumstances, rapid assessment and administration of intramuscular benzylpenicillin within one hour is required. Post antibiotics, PCR testing is required to confirm the diagnosis as blood cultures often fail to grow. In these circumstances a lumbar puncture is not required as treatment for sepsis will also treat meningitis. A throat swab and a wound swab of a disrupted lesion are unlikely to isolate an organism, particularly post antibiotics.

21.16.2 Answer 2

B: Deep tissue sampling for M/C&S and withhold empirical treatment.

The patient has no features of sepsis. Therefore, antimicrobial treatment should be withheld and deep tissue or bone samples taken before starting treatment.

21.16.3 Answer 3

D: Immediately inform the health protection team.

Again, this patient has no features of sepsis. After initial assessment, a stable patient with travel-associated fever and jaundice should be placed in isolation and appropriately investigated. After establishing a diagnosis of hepatitis A, the health protection team should be immediately notified as early immunization of contacts can prevent further transmission.

CHAPTER 22

Pyrexia of unknown origin (PUO)

Mark Melzer

22.1 Defining pyrexia of unknown origin (PUO)

Petersdorf and Beeson defined pyrexia of unknown origin (PUO) in 1961. It is defined as an illness more than three weeks' duration, with a fever > 38.3°C on several occasions and failure to reach a diagnosis after one week of in-patient investigation.

Additional categories have now been added. These include:

- Nosocomial PUO in hospital patients: This is defined as fever of 38.3°C on several occasions caused by a process not present or incubating on admission, where initial cultures are negative and diagnosis remains unknown after three days of investigations. Fever is often related to hospital factors such as surgery, use of biomedical devices (e.g. intravascular devices/urinary catheters), *C. difficile* infection, and decubitus ulcers related to immobilization.
- HIV-associated PUO: This is defined as fever (as in Nosocomial PUO) for four weeks as an outpatient or three days as an in-patient. The commonest causes of fever are typical and atypical mycobacterial infections, cryptococcosis, and Cytomegalovirus (CMV). Lymphoma may cause fever in up to 25% of cases.
- Neutropenic PUO: This includes patients with a fever (as in Nosocomial PUO) with neutrophils < 1.0×10^9/L, with initial negative cultures and an uncertain diagnosis after three days. Bacterial infection is the commonest cause and should be treated empirically.

22.2 Causes of PUO

The causes of a PUO can be categorized as infection (30–40%), neoplasia (20–30%), collagen-vascular and autoimmune diseases (10–20%), and miscellaneous (10–20%).

22.3 Localized infections associated with PUO

The commonest causes of *localized* bacterial infections causing PUO are infective endocarditis, intra-abdominal or pelvic infections, oral cavity infections, osteomyelitis, and infected peripheral vessels. These conditions include:

- Infective endocarditis (IE):
  - Organisms associated with indolent onset (e.g. *Streptococcus viridans*, *Enterococcus* species, coagulase-negative staphylococci).
  - HACEK organisms (e.g. *Haemophilus*, *Aggregatibacter*, *Cardiobacterium*, *Eikenella*, *Kingella*).
  - Culture-negative endocarditis (e.g. *Chlamydia*, *Coxiella*, or *Bartonella*).
  - Non-infective endocarditis:
    - Marantic endocarditis, associated with malignancy.
    - Libman Sacks endocarditis, associated with systemic lupus erythematosus (SLE).
- Intra-abdominal infections.
  - Abscesses:
    - Hepatic (GI tract or biliary in origin).
    - Splenic (associated with IE).
    - Sub-phrenic (associated with previous surgery).
    - Pancreatic (post-pancreatitis).
    - Psoas (associated with terminal ileum disease or lumbar spine osteomyelitis).
  - Pelvic (associated with appendicitis, diverticulitis, or pelvic inflammatory disease).
  - Urinary tract Infection (UTI):
    - Perinephric collection.
    - Intrarenal abscess.
    - Prostatitis, typically tender, boggy, or fluctuant on PR examination.
- Oral cavity/Upper respiratory tract (URT):
  - Periapical dental abscess (often extraction required to eradicate fever).
  - Otitis media/sinusitis.
- Osteomyelitis:
  - Vertebral column.
  - Infected joint prosthesis.
- Infected peripheral vessels.
  - Septic phlebitis (associated with intravenous drug use (IVDU)).
  - Arteriovenous fistulae (associated with haemodialysis).
  - Aneurysms (e.g. non-typhi *Salmonella* infections).

22.4 Generalized infections commonly associated with PUO

Other infectious causes are *generalized* and can be sub-categorized into generalized bacterial infections, mycobacterial, fungal, viral, and parasitic infections. These causes of PUO include:

- Bacterial infections (generalized):
  - Salmonellosis.
  - Brucellosis.

- Chronic meningococcaemia.
- Leptospirosis.
- Borreliosis.
- Q fever (*Coxiella burnetii*).
- Syphilis.
- Disseminated gonococcal infection.
- Mycobacterial infection:
  - *Mycobacterium tuberculosis* (TB):
  - Atypical mycobacterium (e.g. *M. kansasii, M. avium*).
- Fungal infection:
  - Immunocompetent host, where exposure to infection is geographically restricted, often to the Americas (e.g. *Histoplasma capsulatum, Coccidiodes immitis*).
  - Immunocompromised host eg. *Candida albicans, Aspergillus fumigatus, Cryptococcus neoformans.*
- Viral infections:
  - Primary HIV, EBV, and CMV infection.
- Parasitic infections:
  - Malaria.
  - Amoebiasis (usually causes hepatic abscesses rather than GI amoebiasis).
  - Trypanosomiasis.
  - Leishmaniasis.
  - Fascioliasis.

22.5 Types of neoplasia associated with PUO

Neoplasia is the cause of PUO in 20–30% of cases. With the exception of leukaemia, where blood film and bone marrow are key investigations, diagnosis is based upon imaging, tissue biopsy, and, in some cases, tumour markers. The commonest causes of neoplasia causing PUO include:

- Lymphoma.
  - Non-Hodgkin's lymphoma and Hodgkin's lymphoma can be associated with Pel-Epstein fever. This may be difficult to diagnose in the absence of peripheral lymph nodes and may involve extranodal structures (e.g., liver, kidneys, brain).
  - Castleman's disease: Localised or multicentric. This is associated with HHV-8 infection. It remains a difficult diagnosis often requiring multiple lymph node biopsies.
- Leukaemia.
- Solid tumours:
  - Hypernephroma, where fever is present in 20% of cases.
  - Atrial myxoma, where fever is present in 30% of cases. This can mimic infective endocarditis.
  - Adenocarcinoma of breast, colon, or pancreas, as well as liver metastases from any primary site, may also manifest as a fever.

22.6 Autoimmune diseases commonly associated with PUO

The commonest causes of *collagen-vascular* and *autoimmune diseases* causing PUO include:

- Temporal or giant cell arteritis/polymyalgia rheumatica (PMR) is the principle connective tissue aetiology. Characteristically, it is a disease of patients older than sixty-five years of age and is associated with high inflammatory markers.
- Polyarthritis nodosa (PAN) characteristically occurs in patients older than fifty years of age and has a male-to-female ratio of 2:1. There is a higher incidence in patients with hepatitis B and C infection. It is associated with skin lesions, myalgia, abdominal pain, renal impairment, and mononeuritis multiplex.
- Still's disease occurs in patients between sixteen and hirty-five years of age. It is associated with fever, myalgia, arthralgia, and arthritis. Investigations reveal leucocytosis and hyperferritaemia.
- Kikuchi's necrotizing lymphadenitis is often a histological diagnosis. Characteristically, this occurs in women under forty years of age and is associated with fever and enlarged lymph nodes, but no constitutional symptoms. The diagnosis is often made post-lymph node biopsy, which reveals non-granulomatous necrotizing lymphadenitis. Most cases resolve within one to four months.
- Uncommon causes include SLE, systemic-onset juvenile rheumatoid arthritis (RA), sarcoidosis, Wegener's granulomatosis, Takayasu's arteritis, and Cryoglobulinaemia

22.7 Other causes of PUO

There are a variety of less-common *miscellaneous* causes, which include:

- Vascular causes:
  - Approximately one half of patients with pulmonary emboli are febrile. Fever resolves several days following treatment.
  - Haemorrhage into the retroperitoneal space or a dissecting aneurysm are rare causes of a PUO.
- Regional enteritis:
  - Crohn's disease is the most common GI cause.
- Drug fever:
  - The commonest causes are beta-lactam antibiotics, procainamide, isoniazid, alpha-methyldopa, and quinidine. These may be associated with rash or desquamation, providing a diagnostic clue.
- Hereditary causes:
  - Familial Mediterranean Fever is a syndrome characterized by recurrent fever, peritonitis, and leucocytosis. It primarily affects those of Arab, Sephardic Jewish and Armenian descent. Familial Hibernian Fever is a similar syndrome in those of Irish descent.
- Factitious fever:
  - This is commonly encountered in young adults with health care experience and knowledge, and presents more often in females.
- Endocrine disorders:
  - Hyperthyroidism and subacute thyroiditis are the commonest endocrinological causes.

22.8 Assessing and investigating patients with PUO

Particular attention should be paid to the patient's age, gender, ethnicity, country of origin, recent travel, past medical and surgical, family, and drug history. Examination requires careful assessment of the oral cavity, hands, skin, and fundoscopy. A rectal examination should also be considered.

Since 1961 there have been considerable improvements in imaging and interventional radiology enabling easier tissue sampling or drainage of collections. This has expedited the time to detection of abscesses and solid tumours that were once difficult to diagnose.

The commonest investigations yielding a diagnosis include:

- Haematological (full blood count (FBC), blood film and erythrocyte sedimentation rate (ESR));
- Biochemistry (urea and electrolytes (U&E), C-reactive protein (CRP), liver function tests (LFTs), tumour markers);
- Vasculitis screen (urinalysis, auto-antibody screen);
- Microbiology (midstream sample of urine (MSU), blood culture);
- Radiology (chest X-ray, ultrasonography, computed tomography (CT), magnetic resonance (MR), and positron emission tomography (PET) scanning); and
- Histology (lymph node biopsies).

22.9 Managing patients with PUO and their prognosis

This will depend on the underlying diagnosis. No treatment should be started before a cause is found as non-specific treatment is rarely effective and mostly delays diagnosis. Referral to an appropriate specialist is often required.

The prognosis will depend upon aetiology. In the absence of a specific diagnosis patients generally have a benign long-term course.

22.10 Assessment questions

22.10.1 Question 1

A forty-year-old woman of South Asian origin presents with a four-week history of fever and enlarged lymph nodes. She has no constitutional symptoms. A lymph node biopsy is performed, with the following results:
Histology: Necrotizing lymph node
No granulomata.
Microbiology: AFB smear –ve, culture -ve

What is the most likely diagnosis?
A. Kikuchi's disease.
B. Lymphoma.
C. Sarcoidosis.
D. Systemic lupus erythematosus.
E. Tuberculosis.

22.10.2 Question 2

An eighty-seven-year-old Caucasian man is admitted to hospital following a mechanical fall. At presentation there are no signs of infection, although he is prescribed co-amoxiclav for a presumed lower respiratory tract infection. He has a long-term urinary catheter in-situ but no other medical devices. One week later he develops a fever without localizing symptoms.

What is the most likely cause?
A. Catheter-associated UTI.
B. *Clostridium difficile* infection.
C. Drug fever.
D. Hospital-acquired pneumonia.
E. Pressure sore.

22.10.3 Question 3

A sixty-five-year-old man presents with a four-week history of intermittent fever and generalized aches and pains. He has not suffered weight loss. He takes oral allopurinol 100mg once daily for gout. On examination there are no abnormal findings.
Investigations: ESR 97
CRP 121
FBC, U&Es, Lactate dehydrogenase (LDH), and LFTs were normal

What is the most likely diagnosis?
A. Allopurinol-related drug fever.
B. Infective endocarditis.
C. Lymphoma.
D. Polymyalgia rheumatica.
E. Tuberculosis .

22.11 Answers and discussion

22.11.1 Answer 1

A. Kikuchi's disease.
The absence of caseation on histology and the failure to culture TB makes a TB diagnosis less likely. Although tuberculous lymphadenopathy may be asymptomatic, there is often associated fever, night sweats, and weight loss. The age, gender, and ethnicity are in keeping with a diagnosis of Kikuchi's, the most likely explanation for the above presentation. Lymphoma, sarcoidosis, and SLE are other possible causes, but these rarely cause necrotizing granulomata.

22.11.2 Answer 2

A. Catheter-associated UTI.
The presence of a biomedical device, in this case a urinary catheter, makes this the most likely cause in a hospitalized patient. In the absence of diarrhoea, *C. difficile* is unlikely unless the patient has severe infection causing toxic megacolon. Co-amoxiclav is less commonly associated with *C. difficile* infection than cephalosporins and quinolones. The patient should be assessed for hospital-acquired pneumonia and pressure sores, which are less likely causes, as is a drug fever associated with co-amoxiclav.

22.11.3 Answer 3

D. Polymyalgia rheumatica.
As the patient is an elderly Caucasian male, has raised inflammatory markers, and otherwise normal bloods, the most likely diagnosis is polymyalgia rheumatic. In the UK, TB is more common in patients whose country of origin is sub-Saharan Africa or the Indian sub-continent. Lymphoma is possible, but with no weight loss, no abnormal examination findings, and a normal Lactate dehydrogenase (LDH), this too is unlikely. Infective endocarditis is possible but the patient has no peripheral stigmata and normal heart sounds. Allopurinol rarely causes a drug fever.

CHAPTER 23

Blood-borne viruses

C. Y. William Tong and Mark Hopkins

23.1 What are BBVs?

Blood-borne viruses (BBVs) are viral infections transmitted by blood or body fluid. In practice, any viral infection that achieves a high viral load in blood or body fluid can be transmitted through exposure to infected biological materials. In western countries, the most significant BBVs are human immunodeficiency viruses (HIV1 and HIV2), hepatitis B virus (HBV) and hepatitis C virus (HCV). Other viruses that can be transmitted by blood and body fluid include human T cell lymphotropic viruses (HTLV1 and HTLV2), cytomegalovirus, West Nile virus and viruses responsible for viral haemorrhagic fever such as Ebola virus, Lassa virus, and Crimean-Congo haemorrhagic fever virus.

23.2 How BBVs are transmitted

BBVs are transmitted via exposure to blood and body fluid. Some examples of routes of transmission include:

- Sharing needles in people who inject drugs (PWID);
- Medical re-use of contaminated instruments (common in resource poor settings);
- Sharps injuries in healthcare setting, including in laboratories (less commonly through mucosal exposure);
- Transfusion of blood contaminated with BBVs (failure to screen blood donors);
- Transplantation of organs from BBV-infected donors;
- Sexual exposure to BBV-infected body fluid; and
- Exposure to maternal BBV infection: intrauterine, perinatally, or postnatally.

23.3 Post-exposure procedures for BBV

If exposure to a BBV is via a needle stick injury in a healthcare setting, immediate first aid needs to be carried out by gently encouraging bleeding and washing the exposed area with soap and water. Prompt reporting of the incident is required so that an assessment can be done as soon as possible to determine if post-exposure prophylaxis (PEP) is required. The decision may be aided by urgent assessment of source patient infection status (Table 23.1). The British Medical Association has issued guidance for testing adults who lack the capacity to consent. In the case of a sexual exposure to a BBV, immediate consultation to a genito-urinary medicine (GUM) clinic is warranted.

Table 23.1 Initial investigations to aid risk assessment if source and recipient status is not known.

Source	Recipient
• HIV antigen and antibody • Hepatitis B surface antigen • Hepatitis C antibody	• Baseline blood for storage • Hepatitis B surface antibody if known history of vaccination

23.4 Risk factors to be considered

The risk of transmission of BBVs associated with exposure depends on the nature of the exposure and the body fluid involved.

The following factors are important in needle stick injuries:

● Deep percutaneous injury.
● Freshly used sharps.
● Visible blood on sharps.
● Hollow-bore needle used on the source's blood vessels.
● Source patient known to have high BBV-viral load (e.g. during seroconversion illness or in advanced untreated disease)—the risks of transmission of HBV, HCV, and HIV through needle stick injury are usually cited as 1 in 3 (when HBeAg positive), 1 in 30, and 1 in 300, respectively.

High-risk body fluids include blood and all internal body fluids, e.g. pleural fluid, pericardial fluid. Low-risk body fluids include saliva (non-dental), urine, vomit, or faeces that are not visibly blood stained. Contact of body fluid with intact skin is not considered as a significant exposure.

In sexual exposure, viral loads in the genital tract normally correlate with plasma viral loads. However, it is possible for BBVs to remain present in a protected body compartment (e.g. CNS, reproductive tract) while undetectable in the blood. This has been reported for HIV and Ebola virus. The risk of sexual transmission of HIV is dependent on the type of sexual activity, in the following order:

● Receptive anal intercourse (0.042–3%)
● Insertive anal intercourse (0.06–0.065%)
● Receptive vaginal intercourse (0.004–0.32%)
● Insertive vaginal intercourse (0.011–0.38%)
● Receptive oral sex (0–0.04%)
● Insertive oral sex (0%)

Co-existence of a sexually transmitted infection or genital ulcers may increase the risk of HIV transmission.

23.5 Pre-exposure prophylaxis

Pre-exposure prophylaxis (PrEP) is the use of vaccination or chemotherapeutic agents to prevent infection in an individual who is likely to be exposed to the infection as a result of activities related to profession, travel, or sexual behaviour. An example of successful vaccination against BBV is hepatitis B vaccine, which all healthcare workers (HCWs) should have received. The use of antiviral agents such as tenofovir or tenofovir/emtricitabine (Truvada) as PrEP was recently found to be effective in preventing sexual transmission of HIV in individuals with regular high-risk sexual exposures.

23.6 Post-exposure prophylaxis

Postexposure prophylaxis (PEP) (see also Chapter 51) is the use of vaccination or chemotherapeutic agents to prevent transmission of infection (or reduce severity) in an individual who has been exposed to an infective agent. The timing of starting PEP is important as it has to be administered as soon as possible after the exposure to be effective; the acceptable duration is dependent on the particular viral infection concerned.

In the case of a non-immune individual (e.g. not vaccinated or a vaccine non-responder) with exposure to hepatitis B virus, combined active (hepatitis B vaccine) and passive immunizations (hepatitis B immune globulin) can be used as PEP. This is effective within forty-eight hours of exposure, and can be given up to one week after exposure. For individuals with pre-existing vaccine-induced immunity, a booster dose of vaccine is often recommended after exposure. Vaccination of babies born to hepatitis B-positive mother is a form of post-exposure prophylaxis as the transmission in this setting usually occurs perinatally. Vaccine should be administered within 24 hours of birth.

For HIV exposure, the use of combination antiviral agents is recommended as PEP. The efficacy of HIV PEP is supported by animal studies. Also, an observation study on subjects with needle stick injuries demonstrated a reduction in risk of transmission by 80% with the use of zidovudine as prophylactic agent. HIV PEP should be given as soon as possible after exposure and no later than seventy-two hours. The current regimen of choice in the UK is tenofovir/emtricitabine (Truvada) and raltegravir for twenty-eight days. PEP may need to be adjusted if the source patient is suspected of having or known to have resistance against one or more components of the standard PEP.

23.7 Following-up a BBV exposure

Individuals given HIV PEP should be reviewed within seven days to monitor side effects that are present, including full blood count, urea and electrolytes, liver function, bone profile, urine analysis). Baseline HIV testing is recommended and re-tested at six and twelve weeks (from the end of completion of PEP) using fourth-generation HIV Ag/Ab immunoassay.

Individuals receiving a full course of hepatitis B vaccination (+/- hepatitis B immunoglobulin) should be tested for hepatitis B surface antigen (HBsAg) and antibody (anti-HBs) six to eight weeks after completion of the vaccine course.

There is no PEP available for HCV. However, treatment of acute HCV is highly effective with > 90% eradication rate. Individuals exposed to HCV should be vigorously followed up and referred to a hepatologist for active management if found to be infected.

23.8 Screening blood and organ donors

All blood and organ donors need to be screened for infections to prevent transmission. The standard practice in the UK is shown in Table 23.2.

Table 23.2 Viral screening tests for blood and organ donors.

Viruses	Blood donors	Organ donors
HIV	Combined HIV antigen/antibody, HIV RNA	Combined HIV antigen/antibody, (HIV RNA)
HBV	HBsAg, HBV DNA	HBsAg, anti-HBc, anti-HBs, (HBV DNA)
HCV	HCV antibodies, HCV RNA	HCV antibodies, (HCV Ag, HCV RNA)
HTLV	HTLV1/II antibodies	HTLV1/II antibodies
CMV	(CMV IgG, to identify CMV IgG negative blood)	CMV IgG
EBV	Not screened	EBV VCA IgG
West Nile virus	(West Nile virus RNA)[+]	(West Nile virus RNA)[+]
Non-viruses		
Treponema pallidum	*T. pallidum* antibodies	*T. pallidum* antibodies
Toxoplasma gondii	Not screened	*T. gondii* IgG
Trypanosoma cruzi	(*T. cruzi* IgG) [+]	(*T. cruzi* IgG) [+]
Plasmodium spp.	(Malarial antibodies) [+]	(Malarial antibodies) [+]

()—optional dependent on circumstances; [+]—Dependent on travel history

Recently, a high prevalence of hepatitis E virus (HEV) RNA was detected in blood donors (~1:3000). As a result, HEV RNA screening of blood donors has been introduced. The risk of transmission of other infective agents through transfusion is constantly being reviewed.

Individuals who have received blood products, particularly pooled blood products, could have false positive serology test results due to passively-acquired antibodies from the donor.

23.9 Preventing sharps injuries in the healthcare setting

HCWs should receive proper training on how to use sharps safely. The introduction of safer sharp instruments could reduce the risk of injuries. Sharps bin should be used for discarding sharps, which should not be over-filled and should be stored in a safe place, to avoid accidental contact, e.g. by children, visitors. HCWs should practise universal precautions and consider every patient or sample as potentially infectious. Gloves should be used in every procedure that could result in an exposure; mask and eye shield should be used in procedures that may result in splash exposure.

All HCWs should be immunized against HBV and have their immune status checked after completion of the vaccine course.

23.10 How BBV infection can affect the career of a healthcare worker

There are incidents of BBV-infected HCWs transmitting infection to their patients. As a result, there is a restriction of infected HCWs from carrying out exposure-prone procedures.

23.10.1 HIV

HIV-infected HCW with viral load > 200 copies/ml are not allowed to practise exposure prone procedures (EPPs). EPPs are allowed if close monitoring demonstrates that HIV viral load is suppressed by successful combination antiviral therapy.

23.10.2 HBV

HCW with HBeAg-positive hepatitis B are not allowed to practise EPP.

HCW with HBeAg-negative hepatitis B are not allowed to practise EPP if HBV DNA is > 1000 genome copies/ml (equivalent to ~200 IU/ml).

If the baseline HBV DNA level is < 100,000 genome copies/ml (equivalent to ~20,000 IU/ml), and antiviral therapy is successful in suppressing HBV DNA to < 1000 genome copies/ml (~200 IU/ml), return to EPP is permitted.

23.10.3 HCV

EPP is not allowed if HCV RNA is detectable.

EPP is permitted if there is sustained virological response (SVR) after successful antiviral therapy.

23.11 Further reading

BMA_ Needlestick Injuries and Blood-Borne Viruses: Decisions About Testing Adults who Lack the Capacity to Consent.
https://www.bma.org.uk/advice/employment/ethics/mental-capacity/testing-for-bbv-from-needlestick-injuries

Examples of EPP in Different Specialties .http://webarchive.nationalarchives.gov.uk/+/www.dh.gov.uk/en/Publicationsandstatistics/Publications/PublicationsPolicyAndGuidance/Browsable/DH_5368137

Riddell, A., Kennedy, I., Tong, C. Y., 'Management of Sharps Injuries in the Healthcare Setting', *British Medical Journal*, 351 (2015), h3733. http://www.bmj.com/content/351/bmj.h3733

23.12 Assessment questions

23.12.1 Question 1

A surgeon sustains a sharps injury when operating on a known HIV-positive patient. He removes his double gloves and notices a tiny puncture, which bleeds on squeezing.

What is the next most appropriate step in management?
A. Apply alcohol gel to the wound.
B. Apply hypochlorite 1:10,000 to the wound.
C. Call pharmacy for an urgent delivery of PEP.
D. Perform surgical hand scrub with chlorhexidine.
E. Wash with soap and water.

23.12.2 Question 2

A two-year-old child is found to have combined variable immune deficiency (CVID). She is given regular immunoglobulin replacement.

Which of the following blood test results cannot be explained by the immunoglobulin replacement?
A. Detectable CMV IgG.
B. Detectable EBV VCA IgG.
C. Detectable HCV IgG.
D. Detectable hepatitis B core antibody (anti-HBc).
E. Detectable toxoplasma antibody.

Table 23.3 Blood test results of a thirty-year-old HCW found to be infected with hepatitis B virus.

HBsAg	Detected
HBeAg	Not detected
HBV DNA	10,000 IU/ml

23.12.3 Question 3

A thirty-year-old HCW is found to be infected with hepatitis B virus. Table 23.3 shows his blood test results.

Which of the following procedures is he permitted to perform?
A. Arterial cutdown.
B. Deep suturing to arrest haemorrhage.
C. Laparotomy.
D. Repairing of perineal tear after delivery.
E. Venepuncture.

23.13 Answers and discussion

23.13.1 Answer 1

E. Wash with soap and water.

The first step of management after a BBV exposure is to give the exposed area a good wash out. In the case of a sharps injury, the puncture site should be encouraged to bleed gently and wash with soap and water. It is not advisable to scrub the site or use antiseptic agents such as alcohol gel, hypochlorite, or chlorhexidine, as the effect of further physical trauma or exposure to these chemical agents to the wound is not clear. There is a theoretical possibility of inducing further inflammation recruiting inflammatory cells that may be the target of BBV infection. The wound should be covered with an impermeable dressing after cleansing. In the case of mucosal exposure, the exposed area should be copiously washed with water or normal saline. If contact lenses are worn in a splash accident to the eyes, the eyes should be washed with water or normal saline both before and after removing the lenses.

23.13.2 Answer 2

C. Detectable HCV IgG.

Immunoglobulins (such as IVIG, HNIG, or hyperimmune serum such as VZIG) are pooled human blood products. They contain a large variety of immunoglobulins to various infective organisms. Hence, patients receiving these products will be tested positive for antibodies against all these organisms, usually in a high titre. In the UK and many western countries, blood products are universally screened for HIV, HCV, and HTLV antibodies, so these antibodies are not expected to be present in the immunoglobulin preparations, whereas antibodies against CMV, EBV, toxoplasma, or hepatitis B core antigen are not routinely screened and therefore could appear as passive antibodies. Note that although syphilis is routinely screened in many countries, the methods used vary. If the screening method is non-treponemal-specific tests such as VDRL or RPR, the blood product could still have passive antibodies against treponemal-specific antigens resulting in false positive treponemal serology in the recipients of the blood product.

22.13.3 Answer 3

E. Venepuncture.

Exposure Prone Procedures (EPPs) are those procedures where the worker's gloved hands may be in contact with sharp instruments, needles tips, or sharp tissues (e.g. bone or teeth) inside a patient's open body cavity or wound where the hands or fingertips may not be completely visible at all times. Such procedures carry a risk of injury to the worker and may result in exposure of the patient's open tissues to the blood of the worker. This HCW has HBeAg-negative hepatitis B and has a viral load more than the allowed threshold of 1000 copies/ml (200 IU/ml). EPP is therefore not allowed unless the HCW is treated to reduce the viral load to below the acceptable threshold. Of the procedures listed, venepuncture is the only non-EPP procedure.

CHAPTER 24

Tuberculosis and other mycobacterial infections

Simon Tiberi

24.1 The aetiological agent of tuberculosis

Mycobacterium tuberculosis (MTB) is a thin, aerobic, non-spore forming, slow-growing (doubling time twelve hours) non-motile rod-shaped bacteria, belonging to the family Mycobacteriaceae. Mycobacterium tuberculosis complex is made up of several species, including *M. tuberculosis*, *M. bovis*, Bacillus Calmette-Guerin (BCG), *M. africanum, M. canetii, M.caprae, M. microti*, and others.

24.2 The pathogenesis of tuberculosis

Transmission is via inhalation of aerosolized respiratory secretions. After inhalation, majority of bacilli are captured in the upper respiratory tract by mucus and removed through a process called clearance, although bacteria in small droplets can reach the alveoli where the bacilli are ingested by macrophages. If clearance is not effective infection may result. With the involvement of CD4 lymphocytes, interferon-γ and tumour necrosis factor-α, a granuloma is formed, and bacilli may be destroyed. In many cases, the bacilli are not destroyed and can spread into lymphatics or via blood to other sites (any organs) where it can lie dormant for years. This asymptomatic situation is called latent TB infection (LTBI). It may reactivate in 10% of people throughout their lifetime; this increases with immunosuppression and HIV infection. The course of illness is chronic and indolent. However, rapid progression to fulminant disease may result if the host is immunocompromised. Pulmonary TB is the most common and important form of TB because it is the infectious form of the disease. In areas where reactivation predominates (like the UK), there is a higher proportion of extrapulmonary TB.

24.3 Acid-fast bacilli (AFB) and the gold standard test for mycobacteria

Tuberculosis bacilli resist destaining with acid alcohol treatment hence the term. This retention is due to complexing of the carbolfuschin Ziehl-Neelsen stain with mycolic acids present in the waxy cell wall, including lipoarabinomannan (which facilitates survival in macrophages). Microscopy will diagnose TB in 80% of smear-positive patients with a first sputum sample, a further 15% with the second, and 5% with a third. In endemic areas finding acid-fast bacilli in sputum has a 98% specificity, but this is not the case in the UK, a low-prevalence setting, where atypical mycobacteria can have a similar prevalence. In the best settings only 60% of culture-positive patients are also sputum smear-positive as liquid culture, the gold standard, and most sensitive test. When the organism is cultured on solid media (Lowenstein-Jensen) at 37°C, opaque colonies are usually visible after three to six weeks. Culture time is effectively halved with liquid culture and radiometric (BACTEC/MGIT) method using the Middlebrook 7H12 (liquid) medium.

24.4 The GeneXpert™

The Xpert MTB/Rif Ultra™ is a sensitive and accurate test for pulmonary TB; it is a nested PCR test which can identify MTB-DNA and sequences the *rpo* gene for rifampicin resistance and sensitivity for sputum smear. Concordance with culture positive TB is 98.2% and 72.5% for smear negative culture positive TB. Results can be obtained within seventy minutes.

24.5 Multidrug-resistant tuberculosis (MDR-TB)

Multidrug-resistant tuberculosis (MDR-TB) is TB that is resistant to the first-line drugs isoniazid and rifampicin. Extensively drug-resistant TB (XDR-TB) is defined as resistance to isoniazid, rifampicin, plus resistance to a later generation fluoroquinolone (levofloxacin or moxifloxacin) and at least one second-line injectable (amikacin, capreomycin, or kanamycin).

24.6 Incidence of tuberculosis in the UK and worldwide, and its importance

The latest 2017 figures for the incidence of TB in the UK in 2016 was 10.2 per 100,000 and is considered a low-incidence setting for the disease. However, certain inner London areas, e.g. Newham, have an incidence closer to one hundred per 100,000, largely due to re-activation of infection acquired in the remote past, usually abroad. About 3.8% of TB cases in the UK are co-infected with HIV. The risk of developing TB is twenty-six to thirty-one times greater in people living with HIV. In 2016, there were 10.4 million new cases of TB, and 1.64 million deaths (of this, 374,000 were HIV co-infected). TB is a top infectious disease killer worldwide, and the leading cause of death in HIV-infected people: in 2016, one in three HIV deaths was due to TB. Worryingly, drug resistance poses a threat; of 3,516 English patients who tested culture-positive for MTB in 2014, 7% were resistant to isoniazid, 1.7% were resistant to rifampicin, and 1.5% had MDR-TB. In 2016 the global burden of MDR-TB was estimated at 490,000, 3.3% on incident cases and 20% of retreatment cases, and as yet, most MDR-TB cases are undiagnosed and untreated.

24.7 The BCG vaccine, its rationale, and evidence for its use

The Bacillus Calmette-Guerin (BCG) vaccine is derived by the in vitro attenuation of *Mycobacterium bovis*. Despite debate and controversy in its efficacy and mechanism of action, BCG remains widely used. The vaccine is more effective in northern latitudes but less effective in equatorial and tropical areas, perhaps due to interference from circulating non-tuberculous mycobacterial (NTM) strains. The mechanism of action is not known but appears to reduce the incidence of TB meningitis and disseminated/miliary TB in children; it is less effective in preventing pulmonary disease in adults. From this, it can be deduced that the vaccine is effective and prevents the haematogenous spread of TB but affords little protection to the lungs.

24.8 Positive PPD/Mantoux and its significance

The Mantoux test, also called a tuberculin skin test, involves injecting purified protein derivative (PPD) into the skin of the forearm. If there is latent TB infection, a hard red bump will develop at the site of the injection within forty-eight to seventy-two hours (Type IV, delayed hypersensitivity). Prior BCG vaccination or infection with some NTMs may cause a reaction; therefore, the test is not very specific and not useful in populations vaccinated with BCG (healthcare workers).

24.9 Interferon Gamma Release Assay (IGRA)

Interferon Gamma Release Assay (IGRA) is an in vitro test: ELISA (Quantiferon) or enzyme-linked immunospot (ELISPOT). It interrogates lymphocytes with two TB antigens ESAT-6 and CFP-10 (if Quantiferon Gold in Tube also TB 7.7), and these tests measure the interferon gamma released by the T cells in response to these TB antigens. The advantages are that the tests are less subjective than skin testing, require only one visit for testing, and can be used in BCG-vaccinated individuals. Disadvantages include that it cannot differentiate between latent and active disease, samples require processing within thirty-six to forty-eight hours, and cut-offs are not well characterized, with possible indeterminate results.

24.10 Immune Reconstitution Inflammatory Syndrome (IRIS), or TB paradoxical reaction

TB is in itself immunosuppressive. In treating TB, immunocompetence can be reached two to four weeks into therapy and lead to a paradoxical reaction, which is commonly seen in HIV-TB patients initiated on both HIV and TB treatment at the same time (recommendations are now within two weeks if CD4 < 50 or eight weeks if CD4 > 50. This reaction can also occur in immunocompetent patients around 10% of patients and can be effectively treated with NSAIDs and supportive therapy.

24.11 Treating latent tuberculous infection: drug types and duration

Latent TB Infection (LTBI) is asymptomatic and diagnosed by skin test positivity or IGRA testing. Testing programmes are in place to screen persons at high risk for LTBI or progression of the disease.

- Rifampicin and Isoniazid for three months + pyridoxine once daily.
- Isoniazid for six months + pyridoxine once daily.
- Rifampicin alone for four months.

With known exposure to MDR-TB, do not give treatment but follow-up closely and maintain regular observation especially in the first two years after known contact.

24.12 Drug regimen for active pulmonary disease and course of therapy for drug-sensitive tuberculosis

Initial treatment of tuberculosis should consist of four drugs: Isoniazid, rifampicin, ethambutol, and pyrazinamide. If MTB is fully sensitive and patient clinically and radiologically improved then, isoniazid and rifampicin can be used alone after eight weeks and continued for another sixteen weeks to complete a six-month regimen. In patients with extensive cavitary disease who are still sputum culture positive at two months, treatment should be extended to nine months. If isoniazid or pyrazinamide monoresistant treatment should be extended to nine months. With CNS involvement, treatment should be extended to twelve months. Patients with MDR-TB should be referred to a specialized treatment centre and treated for eighteen to twenty-four months, or nine to twelve months with shorter MDR-TB regimen if they qualify. Remember, never add a single drug to a failing regimen because the agent will soon be lost!

24.13 Using corticosteroids in treating tuberculosis

Evidence only supports the use of corticosteroids in CNS TB where studies have shown dexamethasone at the dose of 0.4mg/kg or prednisolone 1mg/kg reduced mortality from 41 to 32% but did not alter morbidity. The use of corticosteroids in pleural, spinal, abdominal, and genital TB, and recent use of steroids in pericardial TB, is no longer recommended.

24.14 Organisms represented by non-tuberculous mycobacteria (NTM)

Organisms represented by non-tuberculous mycobacteria include over one hundred and eighty different species, including M. avium intracellulare complex (including M. chimaera), M. marinum, M. scrofolaceum, M. ulcerans (Buruli ulcer), M. genavense, M. kansasii, M. fortuitum, M. szulgai, M. chelonae, M. ulcerans, M. xenopi, M. simiae, and M. abscessus. They are typically found in soil and water and are ubiquitous.

24.15 Risk factors for NTM infections

Risk factors for NTM infections include immunosuppression, HIV infection, malignancy, transplantation, chronic steroid therapy, COPD, chronic bronchiectasis, prior MTB infection, cancer, bronchiectasis, cystic fibrosis, pneumoconiosis, emphysema, pulmonary aspergillosis, achalasia, silicosis, and impaired cell-mediated immunity. However, NTM infections also occur in immunocompetent hosts.

24.16 Proving an NTM infection without transient colonization

NTM are environmental bacteria that humans encounter on a daily basis. Diagnosis of pulmonary NTM disease is, therefore, challenging: a single positive culture from nonsterile sources including the respiratory or digestive tract need not indicate infection or disease. The American Thoracic Society (ATS) and Infectious Diseases Society of America (IDSA) have issued statements including a set of criteria to differentiate casual NTM isolation from true pulmonary NTM disease. Clinical criteria include pulmonary symptoms, nodular or cavitary opacities on chest radiograph, or high-resolution computed tomographic scan that shows multifocal bronchiectasis with multiple small nodules and exclusion of another diagnosis. Microbiologic criteria include positive culture results from at least two separate expectorated sputum samples or from one bronchial lavage.

A diagnosis of NTM lung disease does not always mandate therapy, which is a decision based on evolution, risk-benefits of therapy for the patient.

24.17 Further reading and useful resources

Griffith, D. E., Aksamit, T., Brown-Elliott, B. A., Catanzaro, A., Daley, C., Gordin, F., et al., 'An Official ATS/IDSA Statement: Diagnosis, Treatment, and Prevention of Nontuberculous Mycobacterial Diseases', *American Journal of Respiratory and Critical Care Medicine*, 175/4 (2007), 367–416.

Nahid, P., Dorman, S. E., Alipanah, N., Barry, P. M., Brozek, J. L., Cattamanchi, A., et al., 'Official American Thoracic Society/Centers for Disease Control and Prevention/Infectious Diseases Society of America Clinical Practice Guidelines: Treatment of Drug-Susceptible Tuberculosis', Clinical Infectious Diseases, 63/7 (2016), e147–e195.

Tuberculosis NICE Guidance 33. Published January 2016. https://www.nice.org.uk/guidance/ng33

World Health Organization Guidelines on Tuberculosis. http://www.who.int/publications/guidelines/tuberculosis/en/

24.18 Assessment questions

24.18.1 Question 1

A twenty-four-year-old man originally from Pakistan attends your clinic concerned about the recent appearance of multiple non-pruriginous hypopigmented macules on his limbs. On questioning he also reports altered sensation in these lesions. His mother recalls he had contact with someone who had leprosy twenty years ago.

Which of the following tests is not useful in the diagnosis of leprosy?
A. Lepromin test.
B. Polymerase chain reaction.
C. Sensation testing.
D. Skin biopsy.
E. Slit smear.

24.18.2 Question 2

A forty-nine-year-old woman presents with nausea six days into the start of her course of treatment for sputum positive pulmonary tuberculosis. She is prescribed correct doses of rifampicin, isoniazid, pyrazinamide, and ethambutol. On routine two-week bloods, full blood count, renal function, and electrolytes are normal. Alanine aminotransferase is 119 U/L. Bilirubin is 32 μmol/L, and clotting is normal. She is negative for blood-borne viruses.

What is the most appropriate next step in management?
A. Add pyridoxine to her medication.
B. Immediately stop all treatment and repeat liver function tests in one week.
C. Keep all medications and repeat liver function tests in one week.
D. Reduce the doses of rifampicin, isoniazid, and pyrazinamide.
E. Temporarily stop rifampicin, isoniazid, and pyrazinamide but continue ethambutol.

24.18.3 Question 3

A twenty-three-year-old, HIV-positive woman with a CD4 count of 45 cells has cervical lymph node and pulmonary tuberculosis. She is commenced on standard anti-quadruple anti-tuberculous treatment and cotrimoxazole, followed by antiretroviral therapy (ART) two weeks later. Four weeks after starting ART, she develops hyperpyrexia, cough, and enlargement of her cervical lymph nodes with ulceration. A chest X-ray shows worsening pulmonary infiltrates.

What is the most likely explanation?
A. Development of non-Hodgkin's lymphoma.
B. Drug reaction.
C. Drug-resistant infection.
D. Immune reconstitution inflammatory syndrome (IRIS).
E. Superadded infection with another opportunistic infection.

24.19 Answers and discussion

24.19.1 Answer 1

A. Lepromin test.
The lepromin test is similar to the Tuberculin test and tests the skin's reaction to Dharmendra antigen, indicating host resistance to *Mycobacterium leprae*. Its results (the delayed hypersensitivity Fernandez reaction and the Mitsuda reaction) do not confirm the diagnosis, but they may be useful in determining the type of leprosy. A positive Mitsuda reaction indicates cell-mediated immunity, expected in tuberculoid leprosy. A negative finding suggests a lack of resistance to disease and is observed in lepromatous leprosy. A negative result may also indicate unfavourable prognosis.

24.19.2 Answer 2

B. Immediately stop all treatment and repeat liver function tests in one week.
Three out of four first-line TB medications (rifampicin, isoniazid, and pyrazinamide) are potentially hepatotoxic, and although a degree of liver enzyme increase is normal it is rarely a problem. The World Health Organization (WHO) recommendations are to stop anti-TB medications with ALT 3x upper limit of normal (ULN) if symptomatic (nausea, vomiting, asthenia, jaundice) or above 5x ULN if asymptomatic. If liver enzymes are raised then liver enzyme levels should be monitored weekly. TB medications if stopped can be re-introduced gradually once liver function tests improved. Treatment can be re-introduced stepwise when liver function tests have normalized.

24.19.3 Answer 3

D. Immune reconstitution inflammatory syndrome (IRIS).

The patient has developed an IRIS. This is commonly seen and is most likely due to the recovery of the immune system (due to the antiretrovirals and anti-TB medications as TB can also immunosuppress) so that it can recognize antigens of agents to which it was failing to respond. It usually presents with tender lymphadenopathy and can also associate with fevers and raised inflammatory markers. IRIS can also occur with the antigens of other infectious agents, for example, cytomegalovirus. Once other infections are excluded, IRIS is usually treated with low-dose steroids if severe or with non-steroidal inflammatory agents if not severe.

Multisystem infections

Mark Melzer

25.1 Bacterial infections that can have multisystem presentation

Many bacterial infections can cause multisystem or metastatic infection, commonly through haematogenous spread, with preferred sites or tropism depending upon specific organism. For example, *Staphylococcus aureus* is a well-recognized cause of infective endocarditis, joint infection, and vertebral osteomyelitis. *Klebsiella pneumoniae* can cause endogenous endophthalmitis in association with a pyogenic liver abscess, a syndrome well described in East Asia. *Streptococcus pneumoniae* typically causes lower respiratory tract infections or bacterial meningitis. The combination of meningitis, pneumonia, and endocarditis is called 'Austrian syndrome' and is strongly associated with hyposplenism or alcohol abuse. Other examples of bacteria that disseminate and cause multisystem infection are covered elsewhere.

25.2 Fungal infections that can have multisystem presentation

25.2.1 Candidiasis

C. albicans or non-albicans species in the blood can metastasize to the eye (causing chorioretinitis or endophthalmitis) or to the heart (causing infective endocarditis). The primary sites of infection are commonly the GI tract or intravascular catheters, and high-risk groups include patients who have recently undergone abdominal surgery, received multiple courses of intravenous antibiotics, and are receiving total parenteral nutrition. Empirical treatment is with either IV liposomal amphotericin or an echinocandin before stepping down to an oral azole, commonly fluconazole at a dose of 400mg od. Because of the risk of metastatic spread, minimum duration is normally two weeks after the first negative blood culture.

25.2.2 Cryptococcosis

Cryptococcosis is caused by one of two species: *Cryptococcus neoformans* or *Cryptococcus gattii*. Unlike *C. neoformans*, *C. gattii* can cause infection in immunocompetent people. The clinical syndrome, Cryptococcosis, is an opportunistic infection for AIDS, but other conditions that predispose to infection are lymphoma, sarcoidosis, liver cirrhosis, and corticosteroids. Following inhalation, cryptococci can disseminate to the cerebrospinal fluid (CSF) and cause meningitis. Occasionally, Cryptococcoma—umbilicated papules on the skin—can occur. Symptoms are often subacute and include fever and dry cough. Following dissemination to the CSF, headache and confusion can occur.

Diagnosis is based upon detection of capsular antigen by latex particle agglutination or culture, typically from blood or CSF. For meningitis, treatment consists of three phases. The induction phase is two weeks of IV liposomal amphotericin and flucytosine, followed by consolidation with eight weeks of oral fluconazole 800mg once daily, then finally secondary prophylaxis, 200mg orally once daily. For HIV +ve patients, combination antiretroviral therapy should be delayed for four to six weeks as earlier implementation results in worse clinical outcomes due to immune reconstitution inflammatory syndrome. Secondary prophylaxis may be stopped when the CD4 count is > 100 x 10^6/l, HIV viral load undetectable for at least three months, and the patient has received a minimum of twelve months of antifungal treatment.

25.2.3 Penicilliosis

Talaromyces marneffei, a thermally dimorphic species of *Penicillium*, is the cause of penicilliosis, a disease similar to disseminated cryptococcosis. It is endemic in SE Asia and associated with bamboo rats. There is a high incidence of disease in AIDS patients in SE Asia. In addition to fever and respiratory symptoms, dissemination to the reticulo-endothelial system include lymphadenopathy, hepatomegaly, and splenomegaly may occur. Diagnosis is based upon culture on Sabouroud agar, yielding a mould at 30°C and yeast at 37°C. Antigen tests for blood and urine are also available. Treatment is with IV amphotericin B for two weeks, then oral itraconazole for ten weeks.

25.2.4 Histoplasmosis

Histoplasma capsulatum is the predominant cause of histoplasmosis, and is found in the soil and often associated with decaying bat guano or bird droppings. It is, therefore, also known as 'Caver's disease' or 'Ohio Valley disease'. It is thermally dimorphic and exists as a brown mycelium in the environment and as yeast at body temperature. Histoplasmosis is predominantly a disease of the lungs but in rare cases dissemination and death may ensue if left untreated. Although in endemic areas the prevalence of infection is high, disease is more common in HIV infected patients. Symptoms typically occur three to seventeen days post-exposure and in the acute phase non-specific respiratory symptoms such as cough occur. Chest X-rays are normal in 40–70% of cases. Chronic disease may resemble TB and disseminated disease may involve the liver, spleen, lymph nodes, adrenals, and retina.

Diagnosis is based upon culture or antigen detection, typically in the blood or urine and the treatment of severe disease is with IV amphotericin, then oral itraconazole.

25.2.5 Blastomycosis

Blastomyces dermatitidis is a dimorphic fungus and the cause of blastomycosis. It is endemic to North America and causes diseases similar to histoplasmosis. The incubation period is thirty to one hundred days and primary lung infections occur in 70% of cases. Sites of dissemination include osteomyelitis (12–60%), genito-urinary tract, including the prostate (25%), and the brain (3–10%), particularly in immunocompromised patients. Types of clinical presentations include:

- Fever, chills, arthralgia, myalgia, headache, and non-productive cough;
- Chronic illness mimicking TB or lung cancer;
- Progressive, severe respiratory disease (e.g. ARDS);
- Wart like skin lesions or ulcers with small pustules at margins;
- Bone lytic lesions causing bone or joint pain;
- Prostatitis. Asymptomatic or causing pain on urinating; and
- Laryngeal involvement causing hoarseness.

Diagnosis is based upon biopsy and culture or urinary antigen detection. Treatment is with oral itraconazole with amphotericin reserved for more severe cases or CNS involvement. Mortality is high in immunocompromised patients (25–40%) and in patients presenting with ARDS.

25.2.6 Coccidioidosis

Coccidiodes immitis is a dimorphic fungus is classified as a Biosafety Level 3 pathogen. It is found in soil in the southwestern US, Northern Mexico, and other areas of the Western Hemisphere. The incubation period is seven to twenty-one days and inhalation may cause lung disease and lesions may mimic a lung tumour. Risk factors for dissemination include primary infection during infancy, primary infection in pregnancy, high inoculum exposure, age > 55 years, immunosuppression (e.g. HIV/AIDS, transplant recipients, and corticosteroids) and comorbidities including diabetes mellitus, cardiovascular, or respiratory disease. Sites of dissemination include skin, bone and joints, lymph nodes, liver, spleen, and the CNS.

Diagnosis is based upon the detection of *Coccidioides* antigens, typically in blood and urine. Treatment of severe disease is with IV amphotericin, then oral itraconazole. Duration of treatment is at least six months.

25.2.7 Paracoccidioidomycosis

Paracoccoidiodes braziliensis is a dimorphic fungus that causes the clinical syndrome paracoccidioidomycosis. It is geographically restricted to Brazil, Colombia and Venezuela and is commonly associated with soil where coffee is cultivated. The route of acquisition is predominantly through inhalation and lung lesions occur in nearly a third of progressive cases. Granulomatous changes also occur in the nasal mucosa sinuses and skin with lymphatic spread to lymph nodes. Two clinical presentations are recognized; the juvenile form characterized by high fever, generalized lymph nodes and pulmonary involvement with miliary lesions, and the adult form, a milder indolent form characterized by reactivation.

Diagnosis is based upon biopsy of affected tissue and fungal culture. Histopathology demonstrates characteristic wheel-shaped yeasts. Sulphonamides (e.g. co-trimoxazole) are as effective as amphotericin and itraconazole.

25.3 Other important infections that can have multisystem presentation

25.3.1 Syphilis

The causative organism is *Treponium pallidum subspecies pallidum*. The most common mode of transmission is sexually, although infection may occur in pregnancy, perinatally or through contaminated blood products. Typically, the primary stage is a painless penile or rectal ulcer occurring three to ninety days after the initial exposure. The secondary phase typically occurs four to ten weeks later and is characterized by fever, lymphadenopathy, and a maculopapular rash involving the palms of the hands and soles of the feet. Highly infectious wart-like lesions known as condyloma lata may appear on mucous membranes. The infection then enters a period of latency, typically three to fifteen years, and may manifest as gummatous syphilis (15%), cardiovascular syphilis (10%), or late neurosyphilis (6.5%). Late neurosyphilis can be categorized as meningovascular syphilis, general paresis, tabes dorsalis, and Argyll Robertson pupils (pupils that accommodate but do not restrict to light).

Within the UK, the prevalence of syphilis is rising, particularly in men who have sex with men (MSM). Common presentations include eye complications, typically anterior uveitis, or otosyphilis, characterized by high-frequency hearing loss. Diagnostic tests include dark ground microscopy of ulcer swabs or lymph node aspirates, but more commonly serological testing. Treponemal IgG is a marker of previous exposure, Treponema pallidum particle agglutination (TPPA) is a confirmation assay, RPR relates to activity, and IgM timing of infection. PCR is also available for use on ulcer swabs. Treatment is dependent upon site and stage of infection but normally involves treatment with a long-acting penicillin, either benzathine penicillin or procaine penicillin, given intramuscularly. For neurosyphilis, treatment is with IV benzylpenicillin, or procaine penicillin and oral probenicid for fourteen days. In those with severe penicillin allergy, doxycycline may be used to treat early or late latent syphilis infection.

25.3.2 Lyme disease

Lyme disease can affect multiple body systems and produce a broad range of symptoms. The causative organism is *Borrelia burgdoferi* and was first described around Lyme, Connecticut in the USA following a cluster of cases misdiagnosed as chronic juvenile arthritis. Infection can occur following exposure to the Ixodes tick which must be attached for thirty-six to forty-eight hours before bacteria can spread. In the absence of treatment, dissemination may occur. The characteristic skin lesion, at the site of the tick bite, is erythema migrans which typically has erythematous margins and central clearing. No rash is apparent in 25–50% of patients. Weeks later (early dissemination), arthralgia (+/- synovitis) occurs and if left untreated CNS involvement (meningitis) or cardiovascular system (CVS) involvement (myocarditis) may ensue. This can manifest as meningitis, facial nerve palsy, and atrioventricular block. After several months (late dissemination) severe and chronic symptoms may occur including polyneuropathy, cognitive impairment, depression, fatigue, and chronic arthritis.

For uncomplicated infection (without CNS involvement) treatment is doxycycline 100mg (o) bd for fourteen days. Alternatives include amoxicillin, cefuroxime, and azithromycin. Chronic fatigue may be a feature of Lyme disease but prolonged treatment does not alleviate symptoms. Diagnosis is based upon symptoms, tick exposure, and serological testing (often negative in the early stages of disease). Serological testing is based upon a two-tier approach, an ELISA screening assay and, if positive or equivocal, more specific Western blot testing.

25.3.3 Leptospirosis

Infection is caused by corkscrewed-shaped bacteria called Leptospira. Up to thirteen different genetic types may cause disease in humans. The spectrum of disease ranges from mild headache, myalgia, and fever to the more severe form (Weil's disease), characterized by fever, severe jaundice, acute kidney injury, and haemorrhage. The incubation period is seven to twelve days and the course of illness classically biphasic, the second phase being characterized by meningitic symptoms at the time of seroconversion. The infection is zoonotic and transmitted by both wild and domestic animals (e.g. rodents). Transmission occurs when animal urine or water or soil containing urine comes into contact with breaks in the skin or mucous membranes. In the developed world, high-risk occupations include sewerage workers and recreational activities such as canoeing.

Diagnosis is based upon direct detection (culture on specialized media takes three weeks so is of little clinical value) and serological testing, the gold standard being the microscopic agglutination test (MAT). For mild disease, treatment is with penicillin G, amoxicillin, and doxycycline. In more severe cases IV ceftriaxone should be used. Organ support may be required, such as haemodialysis, in the ITU setting.

25.3.4 Rickettsiosis

This is a disease caused by intracellular gram-negative bacteria. The pathogenesis of disease is a vasculitic process affecting multiple organs. Most rickettsial pathogens are transmitted by ectoparasites such as fleas, lice, mites, and ticks. Rickettsiosis is divided into the 'spotted fever group' and 'typhus group'. In the UK all infections are travel associated, e.g. scrub typhus acquired while trekking in SE Asia. The incubation period varies from five to fourteen days. Clinical presentations vary and typically develop in one to two weeks. These include fever, headache, malaise, nausea, and vomiting. A vasculitic rash and an eschar at the site of inoculation are tell-tale sign of infection. In cases of scrub typhus, lymphadenopathy, cough, and encephalitis may ensue.

Diagnosis is based upon clinical recognition and serology. Serology requires both acute and convalescent samples. Treatment of choice is doxycycline 100mg (o) bd, although chloramphenicol is a suitable alternative. If left untreated, disease may progress to severe illness and ultimately death.

25.3.5 Q fever

Coxiella burnetii, an intracellular bacterial pathogen, is the causative agent of Q fever. It is morphologically similar to Rickettsia but has a variety of genetic and physiological differences and can persist for long periods in the environment. It is a zoonotic infection and found in cattle, sheep, goats, and other domestic animals. Transmission is via inhalation (low infectious dose) and infection may occur following contact with milk, urine, faeces, and products of conception of infected animals. Q fever is therefore an occupational hazard for vets, farmers, sheep shearers and hide workers. The incubation period is nine to forty days and disease occurs in two phases. The acute phase is characterized by headaches, chills, and respiratory symptoms which may progress to an 'atypical pneumonia'. Less often, Q fever causes a granulomatous hepatitis which may be asymptomatic or cause malaise, fever, right upper quadrant pain, and hepatomegaly. Liver biopsy reveals fibrin ring granulomata. The chronic form, which may occur months after exposure, is often characterized by infective endocarditis. The treatment of acute disease is with doxycycline, typically two to three weeks and doxycycline and hydroxychloroquine should be used in combination to treat infective endocarditis for eighteen months. In pregnancy, treatment of choice is co-trimoxazole.

Diagnosis is based upon serology, with phase I and II antigens distinguishing between acute and chronic infection. In acute infection, antibody response to *C. burnetti* phase II antigen is predominant whereas in chronic infection, phase I IgG > phase II IgG. The gold standard is the indirect immunofluorescent assay (IFA) using *C. burnetti* antigen. Paired samples should demonstrate a fourfold rise in titres.

25.3.6 Bartonella

These are gram-negative intracellular parasites transmitted by ticks, fleas, sand flies, and mosquitoes. The infecting organism is taken up by endothelial cells before being released into the blood stream where they infect erythrocytes. Dissemination to the heart, skin, lymph nodes, liver, spleen, and retina can occur. The commonest species that occur worldwide are *Bartonella henselae* and *Bartonella quintana*. *Bartonella henselae* is the cause of cat scratch fever, characterized by lymphangitis and lymphadenopathy. It can also cause peliosis hepatitis, multiple blood-filled cavities in the liver. Bacillary angiomatosis, vascular lesions of the skin that mimic Kaposi sarcoma in HIV-infected patients is another clinical manifestation as is culture negative endocarditis. It is also a cause of culture negative endocarditis. *Bartonella quintana* is the cause of trench fever, but also bacillary angiomatosis and infective endocarditis. Effective antibiotics for treatment include co-trimoxazole, tetracyclines, and macrolides. Optimal antimicrobial treatment for infective endocarditis is doxycycline (six weeks) and gentamicin (two weeks), although surgical resection is usually required.

25.4 Things to be aware of

This list of infections discussed in this chapter is not exhaustive but infection specialists should be aware that multisystem infections can present to a variety of different specialities where often the differential diagnosis is an 'infectious' or 'non-infectious' cause. For infectious causes, the aetiological agent will depend upon on travel or occupational exposure, host susceptibility, and where within the host the infection has occurred.

25.5 Assessment questions

25.5.1 Question 1

A thirty-seven-year-old HIV seropositive male presents with a two-week history of fever, lymphadenopathy, and hepatosplenomegaly. He was born and lived in Thailand and recently migrated to the UK less than two months ago.

Investigations:

CD4 count	$80 \times 10^6/L$ (430-1690)
Blood cultures	Yeast

What is the most likely organism?

A. *Blastomyces dermatitidis.*
B. *Candida albicans.*
C. *Cryptococcus gattii.*
D. *Histoplasma penicillium.*
E. *Talaromyces marneffei.*

25.5.2 Question 2

A thirty-one-year-old canoeist is admitted to hospital with a ten-day history of fever and myalgia. He is admitted to ITU for ionotropic support and renal replacement therapy.
A diagnosis of leptospirosis is considered.

What is the most appropriate diagnostic test?

A. Antigen detection on EDTA blood.
B. Blood culture.
C. PCR on EDTA blood.
D. Serological testing.
E. Urine culture.

25.5.3 Question 3

A thirty-eight-year-old male Welsh farmer is admitted to hospital with a six-week history of fever, malaise, and weight loss. He has not previously taken antibiotics.

Investigations (Table 25.1):

Table 25.1

Blood culture x3	Negative
Transthoracic echocardiogram	Vegetation seen on mitral valve
Serum total bilirubin	$23\mu mol/L$ (1–22)
Serum alanine aminotransferase	276 U/L (5–35)
Serum alkaline phosphatase	360 U/L (45–105)

What is the most likely cause of his infective endocarditis?

A. *Bartonella quintana.*
B. *Chlamydia psittaci.*
C. *Coxiella burnetti.*
D. *Kingella kingae.*
E. *Streptococcus oralis.*

25.6 Answers and discussion

25.6.1 Answer 1

E. *Talaromyces marneffei.*

This HIV patient has a CD4 count of 80 $\times 10^6$/L and is therefore susceptible to infection with a pathogenic yeast. As the patient was born and had lived in Thailand, *Talaromyces marneffei* is the most likely diagnosis. *Histoplasma capsulatum* and *Blastomyces dermatitidis* are both geographically restricted to North America. *Cryptococcus species*, are more likely to cause meningitis in HIV seropositive patient and candidaemia is less commonly associated with lymphadenopathy and hepatosplenomegaly.

25.6.2 Answer 2

D. Serological testing.

After ten days of symptoms, the diagnosis is based upon serological testing, the gold standard being the microscopic agglutination test (MAT). In the early stages of disease, leptospira may be cultured from urine on specialized media but can take up to three weeks to grow, so is of little clinical value. PCR is not routinely available, nor is an antigen detection assay on EDTA blood. Automated blood culture systems do not detect leptospiraemia.

25.6.3 Answer 3

C. *Coxiella burnetti.*

As a Welsh farmer is likely to be exposed to sheep and cattle, the diagnosis is most likely to be *Coxiella burnetii*. *Kingella kingae* and *Streptococcus oralis* are likely to have been cultured from blood in the absence of previous antibiotic treatment. *Bartonella quintana*, unlike *B. henselae*, is not associated with cats and *Chlamydia psittaci* is an unusual cause of culture-negative endocarditis associated with birds. *C. burnetii* is associated with granulomatous hepatitis.

CHAPTER 26

Cardiovascular infections

Robert Serafino Wani and Satya Das

26.1 Infective endocarditis (IE), its prevalence, and its predisposing factors

Infective endocarditis (IE) is inflammation of the endothelial lining of the heart valves due to infective causes.

IE is a rare condition with an incidence rate of three to nine cases per 100,000 population with a male to female ratio of 2:1. The rate is higher in people with unrepaired cyanotic congenital heart disease, prosthetic heart valves and previous endocarditis. Other risk factors for IE include: rheumatic fever (now accounts for < 10% of IE cases in developed countries), degenerative conditions of heart valves, intravenous drug abuse, diabetes, and HIV infection. One third of the cases are now healthcare associated infection (HCAI), particularly with haemodialysis, cardiac surgery, implantable cardiac devices, intravascular lines, and urinary catheters. In the past decade *Staphylococcus aureus* has replaced viridans streptococci as the leading cause of IE, the rate of enterococcal (mostly *E. faecalis*) and Bartonella IE has increased, while that of culture negative endocarditis has decreased. Untreated IE is a uniformly fatal condition, but the mortality rate can be reduced to 5–40% with appropriate treatment.

26.2 Pathogenesis of IE

There are two important prerequisite steps to the development of IE:

1. *A damaged endothelium* due to high pressure gradient and turbulent blood flow around a heart valve or septal defect. Fibrin and platelet deposition occur on the roughened endothelium forming a non-infective thrombus or vegetation.

2. *Bacteraemia due to endocarditis-prone organisms* resulting from trauma to mucous membranes (e.g. oral cavity, urinary, and gastrointestinal tract) or other colonized tissue or foreign body, which is not cleared by host defence mechanisms.

Micro-organisms then attach to the damaged endothelium through a specific ligand-receptor interaction (hence the predilection for certain organisms to cause endocarditis, e.g. *viridans streptococci* from the mouth), colonize the thrombus, and grow and multiply within it to give rise to a mature/infective vegetation, which is the pathological hallmark of IE. Virulent organisms, classically *S. aureus*, can apparently infect a healthy endocardium.

Damage to the endothelium results in valvular incompetence/regurgitation and symptoms and signs of heart failure and when severe, it is a potentially fatal condition that requires urgent valve surgery, even if the infection has fully responded to antimicrobial therapy.

Vegetation is the source of emboli (and may or may not contain micro-organisms) which can disseminate in the blood stream and occlude small arteries to cause ischaemia and ischaemic necrosis in distant sites in the body, e.g. the central nervous system (commonly manifesting as a stroke), spleen, skin, and other organs.

Immune complex deposition in tissues resulting from the host's antibody response to the invading micro-organisms is probably the basis for some of the clinical presentations of IE, e.g. Osler's nodes and glomerulonephritis.

26.3 Aetiology of IE

The organisms causing IE vary according to whether a native or prosthetic valve is infected, the time of the IE after surgery for prosthetic valve endocarditis, and whether the predisposing condition is people who inject drugs (PWID). IE most commonly affects aortic and mitral valves, i.e. left-sided IE, although in PWID, the tricuspid valve is most commonly affected and less frequently, the pulmonary valve (i.e. right-sided IE due to injection of contaminated drugs directly into the venous system).

The most common organisms causing IE are shown in Table 26.1. In PWID, *S. aureus* is the most common cause of IE (60–70%), followed by β-haemolytic streptococci, *Pseudomonas aeruginosa*, and *Candida albicans*. Polymicrobial infection occurs in 5–25% cases of IE in PWID.

Prosthetic valve endocarditis (PVE) complicates insertion of prosthetic heart valves in about 3% of procedures. Early-onset PVE occurs within one year of valve surgery, and is most commonly due to intra-operative contamination, and has a much higher mortality rate. Late onset PVE occurs after one year of valve surgery and the microbial aetiology more closely resembles that of native valve endocarditis (NVE).

26.4 Presenting features of IE

The clinical presentation with IE is highly variable and depends on the causative organism, the presence or absence of pre-existing cardiac diseases, co-morbidities, and other risk factors for development of IE. It can be an acute and rapidly progressive infection (most commonly due to *S. aureus*), or a sub-acute or chronic condition (usually seen with viridans streptococci and enterococci). The majority of patients (approximately 90%) will present with fever, often associated with systemic symptoms of chills, poor appetite, and weight loss. Heart murmurs are found in 85% of patients. Valvular pathology should therefore heighten the possibility of IE.

Immunological phenomena such as splinter haemorrhages, Roth spots, and glomerulonephritis are less common. Emboli to the brain, lung, or spleen occur in 30% of patients, and are often the presenting feature. IE should be considered in a patient with stroke and fever.

Table 26.1 The aetiology of native valve endocarditis (NVE) and prosthetic valve endocarditis (PVE).

Causes of native valve endocarditis (NVE):

Organism	% of cases Pre 2000	Post 2000
Viridans streptococci (VS)	40	30
Other Streptococci (e.g. Betahaemolytic streptococci/BHS including S.gallolyticus (S. bovis group), Abiotrophia and Granulicatella sp.)	5–15	5–15
Enterococci (mostly E. faecalis)	10	15
Staphylococci:		
S. aureus	25–30	40–45
Coagulase-negative staphylococci (CNS)	< 5	5–10
HACEK group (Haemophilus, Aggregatibacter (Actinobacter) actinomycetemcomitans, Cardiobacterium hominis, Eikenella corrodens, Kingella kingae)	5	< 5
Other organisms (gram-negative bacilli/GNB, Fungi, Polymicrobial)	5	5
Culture negative (CN)	5–25	5–15

Microbial causes of prosthetic valve endocarditis (PVE).

	Early onset PVE (40%)	Late onset PVE (60%)
S. aureus	40%	30%
Coagulase negative		
Staphylococci (CNS)	30%	5%
Viridans Streptococci	<5%	35%
Other Streptococci	<5%	5–10%
Enterococci	10%	15%
Corynebacteria	5%	< 5%
Gram-negative rods (GNR)	6%	< 5%
Fungi (mostly Candida)	5%	< 5%
Mortality rate	60%	10–15%

Atypical presentation (absence of fever) is common in the elderly, the immunocompromised, and in IE caused by less virulent or atypical organisms. High index of suspicion and low threshold for investigations are essential in these and other groups, such as those with congenital heart disease or prosthetic heart valves, to exclude endocarditis and avoid delay in diagnosis.

26.5 Investigating for IE

Elevated C-reactive protein (CRP) or erythrocyte sedimentation rate (ESR), leucocytosis, anaemia, and microscopic haematuria may be present in patients with IE but are non-specific. Imaging, particularly echocardiogram, is important for diagnosis and management of IE. Positive blood cultures (three sets taken aseptically and peripherally) remain a cornerstone in the diagnosis of IE. Minimum inhibitory concentration (MIC) testing should be done for more accurate determination of the organism's susceptibility to antimicrobials and to guide treatment options. Demonstration of micro-organisms in resected valvular tissue/vegetation, intracardiac abscess or embolic fragment by culture, or histology or pathologic lesions showing active endocarditis is the gold standard for diagnosis of IE. Molecular detection of infective organisms on cardiac valves and serology (e.g. for Bartonella and Coxiella burnetti/Q fever) are useful in culture-negative IE. Other imaging modalities such as CT/PET, cardiac MRI, and radio-labelled whole white cell imaging are useful adjuncts in the diagnosis of IE. MRI head is used for detecting cerebral embolic phenomenon in IE such as stroke.

26.6 Diagnostic criteria for IE

The modified Duke criteria is often used for diagnosis of IE, and is shown in Table 26.2.

Table 26.2 Modified Duke Criteria for diagnosis of infective endocarditis.

Major criteria

1. Blood cultures positive for IE
   a. Typical micro-organisms consistent with IE from two separate blood cultures:
      * *Staphylococcus aureus, Viridans streptococci, Streptococcus gallolyticus* (previously known as *Streptococcus bovis*), HACEK group; or
      * Community-acquired *enterococci*, in the absence of a primary focus;
   or
   b. Micro-organisms consistent with IE from persistently positive blood cultures:
      * More than two positive blood cultures of blood samples drawn more than twelve hours apart; or
      * All of three or a majority of four or more separate cultures of blood (with first and last samples drawn more than one hour apart);
   or
   c. Single positive blood culture for *Coxiella burnetii* or phase I IgG antibody titre > 1:800.
2. Imaging positive for IE:
   a. Echocardiogram positive for IE:
      * Vegetation;
      * Abscess;
      * New partial dehiscence of prosthetic valve
   b. Abnormal activity around the site of prosthetic valve implantation detected by 18F-FDG PET/CT (only if the prosthesis was implanted for more than three months) or radiolabelled leukocytes SPECT/CT;
   c. Definite paravalvular lesions by cardiac CT

Minor criteria

1. Predisposition such as predisposing heart condition, or injecting drug use;
2. Fever as temperature > 38°C;
3. Vascular phenomena (including those detected by imaging only):
major arterial emboli, septic pulmonary infarcts, infectious (mycotic) aneurysm, intracranial haemorrhage, conjunctival haemorrhages, and Janeway's lesions
4. Immunological phenomena:
Glomerulonephritis, Osler's nodes, Roth's spots, and rheumatoid factor.
5. Microbiological evidence:
Positive blood culture but does not meet a major criterion as noted above or serological evidence of active infection with organism consistent with IE

Definite IE	Possible IE	Rejected IE
Pathological criteria • Micro-organism demonstrated by culture or histology of a vegetation or intracardiac abscess; • Histology of a vegetation or intracardiac abscess showing active IE. **Clinical criteria** • Two major criteria; or • One major criterion and three minor criteria; or • Five minor criteria	• One major criterion and one minor criterion; or • Three minor criteria	• Firm alternate diagnosis; or • Resolution of symptoms suggesting IE with antibiotic therapy for four or fewer days; or • No pathological evidence of IE at surgery or autopsy; or • Does not meet criteria for possible IE, as above

(adapted from Li et al.)

26.7 Treating IE

IE is difficult to treat because it is an infection in a 'protected site', where the organism is able to multiply unchecked by hiding inside vegetations and thus escaping host defence mechanisms.

Antimicrobial therapy may be unsuccessful due to difficulty in penetrating vegetations and reduced activity as the organisms are mostly in stationary phase of growth. Valve surgery is thus often necessary for cure of the infection. Where this is indicated, the earlier the surgery is performed, the better the outcome usually.

Fundamental steps to successful treatment of IE include:

- The use of bactericidal antibiotics, preferably synergistic in combination (e.g. penicillin/ amoxicillin plus gentamicin for viridans streptococcal and enterococcal endocarditis);
- High dosage given IV for prolonged periods, typically four to six weeks for native valve endocarditis (NVE) and six weeks or longer for prosthetic valve endocarditis (PVE);
- Close monitoring of response to treatment as well as toxicity/adverse drug reactions, including regular testing of serum levels of antimicrobials with low therapeutic index (e.g. aminoglycosides and glycopeptides). NB: For gentamicin, the trough level should be < 1mg/l and peak level 3–5mg/l, which is sufficient for bactericidal synergy. For vancomycin the trough level should be 15–20mg/l;
- A multidisciplinary approach involving cardiologists, infection specialists, and, where necessary, cardiac surgeons in assessing the need for early valve surgery; and
- Regular follow-up of patient after discharging home because of the higher risk of IE in the future. This includes regular dental follow ups and advice about maintaining good oral hygiene.

Table 26.3 summarizes the guidelines for the empiric therapy of IE from the European Society of Cardiology (ESC), the American Heart Association (AHA), and the British Society of Antimicrobial Chemotherapy (BSAC).

Empiric therapy should be adjusted according to culture and sensitivity results and usually follows national guidelines (BSAC in the UK).

26.8 Implantable cardiac electronic devices (ICEDs) and causative agents of ICED infection

ICEDs comprising pacemakers, implantable cardiac defibrillators, and cardiac resynchronization therapy devices have both intravascular and extravascular components. Infection can involve both these components and the tissues surrounding them. ICED infections are life-threatening, particularly when associated with endocardial infection, with a mortality rate of up to 35%. ICED infections can be difficult to diagnose because echocardiography is less accurate, blood cultures less sensitive, and the diagnosis is often not considered. ICED infections are also complex to manage because there are intracardiac and extracardiac components, both of which may become infected and removal of the device can be a major undertaking, with a risk of death or significant complications.

Staphylococci (both S. aureus and coagulase-negative staphylococci (CNS)) are by far the leading cause of ICED-associated infections, accounting for 80–90%. Gram-negative bacilli, Enterococcus species, Streptococcus species, Propiobacterium species, and fungi are less common causes.

Table 26.3 Empiric treatment of IE.

	ESC 2015	AHA 2015	BSAC 2012
Native valve acute	If severely and acutely unwell: ampicillin 12g/day IV in four to six doses + flucloxacillin 12g/day IV in four to six doses or oxacillin 12g/day IV in four to six doses + gentamicin 3mg/kg IV once daily	Ampicillin-sulbactam 12g/day IV in four doses + gentamicin 1mg/kg IV thrice daily	Severe sepsis: vancomycin IV (dose as per local protocol) + gentamicin 1mg/kg IV per each twelve-hour period (ciprofloxacin instead of gentamicin if concerns about nephrotoxicity) If risk of MDR (multi-drug resistant) gram-negative organisms: vancomycin IV (dose as per local protocol) + meropenem 2g IV per each eight-hour period
Native valve indolent			amoxicillin 2g IV per each four-hour period + (optional) gentamicin 1mg/kg IV per each twelve-hour period
Penicillin allergy/ Possible MRSA/ healthcare associated	vancomycin 30mg/kg/day IV in two doses + gentamicin 1mg/kg IV thrice daily + (if possibly MRSA) Rifampicin 900–1200mg by mouth per day in two doses	vancomycin 30mg/kg/day IV in two doses + gentamicin 1mg/kg IV thrice daily + ciprofloxacin 500mg IV twice daily	vancomycin IV (dose as per local protocol) + gentamicin 1mg/kg IV per each twelve-hour period (ciprofloxacin instead of gentamicin if concerns about nephrotoxicity)
Prosthetic valve	Fewer than twelve months post surgery vancomycin 30/mg/kg/day IV in two doses + gentamicin 1mg/kg IV thrice daily + (suggest start rif three to five days later) rifampicin 600mg by mouth twice daily more than twelve months post surgery as native valve	Fewer than twelve months vancomycin IV + gentamicin IV + cefepime 6g/day IV in three doses + rifampicin 300mg by mouth thrice daily More than twelve months As native valve + rifampicin 300mg by mouth thrice daily.	vancomycin 1g IV per each twelve-hour period + gentamicin 1mg/kg IV per each twelve-hour period + rifampicin 300–600mg by mouth/IV per each twelve-hour period If vancomycin intolerant: daptomycin 6mg/kg IV per each twelve-hour period
Duration	Four to six weeks NVE six weeks PVE (two weeks gent)	Four to six weeks NVE six weeks PVE (two weeks gent)	

26.9 Pathogenesis of ICED infection

Contamination of the device could happen during manufacturing or packaging, during implantation (surgical site infection, SSI, is probably the commonest cause), via haematogenous seeding from a distant source, or via contamination after erosion through the skin.

26.10 Clinical features of ICED infection

Clinical features if ICED infection could be localized to the ICED insertion site, such as generator or pocket infection presenting with localized cellulitis, swelling, discharge, dehiscence, or pain. Generator pocket infection and ICED-infective endocarditis (ICED-IE) or ICED lead infections (ICED-LI) often co-exist. Non-specific signs and symptoms of systemic infection, including fevers, chills, night sweats, malaise, and anorexia, may be the only clinical features of ICED-IE/ICED-LI.

26.11 Investigating ICED infection

Chest radiograph, echocardiography (trans-oesophageal more sensitive than trans-thoracic), and at least three sets of blood cultures should be done in all patients with suspicion of ICED infections. After extraction of the device, distal and proximal lead fragments, lead vegetation, generator pocket tissue, and pus from a generator pocket wound should be sent to microbiology for culturing and further microbiological work up.

26.12 Treating ICED infection

Infection immediately post-implantation is likely to be due to *S. aureus* and therefore should be treated with beta-lactams (flucloxacillin) or glycopeptide (vancomycin or teicoplanin) antibiotics, pending culture results. The route of antibiotic administration would depend on the severity of the infection. Duration of therapy should be determined by the type of ICED infection, proposed device management, involvement of other cardiac structures, and the presence of extracardiac foci of infection.

26.13 Antibiotic prophylaxis to prevent ICED infection

Antibiotic prophylaxis can be used to prevent ICED infection. A single dose of appropriate intravenous antibiotic/s is administered within one hour of skin incision during insertion of the device, e.g. IV flucloxacillin and gentamicin.

26.14 Infections affecting the pericardium and myocardium

Certain infections can affect the pericardium and myocardium. Table 26.4 shows some common infectious causes of pericarditis and myocarditis.

26.14.1 Pericarditis

Infection makes up about 16% of disease affecting the pericardium. The clinical features are often confined to the pericardium, as seen in viral pericarditis. Extrapericardial infections can present with

Table 26.4 Common infectious causes of pericarditis and myocarditis.

Viruses	Respiratory syncytial virus (RSV)
	Adenovirus
	Coxsackie virus (types A and B),
	Herpes viruses (CMV, HSV 1&2, EBV, HHV6)
	Parvovirus
	Polio
	Hepatitis B & C viruses
	HIV
	Arboviruses
Bacteria	*Staphylococcus aureus*
	Streptococcus pneumoniae
	Streptococcus pyogenes
	Neisseria meningitidis
	Neisseria gonorrhoeae
	Mycobacterium tuberculosis
	Mycoplasma pneumoniae
	Chlamydia pneumoniae
	Chlamydia psittaci
	Brucella species
Fungi	*Histoplasma sp.*
	Cryptococcus sp
	Aspergillus sp.
	Candida sp.
	Coccidiodes
	Blastomycosis
Others	*Rickettsia rickettsii*
	Borrelia burgdorferi
	Treponema pallidum
	Strongyloides
	Echinococcus species
	Taenia solium
	Paragonimus
	Ascaris

clinical features such as pneumonia and empyema in association with pericarditis. Bacteria and fungi can cause purulent inflammatory exudate (purulent pericarditis).

26.14.2 Myocarditis

Myocarditis is an inflammatory disease of the heart, frequently resulting from viral infections and/or post-viral immune-mediated responses.

Patients tend to present weeks to months after the acute illness, and therefore the utility of viral serology is unproven. Pericardiocentesis and endomyocardial biopsy for histological, microbiological, and molecular work have a diagnostic value. Treatment is supportive and underlying causative agent should be treated if indicated.

26.15 Further reading and useful resources

Gould, F. K., Denning, D. W., Elliott, T. S., Foweraker, J., Perry, J. D., Prendergast, B. D., et al., 'Guidelines for the Diagnosis and Antibiotic Treatment of Endocarditis in Adults: A Report of the Working Party of the British Society for Antimicrobial Chemotherapy', *Journal of Antimicrobial Chemotherapy*, 67 (2012), 269–289.

Habib, G., Lancellotti, P., Antunes, M. J., Bongiorni, M. G., Casalta, J. P., Del Zotti, F., et al., '2015 ESC Guidelines for the management of infective endocarditis: The Task Force for the

Management of Infective Endocarditis of the European Society of Cardiology (ESC). Endorsed by: European Association for Cardio-Thoracic Surgery (EACTS), the European Association of Nuclear Medicine (EANM)', *European Heart Journal*, 36 (2015), 3075.

Li, J. S., Sexton, D. J., Mick, N., Nettles, R., Fowler, V. G. Jr, Ryan, T., et al., 'Proposed Modifications to the Duke Criteria for the Diagnosis of Infective Endocarditis', *Clinical Infectious Diseases*, 30 (2000), 633–638.

Nishimura, R. A., Otto, C. M., Bonow, R. O., Carabello, B. A., Erwin, J. P. III, Guyton, R.A., et al., '2014 AHA/ACC Guideline for the Management of Patients with Valvular Heart Disease: Executive Summary: A Report of the American College of Cardiology/American Heart Association Task Force on Practice Guidelines', *Journal of the American College of Cardiology*, 63 (2014), 2438–2488.

Prophylaxis against Infective Endocarditis: Antimicrobial Prophylaxis against Infective Endocarditis in Adults and Children Undergoing Interventional Procedures (CG64). National Institute for Health and Care Excellence (NICE). http://www.nice.org.uk/guidance/CG64

26.16 Assessment questions

26.16.1 Question 1

A sixty-five-year-old man presents with a four-week history of generalized fatigue. He is found to have bacterial endocarditis caused by *Streptococcus gallolyticus* and is treated with penicillin and gentamicin.

One week after starting the treatment, he has symptomatically much improved. His appetite has returned and he no longer has a fever.

What is the most appropriate next step in management?
A. Colonoscopy.
B. CT scan.
C. Cystoscopy.
D. Dental assessment.
E. Gastroscopy.

26.16.2 Question 2

A sixteen-year-old girl presents with a three-day history of fever and rigors. *Staphylococcus aureus* is isolated from peripheral blood cultures. Her echocardiogram shows aortic valve root abscess. She has undergone an aortic valve replacement. The valve tissue is culture positive for *Staphylococcus aureus* despite being on one week of intravenous flucloxacillin.

What is the most appropriate length of antibiotic therapy for the endocarditis?
A. Four weeks in total including therapy prior to surgery.
B. Four weeks post valve replacement.
C. Six weeks in total including therapy before valve replacement.
D. Six weeks post valve replacement.
E. Two weeks post valve replacement.

26.16.3 Question 3

A sixty-year-old farmer with a history of rheumatic mitral valve regurgitation presents with a six-week history of fever, weight loss, and splinter haemorrhages on his finger nails. Two sets of blood cultures prior to antibiotic therapy are flagged positive. Gram-positive cocci in short chains are seen on microscopy. Pleomorphic gram-variable organisms are seen on the Gram stain from chocolate agar plates, but there is no growth on blood agar plates after twenty-four hours of incubation.

What is the most likely organism?

A. *Bartonella henselae.*

B. *Brucella abortus.*

C. *Coxiella burnetii.*

D. *Granulicatella adiacens.*

E. *Mycoplasma pneumoniae.*

26.17 Answers and discussion

26.17.1 Answer 1

A. Colonoscopy

There is a strong association between group D streptococcus, especially *S. gallolyticus* subspecies *gallolyticus* (*S. bovis* biotype I), bacteraemia and colonic neoplasia. Colonoscopy is recommended, and if negative should be repeated in four to six months' time. Abdominal CT scan may not pick up neoplastic polyps. Patients with recurrent enterococcal bacteraemia or endocarditis should be investigated for pathology in the urinary or gastrointestinal tracts as these are often the portals of entry. Patients with poor dentition should have a dental assessment prior to any valve surgery as oral/viridans streptococci are among the most common causes of IE.

26.17.2 Answer 2

D. Six weeks post valve replacement.

Antibiotic treatment of *Staphylococcus aureus* native valve IE is four to six weeks from the day of negative blood culture. The length of duration of antibiotic therapy post-surgery is dependent upon valve culture result. Positive valve cultures require six weeks of antibiotic therapy from the date of valve surgery. Negative valve cultures will need antibiotic therapy to complete six weeks in total from the date of negative blood cultures.

26.17.3 Answer 3

D. *Granulicatella adiacens.*

Granulicatella and *Abiotrophia* (formerly nutritionally variant streptococci, NVS) have a predilection to cause infective endocarditis in patients with existing valvular pathology. They require pyridoxal and l-cysteine as growth factors; hence, they are difficult to isolate on ordinary culture media such as blood agar plate. The current automated blood culture broths such as BACTEC have pyridol. All the other organisms mentioned are causes of culture negative endocarditis.

CHAPTER 27

Skin and soft tissue infections

Rohma Ghani and Caoimhe Nic Fhogartaigh

27.1 Classifying skin and soft tissue infections (SSTIs)

Skin and soft tissue infections (SSTIs) can be sub-divided based on the anatomical structure(s) affected from superficial to deep (see Table 27.1).

Table 27.1 Skin structures and associated infections.

Structure	Clinical description
Epidermis	Impetigo
Superficial dermis/hair follicles	Folliculitis
Deeper dermis/hair follicles	Furuncle, carbuncle
Dermis and hypodermis	Cellulitis
Superficial subcutaneous tissue (including lymphatics)	Erysipelas
Deeper subcutaneous tissue	Cellulitis
Muscle	Pyomyositis
Superficial and deep fascia	Necrotizing fasciitis

27.2 Clinical features of impetigo

Impetigo affects children more commonly than adults, starting as a macule of erythema and evolving into vesicles that rupture, leaving a golden crusted appearance. Fever and systemic signs are absent. It is highly transmissible and children should be excluded from school until exposed lesions have resolved.

27.3 Hair follicle infections

Folliculitis is a superficial infection presenting with small papules or pustules on an erythematous base around a hair. Fever and systemic signs are absent. If extension into deeper tissues occurs a dermal abscess ('boil' or 'furuncle') may occur, and several lesions may coalesce into a 'carbuncle'. Deeper infection may cause discomfort, fever, and systemic upset. Any hair-bearing area may be affected, but sites most commonly affected include the face, scalp, axilla, inguinal area, thighs, or eyelid ('stye'), and may be associated with shaved or occluded skin.

27.4 Clinical features and grades of cellulitis

Cellulitis is rapidly spreading erythema of the skin associated with pain, swelling, fever, and systemic features such as nausea and malaise. It may be seen as a complication of tinea pedis, superficial abrasions, or insect bites, venous insufficiency, lymphoedema, chronic ulcers, and diabetes. It is almost always *unilateral* and bilateral cellulitis is extremely rare and should prompt consideration of an alternative diagnosis.

The Eron grading system can help guide treatment and admission decisions:

- Class I: the patient has no signs of systemic toxicity and no uncontrolled comorbidities.
- Class II: the patient is either systemically unwell or systemically well *but with a comorbidity* such as peripheral vascular disease, chronic venous insufficiency, diabetes, or obesity, which may complicate or delay resolution of infection.
- Class III: the patient has significant systemic upset such as acute confusion, tachycardia, tachypnoea, hypotension, or unstable comorbidities that may interfere with a response to treatment, or a limb-threatening infection due to vascular compromise.
- Class IV: the patient is septic or has life-threatening infection such as necrotizing fasciitis.

27.5 Differential diagnosis of cellulitis

There are a number of differential diagnoses for cellulitis. For the list below, conditions marked with a '*' may predispose to cellulitis.

- Deep venous thrombosis (DVT): characterized by pain and swelling, usually of the calf with a lesser degree of erythema.
- Ruptured Baker's cyst: may cause unilateral calf swelling with minimal erythema.
- Septic arthritis: if swelling and erythema occurs over a joint, with severe pain on joint movement. Bursitis may present similarly.
- Acute gout: There may be a history of recurrent attacks affecting typical joints such as the first metatarsophalangeal.
- Superficial thrombophlebitis: venous inflammation with thrombus formation.
- Varicose eczema*: dry, scaly, itchy, erythematous skin which occurs as a complication of venous insufficiency.
- Lymphoedema*: subcutaneous swelling due to inadequate lymphatic drainage.

- Oedema with blisters*.
- Lipodermatosclerosis: a painful, red, tender, warm, indurated rash that occurs in the absence of significant systemic upset. It is a panniculitis (inflammation of subcutaneous fat) most likely to occur in the lower limbs of obese women with venous insufficiency.

27.6 Clinical features and classification of necrotizing fasciitis (NF)

In the early stages, necrotizing fasciitis (NF) is indistinguishable clinically from cellulitis. However, rapidly spreading necrosis of superficial and deep fascia is associated with severe pain. *Pain which is disproportionate to the skin examination findings, or rapidly progressive symptoms and signs, should alert the clinician to the possibility of NF.*

Pain, swelling, and oedema may extend beyond margins of erythema, and in late stages ecchymoses, bullae, crepitus (due to gas in the tissues), and cutaneous anaesthesia may be evident prior to skin necrosis. The patient is systemically unwell, haemodynamically unstable, and may develop toxic shock. Laboratory results can be used to aid diagnosis (see Diagnosing SSTIs). When the scrotum or perineum is affected it is referred to as Fournier's gangrene. A microbiological classification of NF is outlined in Table 27.2.

NF can be distinguished from severe cellulitis using the Laboratory Risk Indicator for NF (LRINEC) score (see Diagnosing SSTIs).

27.7 Typical microbiology of SSTIs

The microbiology of SSTI depends on the type of infection, skin barrier, host immunity, and exposures, e.g. environmental contamination, water, animals, etc. It is important to note that the skin is colonized with staphylococci, diphtheroids, and propionibacteria ('normal flora'), and this must be differentiated from infection when isolated in a clinical sample.

S. aureus and beta-haemolytic streptococci (Group A, C, and G) are the main pathogens implicated in community-acquired infection in immunocompetent hosts. Group B Streptococcus may cause SSTI infection in elderly or diabetic patients.

Meticillin-resistant *S. aureus* (MRSA) is increasing and in the United States, community-acquired MRSA (CA-MRSA) is common. Risk factors for CA-MRSA include young age, recurrent skin infection/boils, previous antibiotics, participation in contact sports or gym use, military personnel, male-male sex, imprisonment, and injecting drug use.

In hospital-acquired SSTI, *S. aureus* (including MRSA) is the predominant pathogen, although enterobacteriaceae, *Pseudomonas aeruginosa,* anaerobes, and enterococci may cause infections in surgical wounds or skin ulcers.

As well as staphylococcal and streptococcal infections, patients with diabetic foot ulcers may develop SSTI due to enterobacteriaceae, *Pseudomonas*, and anaerobes. More resistant gram-negative infections may be seen in this group due to frequent courses of antibiotics.

Risk factors and characteristic pathogens (courtesy of Matthew Dryden) include:

- *Recurrent hospital admissions/long-term health-care facility*: MRSA.
- *Contact sports, recurrent boils/abscesses, visiting US*: MRSA; Panton-Valentine leucocidin (PVL)-producing *S. aureus.*
- *Diabetes*: S. aureus, group B streptococci, anaerobes, gram-negative bacilli, P. aeruginosa, MRSA.
- *Neutropaenia*: Gram-negative bacilli, *P. aeruginosa* (ecthyma).

Table 27.2 Microbiological classification of necrotizing fasciitis.

	Organism	Site	Clinical features	Trauma	Comorbidities
Type I	Polymicrobial: including anaerobes, e.g. *Clostridium* spp.	Trunk and perineum	Crepitus may be present; thin, foul-smelling serosanguinous fluid	Often none, or minor	Elderly, diabetes, obesity, peripheral vascular disease, neonate
Type II	Monomicrobial: Group A *Streptococcus* +/– *Staphylococcus aureus*	Limbs	Toxic shock	Yes, Surgical wound	Usually none, injecting drug use
Type III	Gram-negative marine organisms e.g. *Vibrio* spp.	Limbs, trunk, and perineum	Multi-organ failure and shock	Water exposure to open wound / skin abrasion (or ingestion of seafood)	Alcohol excess, liver disease.

- *Bite wounds*:
  - Human: Human oral flora
  - Cat: *Pasteurella multocida*
  - Dog: *Capnocytophaga canimorsus*
  - Rat: *Streptobacillus moniliformis*
  - Consider tetanus and rabies
- *Animal contact*: dermatophyte infection, *Bartonella henselae, Francisella tularensis, Bacillus anthracis, Yersinia pestis.*
- *Water exposure (sea, estuaries, rivers)*: *Vibrio* spp., *Aeromonas hydrophila, Mycobacterium marinum, P. aeruginosa.*
- *Injecting drug use*: MRSA, *Clostridium botulinum, Clostridium tetani, B. anthracis,*
- *Tropical travel*: cutaneous leishmaniasis, cutaneous larva migrans, myiasis.

27.8 Pathogenesis of SSTIs

For an SSTI to occur, several events must take place: disruption of the protective skin barrier (e.g. abrasion or insect bite), adherence of bacteria to host cells, a process of invasion into host tissues, and evasion of the host immune response. Pathogenic bacteria carry a variety of virulence genes encoding proteins which augment the these actions, and Table 27.3 outlines examples. Toxins are some of the most important virulence factors in SSTI pathogenesis, in particular, superantigens.

27.9 Diagnosing SSTIs

The diagnosis of an SSTI is largely a clinical one and laboratory investigations are not required unless there is severe infection, significant comorbidity, or complications. Table 27.4 highlights how laboratory indices may be used to differentiate NF from other complicated SSTIs. Blood cultures are only positive in about 10% of cases, and skin swabs positive in 20–30% where there is evidence of purulence or abscess. Imaging may be helpful to delineate abscess or deeper extension of infection resulting in osteomyelitis but should not delay surgery if NF is suspected.

27.10 Treating SSTIs

Apart from very superficial infection, e.g. folliculitis, or small skin abscesses which may be managed with topical antiseptic or incision and drainage, the patient should receive empirical antibiotic therapy after cultures have been taken. Antibiotic choice should consider the severity of infection, local rates of MRSA, or any risk factors for particular infections (see Typical microbiology of SSTIs).

Eron class I and some class II infections may be treated with oral antibiotics and managed as outpatients or in ambulatory care. Class II infections with no complicating comorbidities should be considered for outpatient parenteral antimicrobial therapy (OPAT) where such facilities exist. Intravenous (IV) therapy is essential where there are signs of systemic toxicity, vomiting, rapidly progressing infection, deterioration following forty-eight hours of oral therapy, or significant immunosuppression. Flucloxacillin is a good choice of first-line therapy where there are no risk factors for MRSA, or clindamycin if there is penicillin allergy. Higher doses should be considered in obese patients. Rest and elevation of the affected limb are also important, and treatment of any predisposing conditions, e.g. tinea pedis, eczema.

Table 27.3 Virulence factors implicated in skin and soft tissue infections.

Classification	Bacteria	Virulence factor	Details
Adherence factors	S. pyogenes	Fimbrillae	Adherence to host epithelial cells.
		M protein	Binds host fibrinogen and blocks complement binding
		Protein F	Allows invasion into epithelial cells to avoid detection
	S. aureus	Clumping factor	Adherence to host epithelial cell
		Protein A	Prevents antibody opsonization and phagocytosis
Exotoxins	S. pyogenes	Haemolysins (streptolysin O & S)	Mediate host tissue damage and immunogenicity (streptolysin O)
		Hyaluronidase & streptokinase	Proteinases which can digest host tissue
	S. aureus	Serine protease	Digest desmosome proteins and cause bullous disease
		Lipases	Digest skin fatty acids to invade through skin barrier
		Panton-Valentine leucocidin toxin (found in 5% of S. aureus isolates)	Membrane pore formation, especially in neutrophils and skin cells leading to cell lysis and skin necrosis
	Clostridium sp.	Collagenases & hyaluronidases	Connective tissue and matrix protein digestion, which can cause rapidly progressive disease
		Alpha-toxin	Cell membrane and nerve sheath degradation; induce metabolic dysfunction through prostaglandin elaboration
Superantigens	S. aureus	Enterotoxins, TSST-1, exfoliative toxin A & B	Bind to T cells resulting in polyclonal T cell activation and massive cytokine release leading to fever, 'toxic shock', organ failure, and 'scalded skin syndrome' and
	S. pyogenes	Streptococcal pyrogenic exotoxins (SPEs)	scarlet fever in infants

Table 27.4 Laboratory Risk Indicator for Necrotizing Fasciitis (LRINEC) scoring system.

Laboratory indices	Results	Score
CRP (mg/L)	< 150	0
	≥ 150	4
Leucocytes (x10⁹/L)	< 15	0
	15–25	1
	> 25	2
Haemoglobin (g/L)	> 135	0
	110–135	1
	< 110	2
Sodium (mmol/L)	≥ 135	0
	< 135	2
Creatinine (mmol/L)	≤ 141	0
	> 141	2
Glucose (mmol/L)	≤ 10	0
	> 10	2

A score ≤ 5 = low risk (< 50%); 6–7 = intermediate risk (50–75%); ≥ 8 = high risk (> 75%).

A review of clinical progress and microbiology results should take place at forty-eight to seventy-two hours and therapy adjusted accordingly. Cover for MRSA (with glycopeptide) or gram-negative pathogens (with co-amoxiclav or ciprofloxacin) should be considered if there has been no clinical improvement in the absence of any microbiology results to guide therapy. Most will require seven to fourteen days' treatment, depending on severity.

More severe SSTIs including NF should have an urgent surgical assessment, and a broader spectrum of antibiotics depending on the site of the infection, e.g. piperacillin-tazobactam plus clindamycin, or ciprofloxacin and clindamycin if penicillin allergic, in combination with a glycopeptide. Urgent and extensive surgical debridement is the cornerstone of management of NF as septic shock and organ failure ensue if necrotic tissue remains. Such cases are likely to require close monitoring and organ support in HDU or ICU settings and should be barrier nursed due to the potential for transmission.

Treatment should again be reviewed regularly and rationalized if an organism is isolated. High-dose benzylpenicillin and clindamycin is the optimal therapy for invasive Group A streptococcal infection. Clindamycin is a protein synthesis inhibitor and inhibits exotoxin production. Intravenous immunoglobulin has also been shown to reduce mortality in streptococcal toxic shock syndrome (TSS), likely due to neutralization of exotoxins. Failure to respond despite adequate antimicrobial therapy should prompt further surgical exploration.

27.11 Further reading

Dryden, M., 'Complicated Skin and Soft Tissue Infection', *Journal of Antimicrobial Chemotherapy*, 65/Suppl 3 (2010), iii35–44.

Lipsky, B. A., Berendt, A. R., Cornia, P. B., Pile, J. C., Peters, E. J. G., Armstrong, D. G., et al., '2012 Infectious Diseases Society of America Clinical Practice Guideline for the Diagnosis and Treatment of Diabetic Foot Infection', *Clinical Infectious Diseases*, 54/12 (2012), 132–173.

Public Health England. Guidance on the Diagnosis and Management of PVL-Associated *Staphylococcus aureus* Infections (PVL-SA) in England. (London, 2008). https://www.gov.uk/

government/uploads/system/uploads/attachment_data/file/322857/Guidance_on_the_
diagnosis_and_management_of_PVL_associated_SA_infections_in_England_2_Ed.pdf

Stevens, D. L., Bisno, A. L., Chambers, H. F., Patchen Dellinger, E., Goldstein, E. J. C., Gorbach,
S. L., et al., 'Practice Guidelines for the Diagnosis and Management of Skin and Soft Tissue
Infection: 2014 Update by the Infectious Diseases Society of America', *Clinical Infectious Diseases*,
59/2 (2014), e10–e52.

27.12 Assessment questions

27.12.1 Question 1

A 72-year-old man presents with a one-day history of feeling unwell. He has diabetes mellitus and
has on-going pain and discharge for a few weeks from his left hallux. He is taking a prolonged course
of flucloxacillin prescribed by his GP. On examination, he is tachycardic and febrile, 39.2°C. There
is a spreading cellulitis around a 3cm ulcer overlying his left hallux and there is bone visible at the
site of the ulcer. Blood cultures are taken.

What is the next most appropriate step in management?
A. Request MRI foot to assess for osteomyelitis.
B. Start IV co-amoxiclav and request urgent vascular review.
C. Start IV flucloxacillin and monitor progress.
D. Withhold antibiotics until blood culture result is known.
E. Withhold antibiotics until tissues has been sent for microbiology.

27.12.2 Question 2

A 25-year-old healthcare assistant has been given a course of antibiotics by his GP for an abscess of
his right middle finger. He has been treated with antibiotics in the community but unfortunately has
re-presented with an infected lesion on his left forearm. This is drained and sent for microbiology
which isolated PVL-*Staphylococcus aureus*.

What is the most appropriate advice after antibiotics and decolonization?
A. Repeat screen one week post-decolonization and return to work once lesion has healed.
B. Repeat screen on last day of treatment and return to work if negative.
C. Repeat screen one week post-decolonization and return to work after three negative screens.
D. Return to work after completion of course of antibiotics.
E. Return to work immediately.

27.12.3 Question 3

A 62-year-old gardener presents with a six-week history of lumps over her left leg. She reports that
the first lesion evolved and had previously ulcerated but now presents as a hard red nodule. She has
further nodules which appear to have a lymphatic distribution. She is not immunocompromised and
has no recent travel history. A biopsy is taken and treatment is started based on the microbiology
and histology results.

What is the most appropriate treatment for this condition?
A. Dapsone for six months.
B. Doxycycline for four to six weeks.
C. Intralesional cidofovir until lesions have resolved
D. Itraconazole for two to four weeks after the lesions have resolved.
E. Pegylated interferon weekly for three months.

27.13 Answers and discussion

27.13.1 Answer 1

B. Start iv co-amoxiclav and request urgent vascular review.

IDSA use PEDIS to grade diabetic foot infections—**P**erfusion, **E**xtent (size), **D**epth (tissue loss), **I**nfection, **S**ensation (neuropathy). This man's infection meets Grade 4, and in this case, broad-spectrum empirical antibiotics are recommended. A foot X-ray is a non-invasive modality to assess early on for underlying osteomyelitis and or soft tissue gas. Vascular input should be sought early as early debridement may decrease the likelihood of future more extensive amputations.

27.13.2 Answer 2

A. Repeat screen one week post-decolonization and return to work once lesion has healed.

PVL-*Staphylococcus aureus* is a notifiable disease. Decolonization followed by repeat screening is appropriate in a healthcare setting due to the risk to patients. Decolonization should take place once skin lesions are healed and repeat screening should occur one week following decolonization. If the repeat screen is positive, then a second round of topical decolonization should occur. Repeated positive screens despite decolonization may be due to persistent shedding from skin lesions, or recolonization from a close contact in the community. A healthcare worker with a persistent positive screen may return to work if no active skin lesions. DNA fingerprinting should be performed in healthcare outbreaks to determine strain relatedness.

27.13.3 Answer 3

D. Itraconazole for two to four weeks after the lesions have resolved.

The diagnosis of this patient is sporotrichosis, which is caused by the dimorphic fungus *Sporothrix schenckii* and itraconazole is the most appropriate treatment. Sporotrichosis usually manifests as a subacute or chronic infection of the cutaneous and subcutaneous tissues. Inoculation via soil is the usual route. Presentation is usually a painless papule appearing at the site of inoculation, which may ulcerate. Similar lesions crop up along lymphatic channels.

CHAPTER 28

Bone and joint infections

Jayshree Dave and Rohma Ghani

28.1 The three most common presentations of bone and joint infections

Patients with bone and joint infections can present with native joint septic arthritis, osteomyelitis, or implant-associated bone and joint infections.

28.2 Presentation of septic arthritis

Patients often present with an acute onset of hot, swollen, painful joint with restricted function in one or more joints over a couple of weeks. On examination the affected joint is painful with a limited range of movement, and fever is present. Risk factors for septic arthritis include an abnormal joint architecture due to pre-existing joint disease, e.g. patients with rheumatoid arthritis, or patients on haemodialysis, with diabetes mellitus, or older than 80 years of age. The differential diagnosis includes reactive arthritis, pre-patellar bursitis, gout, Lyme disease, brucellosis, and Whipples disease.

28.3 Pathogens causing septic arthritis

Staphylococcus aureus is the most common cause of septic arthritis, followed by Group A streptococcus and other haemolytic streptococci including B, C and G. Gram-negative rods such as *Escherichia coli* are implicated in the elderly, immunosuppressed, or patients with comorbidities. *Pseudomonas aeruginosa* is implicated in intravenous (IV) drug users and patients post-surgery or intra-articular injections. *Kingella kingae* causes septic arthritis in children younger than four years of age. *Neisseria gonorrhoeae, Neisseria meningitidis*, and *Salmonella* species can also cause septic arthritis as part of a disseminated infection. Septic monoarthritis commonly occurs in patients with disseminated gonococcal infection.

28.4 Laboratory investigation of a patient with septic arthritis

Blood cultures, white blood cell count, C reactive protein (CRP), electrolytes, and liver function tests are indicated. Serial CRP is useful in monitoring response to treatment. If there is a history of unprotected sexual intercourse, gonococcal testing is recommended. Brucella serology and *Tropheryma whippei* serology may be considered based on the clinical history. Joint fluid aspiration should be performed by a specialist within the hospital. Joint fluid aspirate is processed in the laboratory for microscopy, culture, and sensitivity. Gram stain can show an increase in neutrophils and presence of bacteria.

28.5 Treating septic arthritis

The guidelines provided by the British Society for Rheumatology on the management of hot swollen joints in adults has provided advice for empirical treatment for suspected septic arthritis, but the local antibiotic policy should also be considered. Initial treatment is with intravenous flucloxacillin 2g four times daily, or 450–600mg four times daily of intravenous clindamycin to cover *S. aureus*. A second-generation or third-generation cephalosporin is suggested for gram-negative cover. In patients with suspected meningococcal or gonococcal infection, ceftriaxone is recommended and subsequent length and choices are based upon local policy. Treatment for patients with IV drug use or patients admitted to the intensive care unit should be discussed with the microbiologist. Recommended duration of treatment is two weeks of IV antibiotics followed by four weeks of oral antibiotics. Oral antibiotics such as linezolid and ciprofloxacin with high tissue concentrations can be used after a shorter course of IV therapy. Some studies have demonstrated that recurrences did not occur with a reduced length of treatment, providing adequate drainage had occurred and that the patients were not immunocompromised. Shorter durations varying from seven to twenty-one days may be suitable in immunocompetent patients with a good washout of the joint.

28.6 Defining osteomyelitis

Osteomyelitis is an infective process involving progressive destruction of bone with sequestrum formation. There are currently two classifications of osteomyelitis: the Cierny Mader system and the Lee and Waldvogel system. The Cierny Mader system is useful for guiding therapy and is based upon the assessment of the bone and the physiological status of the individual. Stage one involves infection of the medulla and can be managed with antimicrobial treatment whereas stage four is associated with diffuse osteomyelitis and surgical intervention. The Lee Waldvogel method informs as to whether the infection is acute or chronic, whether the infection is haematogenous or contiguous, and level of vascular insufficiency, and does not provide guidance on treatment.

28.7 Pathogens implicated in osteomyelitis

Over half the infections are caused by *S. aureus* and coagulase-negative staphylococci. However, streptococci, enterococci, and gram-negative bacilli such as *Enterobacter, P. aeruginosa*, and *E. coli* can also cause infection. *S. aureus* is a common cause of osteomyelitis in children with bacteraemia, in the elderly, and in patients with IV catheters. Vertebral osteomyelitis and spondylodiscitis are acquired following bacteraemia or following surgery. Pathogens implicated are *S. aureus*, coagulase-negative staphylococci, *Mycobacterium tuberculosis*, and *Brucella* species.

Children with sickle cell anaemia are at risk of osteomyelitis and septic arthritis particularly with salmonella and *S. aureus*, and often have a history of localized bony pain and a high white cell count, which can be used to distinguish it from a bone infarct. Common pathogens encountered in IV drug users include *S. aureus* and *P. aeruginosa*. Fungal osteomyelitis is uncommon.

28.8 Managing osteomyelitis

Osteomyelitis is a clinical diagnosis with the radiology and microbiology results helping to confirm the diagnosis. X-rays, while inexpensive, have a low negative predictive value, but CT and MRI scans are now routinely used in clinical care. CT-guided biopsy is useful for the diagnosis of infection. Experimental studies have demonstrated that prolonged treatment is crucial in eradicating infection, as *S. aureus* can remain dormant in osteoblasts for a prolonged period of time as it is non–susceptible to antimicrobials. Osteomyelitis in patients with diabetes mellitus is often polymicrobial and may involve an exposed bone or following an ulcer in the overlying skin. Native, acute, and chronic osteomyelitis is treated with antimicrobial therapy for four to six weeks and may necessitate surgical debridement of dead bone and surrounding tissue. The implicated pathogen will guide choice of therapy. Osteomyelitis of a contaminated open fracture requires open surgery, aggressive wound debridement, and insertion of a metal implant. Antimicrobial prophylaxis with co-amoxiclav should be given until soft tissue closure or for a maximum of seventy-two hours only. Children require a shorter parenteral period (minimum forty-eight hours) and up to three weeks of total therapy.

28.9 The two main groups of implant-associated infections

The two main groups of implant-associated infections are peri-prosthetic joint infections (PJI) and internal fixation-associated infections.

28.10 Managing prosthetic joint infections

Implants are at high risk of infection and a low bacterial inoculum can easily cause infection. Biofilm producing-organisms present a challenge and rifampicin (active against gram-positive cocci) and ciprofloxacin are bactericidal. Management of a prosthetic joint infection requires a multidisciplinary approach involving specialists from the departments of orthopaedics, infection, and pharmacy. A patient with PJI may present with acute painful joint post-surgery, sinus, loose prosthesis, erythema or serous discharge post operatively, or wound breakdown. Plain X-rays cannot differentiate between a loosened prosthesis and an infected prosthesis.

There are four treatment options based upon the clinical, laboratory, and surgical parameters. The procedure for debridement and retention of implant (DAIR) involves surgical debridement and radical excision of infected tissue followed by exchange of modular components (femoral head and acetabular liner in total hip arthroplasty) and wound irrigation. This procedure is appropriate for patients with a short duration of symptoms (less than three weeks) or within four weeks of implantation. The implant must be stable, an absent sinus tract, and the organism must be susceptible to commonly used antimicrobial agents. Similar outcomes have been described for antibiotic therapy duration of either six or twelve weeks.

In a single-stage revision surgery all infected tissue and implanted components are removed and a new implant is inserted. This procedure is often considered when there the surrounding soft tissue is healthy and the organism is known. Parenteral antibiotics are given for a minimum of two weeks followed by oral antibiotics for a total period of three months for hip revisions and six months for knee revision surgery.

In a two-stage procedure, the infected tissue and implanted components are removed. Four to six samples are each taken with a new set of instruments and six weeks of antibiotics are given followed by repeat sampling and insertion of the prosthesis to ensure clearance of the infection.

Conservative management is considered when the patient is not fit for surgery and the patient is given antibiotics for life. Deep tissue samples are crucial for determining the antimicrobial susceptibilities for the pathogens for prolonged treatment.

28.11 Further reading and useful resources

British Orthopaedic Association Standards for Trauma http://www.boa.ac.uk/publications/boa-standards-trauma-boasts/

Coakley, G., Mathews, C., Field, M., Jones, A., Kingsley, G., Walker, D., et al., 'BSR & BHPR, BOA, RCGP and BSAC Guidelines for Management of the Hot Swollen Joint in Adults', *Rheumatology*, 45/8 (2006), 1039–1041. https://doi.org/10.1093/rheumatology/kel163a

Chaussade, H., Uçkay, I., Vuagnat, A., Druon, J., Gras, G., Rosset, P., Lipsky, B. A., Bernard, L., 'Antibiotic therapy duration for prosthetic joint infections treated by Debridement and Implant Retention (DAIR): Similar long-term remission for 6 weeks as compared to 12 weeks', *International Journal of Infectious Diseases*, 63(2017), 37–42. doi: 10.1016/j.ijid.2017.08.002.

28.12 Assessment questions

28.12.1 Question 1

A forty-eight-year-old man with renal carcinoma, bilateral nephrectomy, failed renal transplant, on dialysis, and non-insulin dependent diabetes mellitus is admitted with a right hip fracture. Initially he had a right dynamic hip screw insertion, but continues to have pain and serous discharge from the hip. Wound swab grows *Enterobacter cloacae* and coagulase-negative staphylococcus. He has had a hip washout and removal of screw and insertion of a spacer the previous week. Four deep tissue samples from the right hip have grown an *Enterobacter cloacae* sensitive only to meropenem. The patient had been commenced on teicoplanin and meropenem empirically following the wound swab result.

What is the recommended continuation treatment for this patient?
A. Continue meropenem for six weeks and stop teicoplanin.
B. Continue meropenem and switch teicoplanin to co-amoxiclav for four weeks.
C. Continue meropenem and switch teicoplanin to vancomycin for six weeks.
D. Continue meropenem and teicoplanin for six weeks.
E. Stop meropenem and start ciprofloxacin for six weeks.

28.12.2 Question 2

A sixty-eight-year-old man presents with a painful right lower leg. He was involved in a road traffic accident in Morocco when his motorbike collided with a car. His open tibial fracture was debrided and nailed in Morocco, but he continues to have a sharp pain on weight bearing and on examination there is a purulent discharge from the wound. Clinical examination shows a discharging sinus and MRI of the leg shows a collection and sequestrum in the tibia with a non-union and lucency around the nail. Wound swab shows *S. aureus*, which is sensitive to flucloxacillin. The patient is clinically stable.

What is the recommended treatment for this patient?
A. Amputation of the affected limb.
B. Commence co-amoxiclav and fusidic acid for twelve weeks.
C. Commence flucloxacillin for six weeks.
D. Organize a septic screen and start meropenem.
E. Wound exploration, debridement, and excision of dead bone.

28.12.3 Question 3

A seventy-nine-year-old lady underwent a total hip replacement in 2015. She presents to the orthopaedic team with an eight-month history of pain on weight bearing. On examination serous fluid is seen discharging from the wound. An ultrasound guided aspiration grows a coagulase-negative staphylococcus sensitive to glycopeptides, ciprofloxacin, rifampicin, and fusidic acid. She undergoes a single-stage revision and receives high dose IV teicoplanin and oral rifampicin for six weeks. She returns to clinic for her 6-week post operative assessment. She is doing well and the hip is pain free.

What is the most appropriate next step in the management of this patient?
A. Continue teicoplanin and rifampicin for a further 6 weeks.
B. Continue teicoplanin alone for a further six weeks.
C. Stop Teicoplanin and continue rifampicin alone for a further 6 weeks.
D. Give oral ciprofloxacin and rifampicin for a further 6 weeks.
E. Stop all antibiotics.

28.13 Answers and discussion

28.13.1 Answer 1

A. Continue meropenem for six weeks and stop teicoplanin.
This patient had a fracture of his right hip which was ultimately managed as a two-stage procedure. *Enterobacter* is a beta lactamase-producing organism and is often highly resistant to betalactams and cephalosporins, but usually sensitive to carbapenems. For this patient, the treatment was rationalized to meropenem therapy only as no gram-positive organisms were isolated. Treatment is based upon deep tissue samples rather than on wound swabs. It is therefore not necessary to cover the coagulase-negative staphylococcus isolated in the wound swab. The organism can also be resistant to quinolones and as the organism is only sensitive to meropenem, ciprofloxacin cannot be used for treatment of infection. Carbapenem use for the treatment of infections in general is restricted and, in this situation, if the organism was sensitive to ciprofloxacin then providing there were no issues with absorption the patient could have been given oral ciprofloxacin for six weeks. Six weeks' treatment (at least two weeks given intravenously) is indicated between the first and second stage revision arthroplasty.

28.13.2 Answer 2

E. Wound exploration, debridement, and excision of dead bone.
Open fractures of the lower limb require combined management with the orthopaedic team and the plastics team. Open wound fractures can be contaminated with environmental organisms and are managed with open surgery and insertion of a metal implant. Key intervention is to remove the dead bone and send deep samples for culture. Prophylaxis for surgery comprises intravenous co-amoxiclav with the first dose given within three hours. The antibiotic is continued until soft tissue closure or for a maximum of seventy-two hours. If patients are allergic then intravenous clindamycin should be considered. Deep tissue samples or fluids are the mainstay of diagnosis and wound swabs can result in the use of an inappropriate antibiotic as it represents superficial colonization rather than deep infection.

28.13.3 Answer 3

D. Give oral ciprofloxacin and rifampicin for a further 6 weeks.

A single-stage revision surgery is considered when there is good condition of the soft tissue, absence of comorbidities, and the micro-organisms are sensitive to commonly used antimicrobials. There is little evidence to support single-stage versus two-stage exchange and practices vary between centres, probably based upon surgeon experience. For single-stage revision of an infected hip prosthesis, following a two-to-six weeks initial intravenous treatment, a total of three months' therapy is recommended to complete the course. This is extended for six months for single-stage knee implants. In a two-stage exchange, two to six weeks' of antibiotics are given between the first and the second stage and the length of subsequent antibiotics is based upon the culture results of tissues taken at the second stage. Antibiotic options for continuation therapy should include agents that are well absorbed orally and have anti-biofilm activity (rifampicin and quinolones). Rifampicin should never be used as a single agent as resistance develops rapidly.

CHAPTER 29

Upper and lower respiratory tract infections

Simon Tiberi

CONTENTS

29.1 Causes, complications, and management of pharyngitis

Pharyngitis is common with incidence peaking from autumn to spring. Respiratory viruses are most commonly implicated, and are generally self-limiting conditions not requiring diagnostic workup or treatment.

Bacterial pharyngitis is less common, is spread by droplets or direct transmission, and *Streptococcus pyogenes* (Group A strep, or GAS) is the most frequent cause. *Haemophilus influenzae*, *Mycoplasma pneumoniae*, and *Neisseria gonorrhoeae* are less frequent causes.

Rapid antigen detection tests make the point-of-care assessment of GAS pharyngitis possible, although a negative test does not exclude infection. No method can distinguish oropharyngeal colonization from actual infection, but culture can obtain antibiotic susceptibility testing. Suspicion of infection with *Neisseria gonorrhoeae*, *Bordetella pertussis*, *Haemophilus influenzae*, *Mycoplasma pneumoniae*, *Chlamydophila pneumoniae*, or *Corynebacterium diptheriae* should be communicated to the laboratory so that the appropriate culture media is utilized.

The Centor criteria provide a clinical predictive score that can give the likelihood a sore throat is due to a bacterial infection with the following: the presence of tonsillar exudate, tender anterior cervical adenopathy, fever over 38°C, and absence of cough. If three or four of these criteria are met, the positive predictive value is 40% to 60%. The absence of three or four of the Centor criteria has a relatively high negative predictive value of 80%, and may be use to evaluate whether antibiotics can be withheld or deferred. Oral penicillin or macrolide are used to treat streptococcal pharyngitis. Treatment may reduce severity, duration, transmission, and risk of post-infectious sequelae like rheumatic heart disease and post-streptococcal glomerulonephritis. Other complications include scarlet fever, streptococcal toxic shock syndrome, and quinsy.

29.2 Causes and management of otitis media

Otitis media, is frequent in the young children, possibly due to a short and horizontal Eustachian tube. Purulent material buils up leading to a bulging, red tympanic membrane which may rupture and discharge. Intense local pain and fevers may occur. *Streptococcus pneumoniae*, *Moraxella catarrhalis*, and *Haemophilus influenzae* are frequently implicated. Frequently there are no sequelae, although complications include hearing impairment, and less common are mastoiditis, bacteraemia, and meningitis. Diagnosis is clinical based on presentation and otoscopic examination. Microbiological diagnosis is possible through culture of exuate on swab or following tympanocentesis. Treatment is with nasal decongestants and antimicrobial agents (e.g. oral amoxicillin or clarithromycin for ten days). Pneumococcal vaccination has a (modest) role in prevention.

29.3 Causes and treatment of acute sinusitis

Acute sinusitis is the infection of the paranasal sinuses, and in the majority of cases in adults and children it is of viral aetiology and is self-limiting, requiring only symptomatic treatment. If the duration is more than ten days, it is likelier to be bacterial in aetiology, with *Streptococcus pneumoniae*, *Haemophilus influenzae*, and *Moraxella catarrhalis* the major aetiological agents. Diagnosis is guided by symptoms. Imaging can confirm the diagnosis by showing opacification of maxillary or frontal sinuses but is reserved for suspicion of complications. Microbiological diagnosis requires samples from nasal endoscopy. Culture for fungi should also be considered especially in the immunosuppressed or in unresolving cases.

Treatment with nasal decongestants may improve drainage and foster resolution. Amoxicillin, amoxicillin/clavulanic acid, or clarithromycin are used to treat severe forms or immunocompromised patients for ten to fourteen days, with surgery possibly indicated in persistent or severe cases.

29.4 Causes and treatment of bronchitis

Bronchitis can be classified as acute bronchitis, and acute exacerbation of chronic bronchitis.

Acute bronchitis involves a cough and sputum production but no changes on chest X-ray. The large majority of these infections are viral in origin, most commonly caused by rhinovirus, parainfluenzae, and influenza virus. *Mycoplasma pneumonia* and *Bordetella pertussis* are less common but important bacterial causes.

During acute exacerbation of chronic bronchitis, a chronic productive cough changes to become productive of larger quantities of purulent sputum. This may be caused by infection with one of the respiratory viruses, *Streptococcus pneumoniae*, *Moraxella catarrhalis*, or *Haemophilus influenzae*.

Viral swabs for respiratory viruses can be considered. A sputum culture is unlikely to be of true diagnostic value as sputum isolates correlate poorly with the lower respiratory tract, it is therefore not routinely recommended as it may lead to unnecessary or over treatment.

In children, infection of the lower airway causes bronchiolitis, which is typically caused by respiratory syncytial virus (RSV) and results in seasonal outbreaks in temperate climate areas every winter among young children. Premature infants, particularly those with chronic lung or congenital heart disease, are most vulnerable. Monthly administration of a monoclonal antibody (palivizumab) during the epidemic months may serve as passive prophylaxis for these susceptible infants.

Chronic obstructive pulmonary disease (COPD) sufferers may benefit from a few days' treatment with an antibacterial agent (e.g. oral amoxicillin, doxycycline, or macrolide), but many other patients will not experience any benefit from therapy. Patients with high risk of cardiac or respiratory failure should be vaccinated against pneumococcal infection and influenza.

29.5 Managing community-acquired pneumonia (CAP)

CAP is defined as an onset either before or within forty-eight hours of hospital admission. Pneumonia is one of the common causes of death worldwide. A patient will typically present top with a cough and fever. CAP impairs respiratory function. Ideally patients should be assessed with blood cultures, a chest X-ray, and the CURB-65 score, An HIV test should be offered. The identity of the infective agent is frequently elusive, and therefore empirical antimicrobial therapy should be started while microbiological tests are in progress, which varies based on local epidemiology and resistance patterns. Agents should be selected for their action against the most likely pathogens and given by the route and dose that guarantees maximum antimicrobial effect. Response to therapy should be monitored carefully.

CURB-65 is a six-point score based on information available at initial hospital assessment; one point for each for Confusion, Urea > 7 mmol/l, Respiratory rate $\geq$ 30/min, low systolic (< 90mmHg) or diastolic ($\leq$ 60 mmHg) Blood pressure, and age $\geq$ 65 years (CURB-65 score). CURB-65 enables patients to be stratified according to increasing risk of mortality or need for hospital or intensive care admission (Score 0, 0.7%; Score 1, 3.2%; Score 2, 13%; Score 3, 17%; Score 4, 41.5%, and Score 5, 57% mortality).

S. pneumoniae, S. aureus, S. pyogenes, Legionella pneumophila, H. influenzae, Chlamydophila pneumoniae, Mycoplasma pneumoniae, and viruses are common causative agents. Although less common and rare, other possible agents of CAP include Coxiella burnetii, Chlamydophila psittaci, Burkholderia pseudomallei, Paragonimus westermani, Histoplasma sp., Cryptococcus gatti, and Strongyloides stercoralis. Patient history and risk factors are essential for diagnosing these infections.

Aspiration pneumonia follows aspiration of oral or gastric contents, and where initial injury is usually caused by chemical or mechanical insult the infection develops after forty-eight to seventy-two hours—chest X-ray changes either in the lower right lobe or, if supine, the apex of right lower lobe—due to bacterial damage resulting from oral streptococci or anaerobes and will require an agent with anaerobic cover.

Polysaccharide and conjugate polyvalent vaccines can prevent pneumococcal pneumonia and are offered to those at greatest risk: age > 65 years, presence of heart disease, those with chronic renal failure, and the splenectomized.

29.6 Hospital-acquired pneumonia (HAP) and its management

Hospital-acquired pneumonia (HAP) is defined as onset more than forty-eight hours after admission with the following: fever, new pulmonary infiltrate, elevated white cell count, and respiratory symptoms including cough, sputum production, dyspnoea, positive Gram stain, or culture of respiratory secretions.

Pneumonia is the third most common hospital-acquired infection, but the most lethal, with mortality ranging from 8–40%. It is most likely to affect patients with existing respiratory disease or following operations, and ventilated patients (ventilator-associated pneumonia, VAP).

While HAP is pneumonia manifesting forty-eight hours after admission, it also can be further split into early onset HAP with mainly community pathogens, and into late onset HAP after five days of admission, most often caused by P. aeruginosa, S. aureus, and the Enterobacteriaceae via a process of colonization and aspiration from upper GI and oropharynx (most common). Other routes include inhalation of aerosols containing pathogenic organisms from the respiratory equipment or person-person transmission; hematogenous spread from a distant body site; translocation of gut flora; cross-contamination from gloves, hands, devices; and contaminated hospital water supply. Colonization occurs in 30–40% of hospitalized patients and 60–75% of ITU patients. Rarely, Legionella or respiratory viruses are implicated.

Mechanically ventilated patients' respiratory tracts are at risk of colonization with bacteria from the lower GI tract (favoured by reflux and proton pump inhibitor use) and the oropharynx. The organisms enter the trachea along the outside of the tracheal tube. Occasionally, bacteria from the mechanical ventilator and other respiratory support devices get into the lungs via the lumen of the tracheal tube. Most of the infections are Gram negative, and the most common culprits are *Pseudomonas aeruginosa, Staphylococcus aureus, Streptococcus sp., Klebsiella sp., Escherichia coli, Fusobacterium* sp., *Enterobacter sp., Bacteroides sp.,* and *Proteus sp.* Polymicrobial infections are frequent.

The risk of developing pneumonia is twenty times higher than in non-ventilated patients, with a risk of 3% per patient day of developing a chest infection; VAP is the most commonly acquired infection in the ITU. Crude mortality from this condition is from 25–70%. Mortality is highest with *Acinetobacter sp.* and multi-drug resistant (MDR) *Pseudomonas aeruginosa.*

The diagnosis of HAP may be subtler in in-patients with multiple co-morbidities. Chest imaging on acutely deteriorating in-patients is frequently required to rule in or exclude the diagnosis. Making a diagnosis of VAP may be even more challenging, as the presence of radiological infiltrates, increasing oxygen requirement, fever, raised inflammatory markers could point to an infection in another organ or a non-infective process, i.e. pulmonary oedema. Scores like the Clinical Pulmonary Infection Score (CPIS), can be useful to assist in the diagnosis of VAP, it uses temperature, white cell count, tracheal secretions, PO/FiO2 mmHg, chest radiography and tracheal aspirate culture to give a probability score for VAP. Surrogate markers like procalcitonin can also play a role in diagnosis. However, sensitivity is around 80% leading to some false negatives; the test is perhaps more valuable in determining the duration of antibiotics when a reduction in procalcitonin level can be appreciated on effective antimicrobial therapy and can be an effective stewardship tool.

Invasive techniques for diagnosis of VAP are no longer recommended as they may cause trauma and worsen respiratory failure through lavage, only blind bronchoscopy or endotracheal aspiration should be used in intubated patients.

Antimicrobial treatment is commonly tailored to the local susceptibility patterns, anti-pseudomonal coverage should be present in empirical treatment when treating VAP, given mortality rates reaching 27-43% with this pathogen. If there are high rates (>10%) of MDR *Pseudomonas*, two anti-Pseudomonal agents should be used empirically until the isolate and susceptibilities are available before stepping down to one active agent. HAP/VAP in most instances should be treated for no longer than seven days, in certain instances, shorter courses of 5 days may be given.

There is as yet no highly effective preventive strategy against HAP and VAP. However, several measures can be adopted to reduce incidence and mortality.

Once drug-resistant (*Acinetobacter*, MDR *Pseudomonas*) or virulent pathogens (TB, influenza, MERS, SARS) are isolated, infected patients should be isolated to reduce transmission onwards and units. Physicians must continue to have a high index of suspicion of nosocomial pneumonia in order to diagnose and treat them early and minimise the risk of hospital spread.

29.7 Further reading and useful resources

Kalil, A. C., Metersky, M. L., Klompas, M., Muscedere, J., Sweeney, D. A., Palmer, L. B., et al., 'American Thoracic Society, Infectious Diseases Society of America. Management of Adults with Hospital-Acquired and Ventilator-Associated Pneumonia: 2016 Clinical Practice Guidelines by the Infectious Diseases Society of America and the American Thoracic Society', *Clinical Infectious Diseases*, 63 (2016), 1–51.

NICE 191. Pneumonia in Adults: Diagnosis and Management. December 2014. https://www.nice.org.uk/guidance/cg191

Woodhead, M., Blasi, F., Ewig, S., Garau, J., Huchon, G., Ieven, M., et al., 'Guidelines for the Management of Adult Lower Respiratory Tract Infections', *Clinical Microbiology and Infection*, 17/Suppl. 6 (2011), E1–E59.

29.8 Assessment questions

29.8.1 Question 1

A seventy-six-year-old care home resident is admitted with a one-day history of shortness of breath and is apyrexial. Her past medical history includes hypertension, insulin-dependent diabetes, and vascular dementia. She has no known allergies. She is reported to have vomited her lunch the day before, but was well up till then.

Chest X ray:	No consolidation.

What is the most appropriate management for this patient?
A. Intravenous cefuroxime and metronidazole.
B. Intravenous metronidazole.
C. Oral amoxicillin and metronidazole.
D. Oral ciprofloxacin and metronidazole.
E. Supportive care no antibiotics.

29.8.2 Question 2

A twenty-nine-year-old, HIV-positive man, who was born in the UK, attended a drop-in clinic two days after returning from a holiday in Spain. On clinical examination, he is tachycardic 110/min, febrile at 38.5°C with a respiratory rate of 25/min. Blood test shows a white cell count of 17,500/L (Neutrophil 90%). It is known that his HIV was well controlled with a CD4 count two months ago of 550 cells/μL (29%) and undetectable viral load. His urea is mildly raised. A chest X-ray demonstrates right middle and upper lobe consolidation. Urinary antigens have returned showing legionella negative, pneumococcal antigen positive.

What is the most appropriate antimicrobial agent for treating this patient?
A. Amoxicillin/clavulanic acid and clarithromycin.
B. Ceftriaxone.
C. Cotrimoxazole.
D. Levofloxacin.
E. Meropenem.

29.8.3 Question 3

A forty-eight-year-old Canadian woman living in London for the past year develops pneumonia and is admitted following a two-day illness. Her most recent foreign travel was to Ontario twelve months ago.

Investigations performed include blood cultures (before antibiotic), Pneumococcal and Legionella urinary antigens, *Mycoplasma*, *Coxiella burnetii* , and Histoplasma serology.

Which infection can be excluded based on her history and a negative result of her investigations?
A. *Coxiella burnetii*.
B. *Histoplasma capsulatum*.
C. *Legionella pneumophila*.
D. *Mycoplasma pneumoniae*.
E. *Streptococcus pneumoniae*.

29.9 Answers and discussion

29.9.1 Answer 1

E. Supportive care, no antibiotics.
The patient has *ab ingestis* but there is no evidence of pneumonia, and it is likely that the initial chemical insult of the aspiration has led to her symptoms and her admission, although there is

currently no infection to treat. It is likely that the patient may require antibiotic treatment seventy-two hours from the episode. However, antibiotic treatment from the outset does not appear to reduce the frequency of pneumonia and may select for resistant micro-organisms.

29.9.2 Answer 2

B. Ceftriaxone.
Penicillin resistance in the UK varies from 1.7 to 5% in pneumococci. In Europe, Spain has a higher prevalence of penicillin resistance of over 45%. Resistance rates to cephalosporins like cefotaxime and ceftriaxone, however, remain low < 1% in these nations.

The macrolide accompanying the beta-lactam in many empirical regimens may not be effective given significant resistance rates to this class of antibiotics, which is independent of penicillin resistance.

The CD4 count above 500 and compliance with antiretrovirals as well as the chest X-ray findings make *Pneumocystis jirovecii* pneumonia unlikely. The increasing prevalence of pneumococcal isolates resistant to trimethoprim-sulfamethoxazole precludes its use.

Fluoroquinolones are generally sufficient. However, widespread use in certain settings has demonstrated rapid take-up of resistance. Meropenem is effective against *S. pneumoniae*; however, the carbapenems should only be employed in exceptional circumstances (allergy or resistance to other molecules).

29.9.3 Answer 3

B. *Histoplasma capsulatum*.
Although this woman is originally from an area in Canada where she may have contracted histoplasmosis, the incubation period for acute pulmonary histoplasmosis is three weeks. A negative serology result also excludes the infection which would have occurred more than twelve months ago when she last travelled to Canada.

Legionella urinary antigen only detects *Legionella pneumophila* type 1. Though this accounts for 80% of infections with this species, it does not entirely exclude the diagnosis. Blood cultures are positive in 15–30% of patients with *S. pneumoniae* pneumonia, pneumococcal urinary antigen detection being the more sensitive test. Mycoplasma serology may be used, although Mycoplasma PCR is favoured, and a negative result does not exclude mycoplasma infection. Serology for any acute respiratory infection is likely to be negative early in the illness and is best detected some two to four weeks after onset of symptoms. Antibody responses against *C. burnetii* are detectable in patients seven days into infection and a negative result in the early stage of disease does not exclude the diagnosis.

CHAPTER 30

Gastro-intestinal, hepatic, pancreatic, and biliary infections

Anna Riddell, C. Y. William Tong, and Michael Millar

CONTENTS

30.1 Bacterial flora of the gastro-intestinal tract (GIT) and its importance

The gastro-intestinal tract (GIT) hosts the most numerous and diverse reservoir of microbes in humans. There is increasing interest in the relationship between the GIT microbiome and human health. Obesity, diabetes, allergy, and a number of inflammatory diseases have been linked with the human GIT microbiome.

Infections of the GIT arise either as a result of a change in the relationship between the commensal microbes colonizing the GIT (endogenous infection) or entry in to the GIT of a micro-organism which causes disease (exogenous infection). Commensals most commonly invade host tissues as a result of compromised defensive barriers. Disease associated with exogenous infection can be toxin-mediated, or associated with local or systemic invasion of the host. Endogenous infections are usually polymicrobial.

30.2 Common infections in the upper GIT

30.2.1 Infection of the mouth

In the mouth the aetiology, presentation, and anatomical associations have led to the description of a number of syndromes. Peritonsillar infection with involvement of the internal jugular vein is Lemierre's syndrome, which is particularly associated with infection with *Fusobacterium necrophorum*. 'Trench mouth' is a severe form of ulcerative gingivitis, so named because in the absence of oral hygiene it was a relatively common diagnosis among those in the trenches during the First World

War. Ludwig's angina is a severe infection of the floor of the mouth which spreads in to the sub-mandibular and sub-lingual space, often following a tooth-related infection. Deep neck infections are more common in children than adults and can involve the parapharyngeal, retropharyngeal, peri-tonsillar, or sub-mandibular spaces. Children with deep neck infections are more likely than adults to present with cough and respiratory distress.

30.2.2 Infections of the oesophagus

Oesophagitis has a wide range of potential aetiologies. Fungi (particularly Candida species) are probably the most common microbial cause of oesophagitis. Fungal infection of the distal oesophagus is thought to play an important role in the pathogenesis of disseminated fungal infection. Risk factors for fungal infection include poor oral intake, exposure to antibiotics, immunocompromise (HIV, steroids, cancer treatments), gastric acid suppressants, and damage to mucosal integrity (naso-gastric tubes, acid reflux, varices). Bacteria (including Mycobacteria, Actinomycetes, Treponemes), parasites, and viruses (herpes simplex, cytomegalovirus) are rarer infectious causes of oesophagitis.

30.2.3 Gastritis

Helicobacter pylori is one of the commonest causes of gastritis and of human infection globally. Poor socio-economic conditions in childhood seem to be a major determinant of acquisition. The incidence is declining in northern Europe and North America. Infection with *Helicobacter pylori* is a major risk factor for both peptic ulcer disease and for the development of gastric cancer. *Helicobacter pylori* produces considerable quantities of urease and this observation has led to a variety of tests for the diagnosis of infection (breath test, Campylobacter-like organism (CLO)-test). A faecal antigen test is widely used both for diagnosis and as a test for eradication. Treatment of *Helicobacter pylori* is an important element in the effective management of peptic ulcer disease. Eradication usually requires treatment with combinations of antibiotics. NICE provides both diagnostic and treatment algorithms.

30.3 Causes of hepatitis

Enteric transmitted hepatitides hepatitis A (HAV) and hepatitis E (HEV) are both commonly transmitted through the faecal-oral route, though they can also both be transmitted by transfusion of blood or blood products, needles, and sexual contact. The UK blood transfusion service has recently started to screen blood donors for HEV RNA and offers HEV-negative blood to transplant recipients.

Parenteral transmitted hepatitis includes hepatitis B (HBV), hepatitis C (HCV), and hepatitis D (HDV or Delta agent).

Many other viruses can cause hepatic inflammation either as part of the primary infection or due to reactivation, e.g. the herpes viruses (HSV, VZV, EBV, CMV) and flaviruses (e.g. yellow fever). Of these, EBV and CMV are the commonest seen and hepatitis is part of the infectious mononucleosis syndrome. The hepatitis associated with different viruses can be fulminant, especially in the immunocompromised host.

30.3.1 Hepatitis A

HAV infection has been associated with water- or food-borne outbreaks although its incidence worldwide is decreasing. Many people from developing countries have asymptomatic hepatitis A during childhood and therefore will be immune. Hepatitis A is a cause of acute viral hepatitis, and the symptoms are those classical of acute hepatitis of any cause, i.e. jaundice, abdominal pain and fever, anorexia, and dislike of cigarettes. It can be fulminant, although it is a rare cause of liver failure.

Inactivated vaccines are available for HAV. In the UK, vaccination is recommended for people travelling to a high-risk area, patients with chronic liver disease and haemophilia, men who have sex with men (MSM), people who inject drugs (PWID), and individuals at risk of occupational exposure. Vaccination is also recommended as post-exposure prophylaxis in those individuals within seven days of a significant exposure. In higher-risk individuals, combination with passive immunization with human immunoglobulin is recommended.

30.3.2 Hepatitis E

There are four genotypes of HEV: 1 and 2 are associated with large water- and food-borne outbreaks in the developing world and deaths due to fulminant hepatitis. Genotypes 3 (in western countries) and 4 (in the Far East) are zoonoses. Transmission is thought to be due to ingestion of infected pork (or pork products) infected pork, although other meats and foods have been implicated, as have blood transfusion and organ donation. A high mortality due to fulminant hepatitis is observed in pregnant women with genotype 1 HEV.

There is no treatment currently available although there are two commercial recombinant vaccines available. The incidence of HEV is increasing and better understood due to development of serological assays (HEV IgG and IgM) and PCR. In the immunosuppressed population, chronic HEV infection (due to genotype 3 infection) can occur and can lead to the rapid development of cirrhosis. Successful treatment with ribavirin has been described.

30.3.3 Hepatitis B

According to the World Health Organization, hepatitis B is the most common viral hepatitis worldwide with most recent estimates of serologic evidence of HBV infection in 240 million people worldwide. Hepatitis B is endemic in many countries across the world, with high prevalence considered greater than 8% hepatitis B surface antigen (HBsAg) positive. HBV is transmitted by blood or sexual contact, vertical or horizontal transmission. The greatest risk of mother to child transmission occurs during delivery. Many countries have added HBV vaccination in their routine childhood vaccination programme, including the UK since 2017. In high-risk cases (e.g. HBeAg positive and/or high viral load), hepatitis B immunoglobulin (HBIG) as well as HBV vaccination is given to the baby. If the mother has a high HBV DNA level greater than 10^7 IU/ml, tenofovir should also be started during the third trimester to reduce the risk of transmission.

Chronic HBV infection is much more common following infection in childhood, in infancy, or perinatally (95% risk) compared to infection as an adult (5%). However, once exposed to HBV although there may be no serological evidence of active infection or a plasma viraemia, the infection is never full cleared due to the presence of covalent-closed-circular DNA (cccDNA) which acts as a mini-chromosome for latent HBV. There is also evidence of incorporation of HBV DNA into the host genome, which may contribute to development of hepatocellular carcinoma (HCC). Thus even in a patient with no evidence of active viral replication, the potential is for HBV reactivation when immunosuppressed. Please refer to national (NICE) and international (EASL) guidelines for management of the different stages.

30.3.4 Hepatitis D

HDV is a defective virus which depends on the HBsAg outer coat of HBV to enter into hepatocytes. It has a small circular RNA genome which encodes the Delta antigen (HDAg). HDV infection is either acquired at the time of infection with HBV (co-infection) or as a superinfection to an individual already chronically infected with HBV. Co-infection is often self-limiting whereas superinfection increases the risk of chronic HBV with rapid progression to cirrhosis. All newly diagnosed HBsAg positive patients need testing to exclude HDV.

30.3.5 Hepatitis C

The consequences of hepatitis C infection are changing rapidly since the discovery of new antivirals that are extremely effective in treatment. It is a blood-borne virus (BBV) although it can also be transmitted via sexual intercourse (particularly in MSM) and vertically (6%). Unlike hepatitis B in adults, up to 80% of adults develop chronic HCV after acquisition. Like HBV, chronic HCV can lead to cirrhosis and increases the risk of HCC. There are six genotypes identified with worldwide distribution and these genotypes dictate an individual's response to both new and older antiviral therapy. As there is no latent mechanism for HCV, eradication through antiviral therapy is possible. A sustained virological response (SVR) is sought which is usually defined as undetectable HCV RNA six months after cessation of treatment course.

30.4 Other non-viral causes of hepatic infection

30.4.1 Hepatic abscess

Liver abscess can arise as a result of spread of infection from the peritoneal cavity secondary to a procedure (such as endoscopy or surgery), trauma (particularly penetrating injuries, e.g. knife wound), or from the blood. Some enteric infections can spread to the liver through the portal circulation and cause an abscess, e.g. *Entamoeba histolytica*. There is a wide range of potential causative agents, including streptococci of the anginosus (milleri) group, *Enterobacteriaceae*, enterococci, staphylococci, fungi, and protozoa. *Klebsiella pneumoniae* can cause a liver abscess in individuals without evidence of predisposing factors. These infections may involve distant sites including the eye and meninges. Effective management of liver abscesses usually requires remediation of underlying risk factors and drainage of the abscess, in addition to the use of antibiotics. Drainage has the additional advantage of providing samples for microbiology, allowing identification of causal agents, and optimization of treatment.

30.4.2 Cholecystitis and cholangitis

Infection of the gallbladder (cholecystitis) and bile ducts (cholangitis) usually arise in association with an underlying structural abnormality of the biliary tract (e.g. gallstones, cirrhosis, surgery, or cancer). *Enterobacteriaceae*, enterococci, anaerobes, and fungi are common causes of biliary sepsis. There is considerable variation in the concentrations of different antibiotics in the bile when given at conventional doses.

Some antibiotics reach concentrations in bile which exceed blood levels substantially and these include piperacillin/tazobactam, amoxycillin/clavulanate, ceftriaxone, and rifampicin. Metronidazole and cefuroxime reach biliary levels close to those found in blood. Aminoglycosides, vancomycin, and carbapenems do not achieve blood levels in bile, but may still reach supra-inhibitory concentrations. Imipenem is particularly poorly excreted in bile.

The extent of biliary excretion determines the concentration of antibiotics that reaches the bowel and the effects on the bowel flora (gut microbiome) when antibiotics are administered intravenously or intramuscularly.

30.5 Causes of peritonitis

Peritonitis can be primary and spontaneous or secondary to perforation of the bowel. Perforation can follow bowel obstruction or inflammatory, infective, or traumatic damage to the bowel wall. Primary peritonitis is associated with conditions that cause ascites and most commonly seen in association with liver failure. Peritonitis is a complication of peritoneal dialysis most commonly cause by *Staphylococcus spp.* but with a very wide range of less common causes. *Streptococcus pneumoniae* can cause a primary peritonitis as a manifestation of systemic disease. Primary peritonitis in patients without risk factors is most common in women and has been attributed to ascending infection through the female genitourinary tract. The treatment of peritonitis depends on the aetiology.

30.6 Specific GIT pathogens

Diarrhoeal diseases are a substantial cause of illness and death globally, particularly in young children.

30.6.1 Salmonella

There are two species of Salmonella: *Salmonella bongori* and *Salmonella enterica*. *Salmonella enterica* has over 2000 serovars, distinguished by lipopolysaccharide (O) and flagellar (H) antigens. Serovars of this species are responsible for the vast majority of human infections. Salmonella are usually separated into typhoidal and non-typhoidal strains based on the clinicopathological, and epidemiological features. Some of the non-typhoidal Salmonella are highly adapted to specific species of animals (such as Choleraesuis in pigs, and Dublin in cattle), but many can be found colonizing and infecting a range of animal hosts. The non-typhoidal Salmonella, such as *Salmonella* Enteritidis and *Salmonella* Typhimurium, cause gastrointestinal disease in humans following their ingestion in contaminated foods. Person-to-person spread can occur among those who are particularly vulnerable. The risk of disseminated infection depends on the serovar (typhoidal > non-typhoidal; Choleraesuis > Enteritidis). Disease caused by non-typhoidal strains develops twelve to thirty-six hours after ingestion of contaminated foods and is usually a self-limiting gastro-enteritis.

Typhoid (*Salmonella enterica* serotype Typhi) and paratyphoid are adapted to cause invasive infection in humans. The incubation period is usually in the range of one to three weeks. The infective inoculum is much lower than for non-typhoidal strains and person to person transmission is more likely. Diarrhoea may not be a feature of disease. There are a wide range of potential associated complications, including intestinal perforation and abscess formation. Early diagnosis requires that typhoid is considered in patients presenting with a recent travel history to an endemic area (such as the Indian subcontinent) and fever. Treatment with ceftriaxone improves outcomes and reduces the risk of chronic disease. Azithromycin is an effective alternative when isolates are sensitive.

30.6.2 Shigella

There are four species of Shigella: *Shigella dysenteriae*, *Shigella boydii*, *Shigella flexnerii*, and *Shigella sonnei*. *S. dysenteriae* is associated with epidemic disease and a substantial mortality rate. *S. boydii* is particularly associated with the Indian sub-continent. *S. flexneri* and *S. sonnei* are widely distributed causes of sporadic cases and clusters. The infective inoculum for Shigella is exceptionally low, so that person-to-person transmission is common. Shigella can be transmitted sexually, particularly among men who have sex with men (MSM). Resistance to amoxicillin or co-trimoxazole is not uncommon among Shigella isolates, and there is evidence of increasing ciprofloxacin and azithromycin resistance. Azithromycin resistance has been reported in a distinct lineage of *S. flexneri* that is spreading globally in MSM.

30.6.3 Campylobacter

The genus Campylobacter has over twenty species and the taxonomy continues to evolve with new species and sub-species. *Campylobacter jejuni* is the most frequently identified species associated with human gastro-intestinal disease globally. A large number of clinical syndromes have been associated with *C. jejuni*, including inflammatory bowel disease, Guillain-Barré, and Miller

Fisher syndromes, Bell's palsy (unilateral facial paralysis), and reactive arthritis. Gastro-enteritis can be complicated by infection spreading to involve many different organ systems. Risk factors for acquisition include international travel, exposure to contaminated food or water (particularly uncooked or poorly cooked poultry), and contact with farm animals.

Campylobacter fetus is the most frequently associated with blood stream infections. It is not clear that antibiotics provide benefit for patients with campylobacter gastro-enteritis. Disseminated infection does require antibiotic therapy, which may need to be prolonged.

30.6.4 *Escherichia coli* O157:H7

E. coli O157:H7 can cause haemorrhagic colitis through the production of one or more cytotoxins (Shiga toxins). Cattle are the major reservoir for this organism. Other serotypes that can produce Shiga toxins include *E. coli* O26, O111, and O103. The infective inoculum is low so infection can spread to close contacts and cause clusters of infection in households and institutional settings. The spectrum of disease ranges from asymptomatic colonization through to severe colitis, haemolytic uraemic syndrome (HUS), and thrombotic thrombocytopenic purpura. Up to 10% of those infected will develop HUS. The role of antibiotics in the treatment of *E. coli* O157:H7 remains controversial.

30.6.5 Rotaviruses

Although numerous viruses are responsible for diarrhoeal symptoms and diarrhoea can be a feature of systemic viral illness, rotaviruses are the most common cause of severe diarrhoeal disease in young children worldwide. Diarrhoeal disease is the second leading cause of death in children in the developing world and therefore implementation of the rotavirus vaccine is a key public health strategy of the World Health Organization, as this could potentially prevent around 500,000 deaths in under fives per year worldwide. The mode of transmission is similar to bacterial pathogens—via contact with another person or with infected water or food. The two vaccines available (Rotarix and Rotateq) are both live attenuated vaccines and are highly effective in preventing rotavirus. Rotarix is offered in the UK as part of routine childhood immunization and is approximately 85% effective at preventing severe rotavirus in the first two years of life, although this is serotype dependent. Post-marketing surveillance detected a small increased risk of intussusception associated with rotavirus vaccine and so due to the known natural peak in incidence of intussusception at five months of age, it is recommended that the two doses of the vaccine are given within the first six months of life (first vaccine should be given aged < 15 weeks). Despite this, the risks risk of severe diarrhoeal disease and death from rotavirus outweigh the very small risk of intussusception.

30.6.6 Noroviruses

Noroviruses (originally Norwalk-like viruses) lead to gastro-enteritis-like symptoms between twelve and forty-eight hours after being exposed. The infection is normally self-limiting but can be serious in young children and older adults leading to severe dehydration. The required inoculum of virus for transmission is extremely low (< 20 particles) where billions of virions are shed by an infected person and this shedding can continue for weeks beyond the resolution of symptoms. Outbreaks of norovirus are problematic in healthcare institutions or other places for social care. Disinfection of bays/beds/wards is key in interrupting transmission and outbreak and requires the use of chlorine-based, rather than alcohol-containing, disinfectants.

30.7 Protozoa and worms as causative agents in enteric infections

Cryptosporidium spp. (usually C. hominis or C. parvum) cause both sporadic cases and outbreaks of diarrhoeal disease. The infective cysts are resistant to chlorine and removal from drinking water relies on sedimentation or filtration. Even small numbers can cause disease (infective inoculum < 100 oocysts). Infection gives rise to profuse watery diarrhoea. The illness is usually self-limiting. There is no effective treatment. In the immunocompromised host the parasites can become widely distributed outside of the GIT.

Giardia lamblia has a wide range of mammalian hosts. Infective cysts are excreted in stool and infection is usually acquired from contaminated food or water. Diarrhoea and abdominal pain are common symptoms.

Symptoms may recur over ensuing months with Cryptosporidium spp. and Giardia lamblia infection.

Worm infections acquired through contact with contaminated soil are globally very common particularly in areas with poor sanitation (most commonly *Ascaris lumbricoides*, *Strongyloides stercoralis*, *Ankylostoma duodenale*, *Necator americanus*, and *Trichuris trichuria* round worms). *Enterobius vermicularis* (pinworm) infection is common across the world. Eggs laid around the anus are spread on hands into the environment.

30.8 Further reading and useful resources

EASL. Management of chronic hepatitis B virus infection http://www.easl.eu/research/our-contributions/clinical-practice-guidelines/detail/management-of-chronic-hepatitis-b-virus-infection

Green Book Chapter 27b rotavirus https://www.gov.uk/government/uploads/system/uploads/attachment_data/file/457263/Green_Book_Chapter_27b_v3_0.pdf

NICE. Hepatitis B (chronic)—diagnosis and management https://www.nice.org.uk/guidance/cg165?unlid=283063241201621620319

30.9 Assessment questions

30.9.1 Question 1

A 53-year-old male smoker presents with a history of epigastric pain associated with eating and dyspepsia worse after travelling to Pakistan. He has been self-medicating with antacids.

What is the commonest cause of this presentation?
A. Gastric ulceration associated with *H. pylori*.
B. *Giardia lambialis*.
C. Oesophageal cancer.
D. Pancreatitis secondary to alcohol.
E. Ruptured abdominal aortic aneurysm.

30.9.2 Question 2

A 65-year-old man born in the UK presents with a history of malaise, loss of appetite, and upper abdominal discomfort. He is jaundiced at presentation. He has not travelled anywhere, denies recent unprotected sexual intercourse or injecting drug use, and does not have any tattoos.

What is the most likely cause of his illness?
A. Hepatitis A.
B. Hepatitis B.
C. Hepatitis C.
D. Hepatitis D.
E. Hepatitis E.

30.9.3 Question 3

A 25-year-old woman has returned to the UK having visited family in Bangladesh. She presents to the Emergency Department of her local hospital with a recent history of fever, headaches, and lethargy. There is no previous medical history. Some abdominal discomfort is elicited on examination. Blood results show mild anaemia, raised inflammatory markers, and elevated liver transaminases. Blood cultures flag positive with gram-negative rods after twenty-four hours.

What is the most likely cause of her illness?

A. Enteric fever.
B. *Escherichia coli* O157 infection.
C. *Salmonella enteritidis* infection.
D. Urosepsis.
E. *Vibrio spp.* infection.

30.10 Answers and discussion

30.10.1 Answer 1

A. Gastric ulceration associated with *H. pylori*.

This gentleman who has dyspeptic symptoms and epigastric pain after travelling to Pakistan most probably has gastric ulceration associated with *H. pylori* infection. Although the other answers are all possible and he does have risk factors for oesophageal cancer, Option A is the commonest cause of this presentation.

30.10.2 Answer 2

E. Hepatitis E.

This 65-year-old man has clinical features of acute hepatitis and no history of travel or other behaviours increasing his risk of a blood borne virus and so is most likely to have enteric associated acute viral hepatitis E, which currently is the commonest cause of acute viral hepatitis in the UK.

30.10.3 Answer 3

A. Enteric fever

This 25-year-old woman who has recently returned from Bangladesh has characteristic features of enteric fever (due to infection with *Salmonella typhi or paratyphi*). Patients often do not have a history of gastro-intestinal upset but present non-specifically with fever and headaches and characteristically elevated liver transaminases. Diagnosis is usually based on clinical features and positive blood cultures.

CHAPTER 31

Urinary tract and genital infections including sexually transmitted infections (STIs)

Jayshree Dave and C. Y. William Tong

31.1 Causes of urethritis and their treatment

Urethritis, characterized by inflammation of the urethra in men, is caused by *Neisseria gonorrhoeae (gonococcus), Chlamydia trachomatis, Trichomonas vaginalis,* and *Mycoplasma genitalium.* Other causes of non-gonococcal urethritis include ureaplasmas, adenoviruses, and herpes simplex viruses. The presence of urethritis is confirmed by the presence of five or more polymorphs in urethral smear by high-power microscopy.

Symptoms can be minor to profound and vary from clear to mucopurulent discharge. *Gonococcus* is commoner in men who have sex with men (MSM) compared to heterosexuals, and high-risk activities such as chemsex parties increase spread with significant public health consequences. Antibiotic resistance in gonococcus has clinical and public health implications as three cases of extensively drug-resistant *Neisseria gonorrhoeae* with resistance to ceftriaxone (MIC = 0.5 mg/L) and high-level resistance to azithromycin (MIC > 256 mg/L) have been described compromising current treatment recommended by British Association for Sexual Health and HIV Guidelines (BASHH). In England an outbreak of high level azithromycin-resistant gonococcus has also been described by Public Health England (PHE), who alerted clinicians about the need for follow up and test of cure, contact tracing, and treatment failure.

C. trachomatis infection can be treated with azithromycin 1g orally as a single dose or with seven days of oral doxycycline. Risk factors for chlamydia include age younger than twenty-five years, multiple sexual partners, and avoidance of barrier methods for contraception. Metronidazole 2g single dose or 400–500mg twice daily for seven days is recommended for treatment of trichomonas, which can cause a moderate discharge in up to 60% of males. Resistance to azithromycin and doxycycline is common in M. genitalium strains and management of these patients with urethritis requires GUM referral for comprehensive investigation, contact tracing, and public health notification. Molecular methods are used for the diagnosis of these organisms and gonococcal culture is undertaken to obtain antimicrobial susceptibility data from patients with a previous diagnosis by molecular method, in GUM attendees, and their contacts.

31.2 Causes of genital ulcers

Herpes simplex infection results in a painful ulcer preceded by a vesicle. The diagnosis can be confirmed using polymerase chain reaction (PCR) tests of a swab taken from the vesicle or ulcer. Treatment is with aciclovir or valaciclovir. Treponema pallidum subspecies pallidum classically causes a single, painless ulcer (chancre) found in the anogenital or oropharyngeal area and dark ground microscopy or PCR of the lesion can confirm the diagnosis. However, in the absence of the chancre, serology is the mainstay of diagnosis and the organism is exquisitely sensitive to penicillin.

Chlamydia trachomatis serovars L1, L2, and L3 cause lymphogranuloma venereum characterized by ano-genital ulceration. It can be diagnosed using standard chlamydia nucleic acid amplification tests (NAATs) with further specific PCR subtyping of chlamydia-positive samples. Rarely, Haemophilus ducreyi can cause multiple, painful ulceration in the ano-genital regions following an erythematous pustular eruption. It can be treated with macrolides such as azithromycin. The English National Reference Laboratory provides a multiplex PCR test for all these pathogens. Klebsiella granumolatis, which causes granuloma inguinale in the tropics, is rare in the UK and is characterized by painless ulcers in the external genitalia and treated with doxycycline or co-trimoxazole. Other causes of genital ulceration include neoplasia, drug reactions, trauma, and Behçets disease.

31.3 Causes of vaginal discharge

Vaginal discharge is commonly caused by Candida, T. vaginalis, and is also seen in patients with bacterial vaginosis. Risk factors for vulvovaginal candidiasis include oral contraceptives, diabetes mellitus, use of antimicrobials and HIV. The relationship with sexual activity is not defined. Asymptomatic colonization is described in healthy women, especially during pregnancy. Recurrent infection can occur, with most women describing an episode of candidiasis during their life. The vaginal discharge may be thick, curdy, or thin and watery with vulval itching and dysuria. Uncomplicated acute episodes are treated with topical and oral azole therapy, with symptomatic infections in pregnancy treated with topical imidazoles and recurrent infection requiring prolonged treatment with fluconazole.

Bacterial vaginosis is asymptomatic in 50% of women, with symptomatic women complaining of a fishy odour (smell released by using potassium hydroxide preparation (KOH prep) for diagnosis) and a discharge which may be grey and thin. Clue cells on a wet mount microscopy are characteristic of the infection, with epithelial cells packed with gram-negative coccobacilli. Gardnerella vaginalis, Prevotella, Mycoplasma hominis, and Mobiluncus are commonly found in vaginal fluid. However, the presence of Gardnerella is not diagnostic of bacterial vaginosis as it can be found in the vagina of healthy women. In pregnant women the infection is associated with increased risk of HIV acquisition, miscarriage, and preterm premature rupture of membrane. Diagnosis is by using Nugent or Ison/Hay criteria on Gram stain of vaginal fluid and observing the relative numbers of lactobacilli, Mobiluncus, and Gardnerella. Treatment is with metronidazole 2g stat or 400mg twice daily for seven days.

Up to half of women with trichomonas are asymptomatic and the rest have non-specific symptoms such as itchy, vaginal discharge, and dysuria. The classic frothy discharge is seen in a third of the women and up to 70% of women have a thin or thick discharge. Sixty percent of men can have a discharge with or without dysuria. Infection in pregnancy is associated with preterm delivery and low birth weight. Infection may enhance HIV transmission. Increasingly, NAATs are available for diagnosis, although many laboratories still use microscopy and culture. Metronidazole is used for treatment. Contacts require treatment and management of these patients by GUM is recommended so that cases and contacts are investigated for co-existing STIs.

31.4 Human papilloma virus (HPV)

There are > 100 different subtypes of HPV with two major phylogenetic branches targeting either keratinized squamous epithelial cells or mucosal non-keratinized squamous epithelial cells. The former causes common cutaneous warts which are transmitted by physical contact, whereas the mucosal types are most commonly sexually transmitted. The mucosal types are further subdivided into low-risk (e.g. HPV 6,11—causes of genital warts) and high-risk types (e.g. HPV 16, 18, 31) dependent on their association with malignancy. HPV is highly contagious and almost 40% of women get infected within two years of sexual experience. Most women will clear the infection within one year. However, persistent infection with high-risk types can predispose to malignant transformation (in combination with other co-factors such as genetics or smoking). HPV 16 is responsible for almost 60% and HPV 18 for > 15% of all cervical cancers in Europe. In addition, high-risk HPVs are also associated with cancers of vulva, vagina, penis, anus, mouth, and throat. The conventional cervical cancer screening programme depends on cytology. Increasingly, HPV DNA is used as a second-line testing after cytology. In the future, it is likely that HPV testing will be used as the first-line screening tool. Virus-like particles have been developed and used as vaccines for HPV. Currently, a quadrivalent HPV vaccine targeting HPV 6, 11, 16, and 18 are offered in the UK to all twelve- to thirteen-year-old females. This programme is recently extended to MSM.

31.5 Managing urinary tract infection (UTI) in healthy women

Urine turbidity and microscopy are poor measures for determining whether a patient has a urinary tract infection (UTI). While the evidence for dipstick tests is limited and flawed, it is reasonable to assume a dipstick test that is positive for leucocyte esterase or nitrites in a woman with a symptom of UTI such as dysuria or frequency has a high probability of UTI. A negative dipstick test in these women has a probability of less than 20% of UTI, but evidence suggests treatment with a three-day course of antibiotics reduces symptoms. Therefore, in these situations it may be that following a midstream urine (MSU) sample, treatment can be considered or the patient can return if symptoms persist. Empiric treatment with either trimethoprim or nitrofurantoin for three days is suggested for women presenting with dysuria, urgency, or frequency as evidence suggests these symptoms are associated with bacteriuria, and patients with a previous probability of bacteriuria of 50% have a 90% probability of having a lower UTI. Note that nitrofurantoin can cause toxicity in the elderly and should not be given with potassium citrate, which is an alkalizing agent. Women presenting with back pain and fever as well as lower urinary tract symptoms such as dysuria and frequency, which is suggestive of pyelonephritis, can be treated with empirical oral antibiotics in the community, after an MSU, providing that the patient does not have sepsis or is able to tolerate medication and fluids. Scottish Intercollegiate Guidelines Network (SIGN) guidance suggests hospitalization if the patient does not improve after twenty-four hours. Treatment is with seven days of ciprofloxacin or fourteen days of co-amoxiclav. Asymptomatic bacteriuria in healthy and elderly women, even in patients with diabetes mellitus, does not require treatment. Risk factors for asymptomatic bacteriuria include female sex, sexual activity, diabetes, age, institutionalization, and presence of a catheter.

31.6 Managing UTI in pregnant women

Management of both symptomatic and asymptomatic UTI is important to reduce morbidity and mortality in pregnant women. Evidence suggests that treatment of asymptomatic infection in pregnancy is associated with reduced risk of upper UTI, preterm delivery, and low birth weight. Treatment with three to seven days of antibiotics is recommended and this can include penicillins and cephalosporins. Trimethoprim should be avoided in the third trimester of pregnancy. A pregnant woman presenting at the antenatal clinic should have an MSU (avoid dipstick tests, which have a low sensitivity) and if bacteriuria is detected then a repeat MSU is taken.

Symptomatic bacteriuria is associated with premature rupture of membranes and preterm labour, and the infection is treated with a seven-day course of appropriate antibiotic with repeat MSU taken after a week to show that the infection has cleared. For more information, interested readers are referred to Chapter 37, Pregnancy-associated infections.

31.7 Managing UTI in male patients

UTI in a male is regarded as complicated as it may follow an underlying urinary tract abnormality or following instrumentation of the urinary tract. Patients who do not respond to treatment, have recurrent infections, or who present with fever and back pain and urinary symptoms require urology referral. Following an MSU, treatment is with trimethoprim or nitrofurantoin for seven days. Fever and back pain reflects a lower UTI and patients with recurrent infections or febrile UTI may have prostatic involvement and treatment with ciprofloxacin for a month is suggested in patients with prostatic symptoms.

31.8 Managing UTI in patients with catheters

Catheter-associated UTI is common bearing in mind that UTI is the most common hospital-acquired infection in the UK. Diagnosis of infection is not straightforward as bacteriuria increases with catheter dwell time and the presenting signs and symptoms are poor predictors of catheter associated infection. However, a catheterized patient with fever may present with back or suprapubic pain and clinical features of sepsis. Rigors, altered mental state, and costovertebral angle tenderness are positive predictors once other causes for infection are excluded. A urine sample should be sent for culture and empiric antibiotic therapy should be commenced based upon clinical features and severity of infection. Urine dipstick test and microscopy do not have a role in the diagnosis of infection. Current evidence suggests that antibiotic prophylaxis to prevent catheter-associated infections is not recommended for routine use; however, gentamicin prophylaxis is reserved for patients with a history of recurrent catheter-associated infections or patients who have developed infection post catheter change. Readers are referred to Chapter 34, Device-associated infections for more information.

31.9 Further reading and useful resources

Australian Government. Department of Health. Multi-drug resistant gonorrhoea 2018. Available from: http://www.health.gov.au/internet/main/publishing.nsf/Content/mr-yr18-dept-dept004.htm.

British Association for Sexual Health and HIV Guidelines.
https://www.bashh.org/guidelines

Public Health England. High level azithromycin resistant gonorrhoea in England. Microbiological and epidemiological information related to an outbreak diagnosed amongst residents of England since November 2015. PHE publications gateway number 2016039. https://www.gov.uk/government/publications/high-level-azithromycin-resistant-gonorrhoea-in-england

Public Health England. UK case of Neisseria gonorrhoeae with high-level resistance to azithromycin and resistance to ceftriaxone acquired abroad. Health Protection Report Volume 12, Number 11. 2018.

Scottish Intercollegiate Guidelines Network. *Management of Suspected Bacterial Urinary Tract Infection in Adults.* (Edinburgh, 2012). http://www.sign.ac.uk/assets/sign88.pdf

31.10 Assessment questions

31.10.1 Question 1

A thirty-four-year-old man who has sex with men presents to the GUM clinic with a one-day history of a painless ulcer on his penis. The lesion is firm and round. There is no associated systemic symptom, urethral discharge, or skin rash. There is no history of recent travel.

What test is the most likely to provide a rapid diagnosis for this patient?
A. Chlamydia nucleic acid amplification test.
B. Dark ground microscopy of swab from the lesion.
C. Herpes simplex PCR.
D. Light microscopy of swab from the lesion.
E. Rapid plasma reagin test (RPR).

31.10.2 Question 2

A twenty-three-year-old pregnant woman presents at 28-weeks gestation to the antenatal clinic with a two-day history of several painful genital ulcers. There is no previous history of similar lesions. A viral swab is taken and herpes simples virus type 2 (HSV-2) DNA is detected.

What test is the most useful to assess the risk of transmission of HSV-2 to her baby?
A. Herpes simplex virus DNA load of her lesion.
B. Herpes simplex virus DNA testing of her blood.
C. Herpes simplex virus susceptibility test for aciclovir.
D. Herpes simplex virus type specific antibody of her partner.
E. Herpes simplex virus type specific antibody of her booking blood.

31.10.3 Question 3

A twenty-two-year-old primigravida attends the antenatal clinic for a routine visit at forty weeks. She complains of tiredness but does not report any other symptoms.
   Investigations:

Urine microscopy	20 white blood cells, no red blood cells
MSU Culture	10^5 E. coli
Sensitive to	amoxicillin, trimethoprim, cephalexin, and nitrofurantoin

What is the most appropriate management of this patient?
A. Prescribe amoxicillin for seven days.
B. Prescribe nitrofurantoin for seven days.
C. Send a repeat midstream urine for analysis.
D. Take blood for renal function.
E. Test the urine sample with a dipstick test.

31.10.4 Question 4

A seventy-year-old lucid woman is admitted from a nursing home to the general medical ward following a fall.

Investigations:

Urine dipstick test	positive for nitrites
Culture (clean catch urine)	E. coli isolated

What is the most appropriate management of this patient?
A. Ask for a repeat urine.
B. Empirically treat her with antibiotics regardless of symptoms.
C. Repeat the urine dipstick test the next day.
D. Send the urine for microscopy.
E. Treat with antibiotics only if there is exacerbation of urinary symptoms.

31.11 Answers and discussion

31.11.1 Answer 1

B. Dark ground microscopy.

This patient presents with a painless genital ulcer with no other systemic or urethral symptoms. The most likely diagnosis is a chancre of primary syphilis. The quickest way to establish this diagnosis is by performing dark ground microscopy of a sample taken from the lesion. The organism, *Treponema pallidum*, can be seen teeming under the microscope in the case of primary syphilis. The organism is not visible using routine light microscopy. RPR or venereal disease research laboratory (VDRL) test is a very useful serological marker for secondary syphilis. However, the antibody titre may not have been detected in early primary syphilis. Genital lesions caused by HSV are more likely to be painful, although it is still important to exclude genital herpes by sending a sample for HSV PCR. However, the result is not likely to be quick and will take at least one day to turn around. Chlamydia can occasionally cause genital ulceration, particularly those in the LGV serovars. LGV lesions in MSM tend to cause proctitis rather than penile ulceration. Although a chlamydia test needs to be performed as part of the STI work up, this is a less likely diagnosis.

31.11.2 Answer 2

E. Herpes simplex virus type specific antibody of her booking blood.

The greatest risk of mother-to-child transmission of HSV in the perinatal period is primary infection of the mother during the late trimester. There won't be sufficient time for the mother to develop antibodies and the baby will not have received enough passive maternal antibodies to help to resist the infection. Lack of a previous history does not exclude herpes reactivation. Testing of an earlier maternal blood sample, such as the booking blood, can help to distinguish primary infection from secondary infection. While the amount of virus shed by the mother is likely to be important as well, under current guidelines, this patient should receive aciclovir therapy to suppress the virus until delivery. Aciclovir resistance is extremely unlikely in someone who has not previously been treated with the agent. The obstetric team will inspect the genital area for lesions at delivery and make a decision on whether the baby should be delivered by Caesarean section rather than vaginally to avoid exposing the baby to HSV in the genital tract.

31.11.3 Answer 3

A. Prescribe amoxicillin for seven days.

The foetus is potentially at risk in a pregnant woman with asymptomatic bacteriuria or with symptomatic UTI. Asymptomatic and symptomatic bacteriuria requires treatment with antibiotics based upon culture susceptibility results. Amoxicillin for three to seven days is a reasonable choice and an antibiotic beyond seven days is unnecessary. Nitrofurantoin should be avoided at term because of the risk of haemolysis in the neonate. The first step in antenatal management is to obtain a careful history to determine the presence of symptoms. This will then be followed by taking an MSU and then determining whether the results show asymptomatic or symptomatic bacteriuria. Urine dipstick testing has a low negative predictive value and has no role in the investigation of UTI in pregnancy. Pyelonephritis should be considered if the patient has loin pain and fever.

31.11.4 Answer 4

E. Treat with antibiotics only if there is exacerbation of urinary symptoms.

Asymptomatic bacteriuria is common in the elderly. Elderly, nursing home patients often have dysuria, nocturia, and frequency because of physiological changes and treatment should be considered only if the patient reports exacerbation of symptoms. Urine dipstick testing is not useful in this clinical situation and a careful history is important. If the patient presents with delirium, confusion, and fever then the possibility of a UTI should be considered and empiric treatment commenced.

CHAPTER 32

Infection of the central nervous system

Caryn Rosmarin

32.1 Common terms used to describe CNS infections

Meningism is the syndrome of the triad of symptoms of headache, neck stiffness, and photophobia caused by irritation of the meninges. While it is often associated with a diagnosis of meningitis, it is also present in other conditions causing meningeal irritation such as subarachnoid haemorrhage, trigeminal neuralgia, migraine, or febrile illness in children.

Meningitis is process of inflammation of the meninges, which may or may not be due to an infectious agent. Strictly speaking, it is a pathological diagnosis, but in lieu of the impracticability of biopsying the meninges, surrogate markers are used to infer inflammation. These include raised cerebrospinal fluid (CSF) white cell count and protein; and meningeal enhancement using contrast enhanced MRI or CT of the brain.

Encephalitis is process of inflammation of the brain parenchyma. Strictly speaking, it is again a pathological diagnosis, and again surrogate markers are used to infer this inflammation, although it is slightly more difficult due to the protected nature of the brain. CSF white cell count and protein are expected to be elevated and parenchymal inflammation may be seen on contrast enhanced MRI.

Meningoencephalitis is a combination of the above with inflammation of both the meninges and the adjoining brain parenchyma.

Aseptic meningitis is said to be present when there is meningism and signs of meningeal inflammation on CSF and imaging, but no bacterial cause is found on culture or molecular diagnostics. Viral meningitis is the commonest cause, although post-neurosurgical aseptic meningitis is often chemical in nature.

32.2 Clinical features of meningitis

Meningism plus fever are the classic symptoms of meningitis. The onset may be acute, subacute, or chronic, depending on the cause.

Neck stiffness may range from mild discomfort to an almost rigid neck and is not a sensitive test in young children or elderly. While not used routinely and with low sensitivity particularly in young children and elderly, Kernig's and Brudkzinski's signs, both of which stretch the meninges worsening the irritation and increasing pain, have a good positive predictive value.

Non-specific signs of intracranial pathology may be present, such as signs of raised intracranial pressure (ICP), vomiting, reduced level of consciousness, focal neurological signs, seizures, or irritability, especially in the immunocompromised, elderly, and young children who may not have classic signs and symptoms. There are often associated symptoms such as respiratory tract infection, gastro-intestinal symptoms, or a rash, which may link to the causative pathogen.

32.3 Causes of acute meningitis

The incidence and aetiology of meningitis vary in time, by geographic region, with age, comorbidities, and vaccination status.

The aetiology of acute meningitis is more often viral than bacterial, with enteroviruses such as coxsackie and echoviruses being the cause in most cases. Symptoms are often mild or asymptomatic and associated with additional symptoms such as sore throat, cold and flu-like illnesses, and diarrhoea. Other viral aetiologies include the herpes viruses, mumps, measles, adenoviruses, lymphocytic choriomeningitis, and early HIV infection. *Herpes simplex* viruses (HSV) can cause meningitis or encephalitis and it is important to distinguish between these as treatment and prognosis differ. Meningitis is more often caused by HSV-2 (the cause of most genital herpes). HSV has been linked to a syndrome called recurrent lymphocytic meningitis (which includes Mollaret's meningitis) that is characterized by sudden attacks of meningitis symptoms that usually last for two to seven days and are separated by symptom-free intervals lasting for weeks, months, or years. Mumps was the most common cause of viral meningitis in the UK before the measles, mumps, and rubella vaccine (MMR) was introduced, and occurred in ±15% of patients with mumps. Resurgence in cases in the UK has largely affected teenagers and young adults who did not receive the MMR vaccine.

Bacterial meningitis, while less common, is more devastating in its morbidity and mortality. Causative bacteria differ by age, risk factors and immune status as in Table 32.1.

Table 32.1 Common causes of bacterial meningitis.

Neonates	Group B streptococcus (*Streptococcus agalactiae*) *Escherichia coli* *Listeria monocytogenes*
Neonates in NICU	Group B streptococcus (*Streptococcus agalactiae*) *Escherichia coli* *Listeria monocytogenes* Plus risk of outbreaks from gram-negative rods such as *Serratia,* *Citrobacter, and Klebsiella* species
Infants and Children	*Streptococcus pneumoniae* *Neisseria meningitidis* *Haemophilus influenzae* type B in the non-immunized *Mycobacterium tuberculosis**
Older children to Adults	*Streptococcus pneumoniae* *Neisseria meningitidis* *Mycobacterium tuberculosis**
Pregnant women	Additional risk of— *Listeria monocytogenes*
Elderly	*Streptococcus pneumoniae* *Listeria monocytogenes*
Immune-compromised	Additional risk of— *Listeria monocytogenes* *Cryptococcus neoformans*** In those with complement deficiency, additional risk of recurrent infection with encapsulated organisms— *Streptococcus pneumoniae* *Neisseria meningitidis* *Haemophilus influenzae*
Post neurosurgery	*Staphylococcus aureus* Coagulase-negative staphylococci Corynebacteria *Propionibacterium acnes* Gram-negative rods including *Pseudomonas sp.*
Post open trauma	*Staphylococcus aureus* *Pseudomonas sp.* Gram-negative rods

Post closed trauma, base
    of skull fracture or in
    association with sinusitis
    or otitis media
	Streptococcus pneumoniae
	Other streptococci and oral flora
	Haemophilus influenzae
	Non-sporing anaerobes
	Gram-negative rods including *Pseudomonas sp.* if causing ear or sinus
	    infection

* = in high risk population groups
** = not bacterium but added for completeness

32.4 Pathogenesis of bacterial meningitis

Bacteria breach the protection of the meninges and blood-brain barrier and reach the subarachnoid space most often via haematogenous spread or, less often, by extension from contiguous structures such as the sinuses or ears, or direct inoculation following trauma or surgery. In primary bacterial meningitis, nasopharyngeal colonization is usually the first step before bloodstream invasion. The exact mechanism of entry into the CNS is not known, but bacteria pass through the vascular endothelial cells of the CNS and the capillaries of the choroid plexus. Infection is usually confined to the subarachnoid space, causing inflammation of the surrounding meninges. The inflammatory response contributes to the pathophysiology and morbidity of the disease. Additional damage due to oedema and vascular inflammation increases ICP and may lead to cerebral herniation and infarcts.

32.5 Diagnosing meningitis

Unless contraindicated, a lumbar puncture (LP) should be performed as soon as possible. The opening pressure and appearance of CSF should be noted and it should be sent for urgent microscopy, culture, and sensitivity (MC&S), viral PCR, protein, and glucose. A simultaneous blood glucose should be obtained for comparison with the CSF glucose. Blood cultures should also be taken, as well as a throat swab and blood for molecular diagnostics, especially when an LP is contra-indicated. CSF findings can help to suggest a broad aetiology of meningitis as in Table 32.2. No finding is absolute, and there will always be exceptions, but interpretation acts as a guide. Bacterial meningitis usually has a very high white blood cell count, the majority of which are neutrophils, while viral meningitis has a lower count with a predominance of lymphocytes. If CSF is obtained very early in the infection the predominant cell type might be inverted or mixed. Aside from bacterial culture, CSF is usually accurate up to several hours after antibiotics are started and should still be performed even if delayed. Antibiotics should not be unreasonably withheld while waiting to do an LP. Contrast CT scan or MRI is sometimes performed to rule out other causes, particularly if signs of raised ICP are present.

Table 32.2 Interpretation of CSF findings in adults.

	Opening Pressure (cmH$_2$O)	Appearance	Cells/ul	Major cell type	Protein (g/L)	CSF:Blood glucose ratio
Normal values	12–20	clear	< 5	lymphocytes	< 0.4	> 0.6
Bacterial meningitis	normal/high	turbid	500–10000	neutrophils	high/very high	very low
Viral meningitis	normal	clear	50–1000	lymphocytes	normal/high	normal
Tuberculous meningitis	high	opalescent/ fibrin strands	50–500	lymphocytes ± neutrophils	high/very high	very low
Cryptococcal meningitis	high/very high	clear	0–500	lymphocytes	normal/high	low
Encephalitis	normal	clear	5–100	lymphocytes	normal/high	normal

32.6 Treating meningitis

Due to the potential morbidity and mortality associated with meningitis, initial intravenous (IV) treatment should start before the causative organism is confirmed. Empiric treatment outlined in Table 32.3 is based on the common causes as outlined in Table 32.1. Treatment of viral meningitis without any signs of encephalitis is not routinely recommended.

In severe beta-lactam allergy in non-pregnant women, chloramphenicol + vancomycin is the first line therapy, with additional cotrimoxazole to cover for *Listeria monocytogenes* when suspected. In pregnant women a risk-benefit discussion needs to occur as some of these drugs may harm the foetus.

Table 32.3 Empiric treatment of suspected bacterial meningitis.

Clinical situation	First-line IV treatment	Additional treatment
Neonates	Cefotaxime + ampicillin OR Ampicillin + gentamicin	
Neonates in NICU	Meropenem	
Infants and children	Cefotaxime OR ceftriaxone	Add vancomycin if penicillin or cephalosporin resistant *Streptococcus pneumonia* suspected
Older children to adults	Ceftriaxone	Add vancomycin if penicillin or cephalosporin resistant *Streptococcus pneumonia* suspected
Pregnant women	Ceftriaxone + ampicillin	
Elderly	Ceftriaxone + ampicillin	
Immunocompromised	Ceftriaxone + ampicillin	
Post neurosurgery	Meropenem + vancomycin	Add intrathecal antibiotic if EVD *in situ*
Post open trauma	Ceftriaxone + metronidazole + aminoglycoside	Alternative = meropenem + vancomycin
Post closed trauma, base of skull fracture, or in association with sinusitis or otitis media	Ceftriaxone	

Once a gram stain, culture, or PCR result has confirmed the identity of the pathogen, definitive treatment can be instituted as in Table 32.4.

32.7 Steroid use

As some of the clinical features and complications of meningitis are due to the inflammatory process of the disease, made worse by the killing and degradation of the bacteria, steroids have been recommended in attempt to reduce the inflammatory response. They were initially successful in reducing the complications of deafness and neurologic deficit seen in children with *H. influenzae* meningitis. Although results are conflicting in its effect on other forms of meningitis, particularly in those with underlying HIV infection, a Cochrane review found it reduced mortality in *S. pneumoniae* meningitis and deafness and neurologic deficit from all causes of meningitis. There was also no harm found in those who were given steroids. Thus, the current UK recommendation is to give dexamethasone empirically before or soon after antibiotics are started and continue for four days when *S. pneumoniae* is either proven or suspected.

32.8 Those needing prophylaxis in cases of meningitis

Prophylaxis against *N. meningitidis and H. influenzae* is aimed at eradicating nasopharyngeal colonization rather than directly preventing disease. Only those who come into regular or prolonged contact with a patient during the infectious period, or those with significant mucosal exposure to a patient's secretions without personal protective equipment, require prophylaxis. This is usually limited to those at risk in the patient's household contacts, occasional work or school contacts, and very few hospital contacts. Prophylaxis should be given as soon as possible after contact. Ciprofloxacin is the agent of choice. If unable to take ciprofloxacin, rifampicin or

Table 32.4 Definitive treatment of bacterial meningitis.

Organism	Treatment	Duration
Neisseria meningitidis	High-dose cefotaxime or ceftriaxone OR ampicillin OR benzyl penicillin Severe penicillin allergy: High-dose chloramphenicol	5–7 days
Streptococcus pneumoniae	High-dose cefotaxime or ceftriaxone Add vancomycin if: Clinical deterioration Penicillin or cephalosporin-resistant pneumococcus Recent travel from region with high level of penicillin- or cephalosporin-resistant pneumococcus Severe penicillin allergy: High-dose chloramphenicol	10–14 days
Listeria monocytogenes	High-dose ampicillin + gentamicin Penicillin allergy: High-dose cotrimoxazole	21–28 days
Group B streptococcus (Streptococcus agalactiae)	High-dose ampicillin + gentamicin OR High-dose benzyl penicillin + gentamicin OR High-dose ceftriaxone + gentamicin Gentamicin use is for the first week only Severe penicillin allergy: High-dose chloramphenicol	21 days
E. coli and other gram-negative rods including Pseudomonas sp.	High-dose meropenem OR ceftazidime ± aminoglycoside Amend according to susceptibility	21–28 days
Staphylococcus aureus	High-dose flucloxacillin or ceftriaxone ± rifampicin Severe penicillin allergy: High-dose vancomycin ± rifampicin	28 days

ceftriaxone can be used. Even if prophylaxis is taken, contacts of patients with invasive infection still have an added risk for at least six months. Vaccination should also be offered to contacts at risk.

32.9 Clinical features of encephalitis and its diagnosis

In addition to headache and fever, patients may have reduced levels of consciousness, altered behaviour, focal neurology, or seizures. Diagnosis is based on laboratory and typical MRI findings. Viral PCR of the CSF is the mainstay of diagnosis, although it may be negative early in infection. If highly suspicious in the face of a negative result a repeat sample should be tested.

32.10 Causes and treatment of encephalitis

Most cases of encephalitis are viral (see Table 32.5) with many viruses causing encephalitis as their primary disease, or as part of a systemic infection. The arboviral encephalitides are mostly epidemic (often in summer) while the others are mostly sporadic. Travel history is important as arboviruses are often geographically specific. Because the clinical findings are similar in many cases

Table 32.5 Common causes of viral encephalitis.

Arbovirus infections	Dengue
	Yellow Fever
	West Nile virus
	Tick-borne encephalitides
	Japanese B encephalitis
	Equine encephalitides
	St. Louis encephalitis
Enterovirus infections	Coxsackievirus
	Echovirus
	Poliomyelitis
Myxovirus infections	Mumps
	Measles
	Rubella
	Influenza
	Hendra
	Nipah
	Rabies
Herpesvirus infections	Herpes simplex virus
	Herpes zoster virus
	Cytomegalovirus
	Human Herpes 6 virus
	Virus B (Herpes simiae)
Polyomavirus	JC virus

Table 32.6 Non-viral causes of encephalitis.

Bacteria (including spirochaetes)	*Listeria monocytogenes*
	Mycobacterium tuberculosis
	Mycoplasma pneumoniae
	Legionella pneumophila
	Bartonella sp.
	Salmonella typhi
	Brucella sp.
	Leptospirosis
	Treponema pallidum
	Borrelia burgdorferi
	Tropheryma whipplei
Rickettsia	Q fever
	Endemic and Epidemic typhus
	Rocky mountain spotted fever
	Ehrlichiosis
Fungi	Cryptococcosis
	Histoplasmosis
	Coccidioidomycosis
	Blastomycosis
Parasites	*Toxoplasma gondii*
	Cerebral malaria
	African trypanosomiasis
	Hydatid disease
	Cysticercosis
	Amoebic meningoencephalitis (*Naegleria fowleri, Acanthamoeba,* and *Balamuthia*)
	Schistosomiasis

of encephalitis, the diagnosis of the offending agent must be made in the laboratory. Herpes simplex encephalitis (HSE) is the most common sporadic (nonepidemic) form of encephalitis. Aciclovir should be started as empiric therapy in all patients with suspected encephalitis while awaiting results. Directed treatment will follow further recommendations once cause of encephalitis is known.

Subacute sclerosing panencephalitis (SSPE) is a rare and chronic progressive form of encephalitis caused by a persistent infection with measles virus. It presents many years to decades after primary infection and should not be confused with acute disseminated encephalomyelitis (ADEM), which is an immune-mediated inflammatory demyelinating condition predominately affecting the white matter of the brain and spinal cord. ADEM occurs on the background of a previous, but recent, viral infection (respiratory, gastrointestinal infection, or childhood exanthematous infection such as measles, rubella, or chickenpox), or following recent vaccination.

Encephalitis or an encephalitis-like picture can also be caused by bacteria, fungi, and parasites as part of a primary or systemic disease (see Table 32.6). Autoimmune encephalitis is also increasingly being recognized, e.g. anti-NMDA receptor encephalitis and voltage-gated potassium channel antibody encephalopathy.

32.11 Causes of chronic meningitis

Chronic meningitis is more slowly evolving and is defined as meningitis that persists for more than four weeks. The signs of meningeal inflammation are usually not as marked as in acute meningitis and there are more findings of debilitation, altered mental state, and focal neurologic damage, including cranial nerve damage, hydrocephalus, and stroke. Causes are classed into three broad categories; infectious, autoimmune, and neoplastic. Fungal, bacterial, viral, and parasitic organisms can cause chronic meningitis. With increasing use of immunosuppressant medications, as well as predisposing conditions such as impaired cellular and humoral immunity, there is a larger population at risk of chronic meningitis. The most common causes of chronic infectious meningitis include *Mycobacterium tuberculosis, Cryptococcus* species, *Aspergillus species*, and syphilis. Autoimmune causes include sarcoidosis, lupus, vasculitis, and Behçet's, while neoplasms, especially lymphoma, cause carcinomatous meningitis.

32.12 Cerebral abscess or empyema risk factors and causative organisms

Most of these have an identifiable risk factor including neurosurgery, head trauma, a contiguous parameningeal focus (otitis, sinusitis, mastoiditis, dental abscess), or a distant focus with haematogenous spread (bronchiectasis, lung abscess, endocarditis). Cyanotic congenital heart disease and pulmonary arteriovenous malformations increase the risk because bacteria reaching the right side of the heart are shunted to the left side of the heart and systemic circulation. Single or multiple abscesses can occur depending on the clinical source.

Bacteria are the commonest cause and depend on the risk factor and source. Those coming from contiguous sites are often caused by upper respiratory tract or dental flora, while those post trauma and neurosurgery are more likely to be skin flora, *S. aureus*, and gram-negative bacilli. About half are polymicrobial and include aerobic and anaerobic bacteria.

32.13 Diagnosing and treating cerebral abscesses or empyema

Clinical presentation is usually due to the pressure effect of the abscess and includes headache, focal neurologic signs, seizures, or behavioural change. Fever may be present depending on aetiology.

Ring-enhancing lesions on contrast CT or MRI scanning are usually diagnostic. Other causes of intracerebral-enhancing lesions include tumours, tuberculomas, cryptococcomas, toxoplasmosis, cysticercosis, or hydatid disease.

Abscesses should be managed both medically and surgically. Drainage or aspiration of the abscess reduces morbidity and mortality and aids in diagnosis of the causative organism(s). Empiric antibiotic treatment should cover the likely micro-organisms, and so depends on the risk factor and source. Ceftriaxone plus metronidazole is the recommended choice until therapy can be guided by MC&S.

32.14 Presenting features of spinal epidural abscess

This is one of the most missed diagnoses when it comes to CNS infections, and can be devastating in its morbidity. It can evolve as an acute, subacute, or chronic infection, the latter being the more difficult to diagnose. There is most often pain over the infected area of the spine and fever is usually present. Nerve root pain is followed by spinal cord symptoms such as urinary retention that occurs as a result of compression or infarction of the cord due to accumulation of pus in the tight epidural space of the vertebral canal. If treatment can be instituted before the spinal cord is affected, the outcome should be good, otherwise irreversible cord damage and paralysis often result.

32.15 Aetiology and treatment of spinal epidural abscess

The source of infection is either haematogenous spread (50%) from a distant site (skin, soft tissue, urinary, or respiratory tract), local invasion (30%) from a contiguous site of infection (vertebral osteomyelitis, psoas abscess) or iatrogenic inoculation (surgery, lumbar drains, epidurals).

Most patients have at least one underlying risk factor, the most common being diabetes, IV drug use, spinal trauma, and underlying spinal abnormalities.

Treatment is both surgical and medical with urgent drainage being the most crucial, especially before any neurologic symptoms appear. Surgery after neurologic symptoms have been present for more than twenty-four hours has minimal effect on reversing this. S. aureus is the most common cause and empiric treatment should cover for this. If the urinary tract is thought to be the source, cover for gram-negative rods should be included.

32.16 Post-neurosurgical infection

Post-surgical infection follows any neurosurgical procedure, especially those complicated by a persistent CSF leak or where prosthetic material is placed, including drains, shunts, and cranioplasty.

Infections include superficial wound infection, osteomyelitis, empyema, abscess, post-operative meningitis, ventriculitis, CSF shunt, and external ventricular drain (EVD) infection.

Post-operative meningitis can be either infective or aseptic, although they are often difficult to distinguish. The latter is secondary to blood, tumour, or surgical material irritating the meninges and causing inflammation. In the former, organisms differ from community-acquired ones, with staphylococci and gram-negative bacteria being more common than upper airway flora. In this light, empiric treatment should cover more broadly to include the range of possibilities. Most other forms of post-neurosurgical infection require both antibiotic and surgical management. Collections of pus need to be drained, and infected prostheses, drains, and shunts removed.

Not surprisingly, the most common post-neurosurgical infections are related to CSF shunts and EVDs. CSF shunts are semi-permanent closed drainage systems in patients with hydrocephalus, with most being ventriculoperitoneal (VP) shunts. The source of infection is usually bacterial contamination at the time of surgery with biofilm formation on the shunt catheter. Removal of the shunt is almost always needed, and treatment with intraventricular ± IV antibiotics. EVDs are temporary external drainage systems used for CSF drainage or ICP monitoring post haemorrhage or trauma. They can also be inserted as an interim drainage and antibiotic delivery system in those whose permanent shunts are removed for shunt infection. The main sources of infection of EVDs are bacterial contamination both at the time of surgery and with continual manipulation of the drain. Removal of the EVD is almost always needed, followed by replacement and treatment with intraventricular antibiotics. IV antibiotics are only needed if patients are systemically unwell, or no EVD is *in situ*. Coagulase-negative staphylococci are the commonest cause of infection in both VP shunts and EVDs.

32.17 Further reading and useful resources

McGill, F., Heyderman, R. S., Michael, B. D., Defres, S., Beeching, N. J., Borrow, R., et al., 'The UK Joint Specialist Societies Guideline on the Diagnosis and Management of Acute Meningitis and Meningococcal Sepsis in Immunocompetent Adults', *Journal of Infection*, 72 (2016), 405e–438e; and Corrigendum to the above, *Journal of Infection*, 72 (2016), 768e–769e.

Tunkel, A. R., Hartman, B. J., Kaplan, S. L., Kaufman, B. A., Roos, K. L., Scheld, W. M., Whitley, R. J., 'Practice Guidelines for the Management of Bacterial Meningitis', *Clinical Infectious Diseases*, 39 (2004), 1267–1284.

Tunkel, A. R., Glaser, C. A., Bloch, K. C., Sejvar, J. J., Marra, C. M., Roos, K. L., et al., 'The Management of Encephalitis: Clinical Practice Guidelines by the Infectious Diseases Society of America', *Clinical Infectious Diseases*, 47 (2008), 303–327.

32.18 Assessment questions

32.18.1 Question 1

A 45-year-old women presents to A&E with a three-day history of fever, headache, vomiting, and a rash. She is normally healthy, has no significant medical history, and has not travelled recently. She mentions she has had a few episodes of diarrhoea two days prior to onset of illness, which she thought was possibly just 'something she ate'. Paracetamol has not helped the headache much.

On examination her temperature is 37.9°C, heart rate 102b/min, and blood pressure normal. She has a faint disappearing rash on her torso, no lymphadenopathy, and her upper and lower airways are clear. Her abdomen is soft with mild generalized tenderness but no masses nor organomegaly. She has some pain with flexion of her neck and mild photophobia but no focal neurologic signs (see Table 32.7 for a full list of investigation results).

What is the most appropriate next step in her management?
A. Isolate the patient in a side room.
B. Send the CSF for TB culture.
C. Send the CSF for viral PCR.
D. Start iv aciclovir.
E. Start iv ceftriaxone and aciclovir.

Table 32.7 Investigation results from 45-year-old women presenting to A&E with a three-day history of fever, headache, vomiting, and a rash.

White cell count	$8.6 \geq 10^9/L$ (4.0–11.0)
Serum C-reactive protein	24 mg/L (<10)
Cerebrospinal fluid:	
Total protein	0.50 g/L (0.15–0.45)
Glucose	4.1 mmol/L (3.3–4.4)
Cell count:	
White cell count	183 /μL (<5)
Red cell count	26 /μL (0)
Lymphocyte count	118 /μL (<3)
Neutrophil count	65 /μL (0)
Gram stain	No organisms seen

32.18.2 Question 2

A 24-year-old pregnant woman presents to A&E with a two-day history of fever, headache, nausea, vomiting, and mild confusion. She has no medical history of note, and recently returned from France where she went for a wedding and cheese-tasting tour. An MRI brain was normal (see Table 32.8).

Table 32.8 Investigation results from a 24-year-old pregnant woman presenting to A&E with a two-day history of fever, headache, nausea, vomiting, and mild confusion.

White cell count	$12.6 \geq 10^9/L$ (4.0–11.0)
Serum C-reactive protein	82 mg/L (<10)
Cerebrospinal fluid:	
Total protein	0.98 g/L (0.15–0.45)
Glucose	2.1 mmol/L (3.3–4.4)
Cell count:	
White cell count	513 /μL (<5)
Red cell count	<5 /μL (0)
Lymphocyte count	125 /μL (<3)
Neutrophil count	388 /μL (0)
Gram stain	Not yet available

What empiric IV treatment would you prescribe for this patient?
A. Ampicillin + aciclovir.
B. Ampicillin alone.
C. Ceftriaxone + aciclovir.
D. Ceftriaxone + ampicillin.
E. Ceftriaxone + ampicillin + aciclovir.

32.18.3 Question 3

A 15-year-old boy presents with a two-day history of headache, fever, and a few non-blanching lesions on his legs and abdomen. An LP is performed and Table 32.9 shows his CSF sample.

Table 32.9 Investigation results from a 15-year-old boy presenting with a two-day history of headache, fever, and a few non-blanching lesions on his legs and abdomen.

White cell count	$15.6 \geq 109/L$ (4.0–11.0)
Serum C-reactive protein	182 mg/L (<10)
Cerebrospinal fluid:	
Total protein	1.28 g/L (0.15–0.45)
Glucose	1.8 mmol/L (3.3–4.4)
Cell count:	
White cell count	1154 /μL (<5)
Red cell count	<5 /μL (0)
Lymphocyte count	58 /μL (<3)
Neutrophil count	1096 /μL (0)
Gram stain	Gram-negative diplococci

The most likely cause of his meningitis is:

A. *Haemophilus influenzae.*
B. *Listeria monocytogenes.*
C. *Neisseria meningitidis.*
D. *Streptococcus agalactiae.*
E. *Streptococcus pneumoniae.*

32.19 Answers and discussion

32.19.1 Answer 1

C. Send the CSF for viral PCR.

The CSF result is suggestive of a viral, rather than bacterial or tubercular, infection as the protein and glucose are normal. The cell count has a lymphocytic predominance, again suggestive of viral, rather than bacterial, aetiology. The most common cause of meningitis in otherwise healthy individuals is enterovirus; therefore, viral PCR is required to confirm this diagnosis. Although less likely, HSV cannot be excluded clinically in this case, but treatment is not indicated unless signs of encephalitis are present.

Most people who are infected with enteroviruses are asymptomatic or have a mild flu-like illness, including fever and rash. Their normal site of replication is the gastrointestinal tract, where the infection can be subclinical or result in a mild gastro-intestinal disorder. However, in a proportion of cases, the virus spreads to other organs, causing severe disease typical of individual enterovirus types (of which there are over 70). Clinical and severe infections include neonatal infection, herpangina (coxsackievirus A), hand, foot, and mouth disease (coxsackievirus A16 or enterovirus 71), haemorrhagic conjunctivitis (coxsackievirus A24 and enterovirus 70), severe respiratory infection (enterovirus 68), meningitis (many), encephalitis (many), myocarditis (coxsackievirus B), pericarditis, myositis, and paralysis (enterovirus 68, poliovirus).

Enteroviral transmission is most often faecal-oral but can also be through fomites or contact with eyes, nose, and mouth as they are often found in the respiratory secretions (e.g., saliva, sputum, nasal mucus) and stool of an infected person. Outbreaks occur particularly in summer.

There is no specific treatment for enteroviral infection other than supportive. Prevention in the form of vaccination is only available for poliovirus. For the others, good hand hygiene and avoiding contact with infectious people is the best strategy.

32.19.2 Answer 2

D. Ceftriaxone + ampicillin.

The CSF findings are consistent with bacterial meningitis. As the patient is pregnant, and a possible history of eating unpasteurized cheese, *Listeria monocytogenes* is high on the differential. Listeriosis is a food-borne disease acquired through eating contaminated food or drink. Vegetables can become contaminated from the soil or from manure used as fertilizer. Animals can carry the bacterium in their gut without appearing ill and can contaminate foods of animal origin such as meat and dairy products. The organism is destroyed by cooking and pasteurization, and hence is most often found in those foods that are unpasteurized, undercooked, or contaminated after the cooking process. As a disease it is most often associated with dairy products made with raw, unpasteurized milk, particularly soft cheeses. Other implicated food products include cold meats, sausages, pates and meat spreads, undercooked chicken, raw vegetables, and salad ingredients such as sprouts. It has the ability to survive and grow at low temperatures and will happily multiply in contaminated food in your (or the supermarket's) fridge. It is also tolerant of high salt, nitrate, and acidic environments, and will therefore grow in cured or smoked meats and fish. Outbreaks of listeriosis occur not infrequently, although they can difficult to recognize, especially if the source is a production plant with a wide national or international distribution.

Pregnant women are at significantly higher risk than other healthy adults of listeriosis. Despite the fact it usually causes a mild flu-like illness, pregnant women should always be treated as the organism can cause chorioamnionitis and be vertically transmitted resulting in stillbirth, foetal infection, or serious neonatal infection, where it can cause both early and late neonatal infection. In pregnant women and non-pregnant individuals, particularly at extremes of age and in the immunocompromised, it can progress to a more severe form of disease including meningitis. As most infections in healthy individuals cause only a mild flu-like illness, the incidence of the disease is not well known.

L. monocytogenes is a small, motile, gram-positive rod that can grow both aerobically or anaerobically. The gram stain and growth on culture plates can be very similar to that of *Streptococcus agalactiae*, both of which cause severe neonatal disease. The two organisms are distinguished by the catalase test, with *L. monocytogenes* being positive. Another important difference is their antibiotic susceptibility, with *L. monocytogenes* being susceptible to penicillin-based antibiotics but resistant to cephalosporins, which are the usual first choice for empiric treatment of community acquired meningitis. Treatment for listeria meningitis therefore needs to be added in those with any risk factor for the disease.

32.19.3 Answer 3

C. *Neisseria meningitidis.*

Infection with *N. meningitidis* can cause septicaemia with multiorgan failure or acute fulminant meningitis. Recurrent meningococcal infection occurs in patients with terminal complement deficiency or asplenia. There are at least twelve serogroups identified classified according the polysaccharide capsule, but only five of these (A, B, C, Y, and W-135) are responsible for the majority of epidemic meningococcal disease. *N. meningitidis* is the most common cause of meningitis in children from two to eighteen years of age. Risk factors include living in close quarters, smoking, and a recent upper respiratory tract viral infection. Nasopharyngeal carriage of meningococcus in the throats of the public is common (5–10%) and droplet spread or close mucosal contact forms the source of much of the transmission. More than 95% of cases have no obvious contact, yet close household contacts of a case of invasive disease have a significantly higher risk of disease. In a small percentage of colonized individuals the meningococcus invades the mucosa and enters the bloodstream and spreads to many organs, including the brain. Vaccination against meningococcus is part of the routine vaccine schedule in children in the UK. Close contacts of cases that have been given chemoprophylaxis can later be offered appropriate vaccine once the serogroup has been confirmed. This will extend the period of protection. Travellers to high-risk areas are also offered vaccination.

CHAPTER 33

Ocular infections

Ruaridh Buchanan and Caryn Rosmarin

33.1 Infections affecting the eye

Pathogens of every type can affect the eye—bacterial, fungal, viral, protozoal, and parasitic.

33.2 Parts of the eye

The eye is a complex structure but for the purposes of categorizing infections it can be viewed as a series of layers, which are:

- Conjunctiva
- Cornea
- Vitreous humour
- Retina

33.3 Common conjunctival infections

The bulk of acute conjunctivitis is viral—up to 90% of infection will be due to adenovirus. Enterovirus species can cause acute epidemic haemorrhagic conjunctivitis, e.g. coxsackie A 24 virus, enterovirus 70. Bacterial causes are more common in children than adults and include *S. aureus*, *S. pneumoniae*, and *H. influenzae*. *Pseudomonas aeruginosa* and other Gram negatives may cause conjunctivitis in contact lens wearers.

It is sometimes possible to differentiate viral from bacterial disease clinically. Where viral conjunctivitis usually results in watery eyes and often comes in concert with a more generalized viral illness, bacterial infection usually occurs in the absence of systemic features and is more likely to be associated with purulent discharge or matting of the eyelids.

33.4 Does conjunctivitis require treatment?

Viral conjunctivitis does not require specific treatment save in the rare instances where herpes simplex virus is the causative agent—topical aciclovir can then be used. Bacterial infections, however, will resolve more rapidly with topical therapy. A wide range of preparations are available but topical chloramphenicol is the mainstay of treatment.

33.5 Is systemic treatment ever required in conjunctivitis?

Purulent conjunctivitis in the neonate is often a result of congenitally acquired *N. gonorrhoeae* or *Chlamydia trachomatis* infection. In these circumstances conjunctivitis can be the herald of systemic infection and it is therefore wise to treat both systemically and topically. Swabs can be sent for PCR and culture to identify the pathogen. *Chlamydia* can be treated with topical and oral azithromycin; gonococcal infection can be treated with topical chloramphenicol and a systemic cephalosporin chosen based on local sensitivity patterns. Sexually active adults can also occasionally suffer from these infections and should be treated similarly.

33.6 Common corneal infections

Herpes simplex virus is a relatively common cause, usually inoculated directly into the eye by contaminated fingers. The classic presentation is with a unilateral dendritic ulcer, easily visualized on fluorescein dye staining. Herpes zoster virus can also affect the cornea—reactivation in the distribution of the ophthalmic branch of the trigeminal nerve (CN V) results in ophthalmic shingles. Patients presenting with ophthalmic shingles should always be referred for an ophthalmology opinion to exclude keratitis. In the absence of obvious eye involvement, Hutchinson's sign (involvement of the tip of the nose) is suggestive of higher risk of corneal involvement as the nasociliary branch of the trigeminal nerve supplies both the cornea and the tip of the nose. In both cases the diagnosis is predominantly clinical, though PCR can be performed for confirmation.

Bacterial keratitis results from direct inoculation of the cornea. There is often a preceding insult which becomes secondarily infected; contact lens wearers are at increased risk. Common pathogens include *S. aureus* and *P. aeruginosa*. The same can be said of fungal keratitis, which can be due to *Candida* species or filamentous fungi such as *Fusarium*. Corneal scrapings, inoculated directly onto culture media, can yield a microbiological diagnosis.

A rare but important infection is *Acanthamoeba* keratitis. This almost exclusively affects people who wear contact lenses, specifically those who use non-sterile water to clean their lenses. The waterborne amoebae contaminate the lenses and then transfer to the cornea when they are worn. Diagnosis requires a high degree of suspicion as corneal scrapings must be placed onto culture media with a lawn of *E. coli* growth—*Acanthamoeba* are detected by lines of clearance where the mobile amoebae have ingested the bacteria as they travel.

33.7 Treating corneal infection

Keratitis is a sight threatening condition and must be treated aggressively; treatment should always be supervised by an ophthalmologist. Herpes virus infections are treated with topical antivirals (aciclovir); ophthalmic shingles patients can also be treated with oral aciclovir/valaciclovir if their condition is severe. Empiric treatment for bacterial keratitis must cover *S. aureus* and *P. aeruginosa*—ciprofloxacin and levofloxacin are common first line agents, but preparations of fusidic acid and aminoglycosides are also available. Treatment should be tailored based on the results of any corneal culture. Topical antifungal agents include natamycin, amphotericin, and voriconazole. Patients with *Acanthamoeba* keratitis must be referred to a tertiary centre with experience of the condition and access to specialist pharmacy support as topical amoebicidals often need to be prepared on a patient-by-patient basis. Agents used include biguanides and chlorhexidine.

33.8 Common vitreous chamber infections

Endophthalmitis is caused by a variety of bacterial and fungal species. Classically these infections are classified as being either exogenous or endogenous in nature.

33.8.1 Exogenous

These infections are inoculated into the eye from an external source. This can either result from accidental trauma or be iatrogenic following surgical procedures.

The risk of endophthalmitis following ocular surgery is low—estimated at approximately 1:300 following cataract surgery and about 1:3000 following intraocular injections, although these numbers vary by the complexity of the procedure. These infections are usually caused by coagulase-negative *Staphylococci*, although other organisms can be responsible.

Trauma to the eye can result in infection with a wide variety of different pathogens, depending on the nature of the injury. Environmental Gram negatives, including *Pseudomonas* species, are common, and fungal infection can also occur. This is a situation where culture results can be of real benefit in guiding therapy.

33.8.2 Endogenous

These infections occur as a result of haematogenous spread from an infection elsewhere within the body. As a result, a wide variety of pathogens can be responsible. Certain patient factors, such as diabetes, infective endocarditis, and severe immune suppression associated with chemotherapy and transplant are associated with an increased risk of endogenous ophthalmitis. Of particular concern are *Candida* species, which frequently spread to the eye—a formal ophthalmology review should be considered in all patients with candidaemia but is especially important if there is a prolonged interval before diagnosis or a source cannot readily be identified. This is particularly true for neonates with candidaemia. *Klebsiella pneumoniae*, particular the aggressive K1 strain, is becoming more prevalent, especially in South East Asia where it is the most common cause of both endophthalmitis and liver abscess.

33.9 Treating endophthalmitis

Like keratitis, endophthalmitis is a sight-threatening condition, and thus an ophthalmic emergency. In severe cases the treatment may be surgical as well as medical and vitrectomy or enucleation of the affected eye may be required. The mainstay of treatment is early direct intravitreal administration of antibiotics—usually ophthalmology will perform a vitreous biopsy for culture and instil antibiotics immediately thereafter. Empirical treatment should cover Gram positive and Gram negative organisms, including *Pseudomonas species*—the combination of vancomycin and ceftazidime is the most commonly used treatment, although amikacin may be used in place of ceftazidime. Fluoroquinolones and clindamycin are also available. Concomitant systemic therapy should be given for endogenous endophthalmitis and considered in severe cases of exogenous infection, or when the source cannot easily be determined. Fungal endophthalmitis always requires prolonged systemic treatment whether endogenous or exogenous. If the pathogen is already known then targeted therapy can be used, otherwise empiric therapy with liposomal amphotericin B is employed. Intravitreal injections of amphotericin B and voriconazole can also be used. Referral to a centre with experience of managing such infections is advisable.

33.10 Common retinal infections

The retina is a highly vascular structure and as a result is a potential site for seeding by any endogenous bacterial or fungal infection. However, the majority of severe infections occur in the immunocompromised, particularly those with advanced HIV infection. Of particular importance are toxoplasma retinitis and cytomegalovirus (CMV) retinitis.

33.10.1 Toxoplasma retinitis

This is the commonest cause of retinitis. Classically regarded as a congenital infection, it can also occur in adults as a late manifestation of congenital infection or as a result of being immunocompromised. In adults, the most common presentation is with unilateral decreased visual acuity; in children, it may be part of a more complex syndrome.

Serological testing for toxoplasma-specific IgG can confirm that a patient has been exposed to toxoplasma at some time but cannot prove current infection; in congenital cases it may only represent maternal antibody. IgM is more useful in identifying active infection but depending on the assay used can remain positive for as long as two years after acute infection. Along with IgA testing, it can be useful in diagnosing congenital cases. IgG avidity testing can ascertain whether infection occurred more or less than six months previously but cannot prove active infection. As the eye is an immune privileged site, antibody production is often much higher within the eye than systemically; thus, comparing immunoglobulin levels in the eye and the blood can be helpful in proving the diagnosis. The PHE Toxoplasma Reference Laboratory in Swansea can advise on this, as well as perform PCR on vitreal samples.

Ocular toxoplasmosis is treated similarly to CNS disease with systemic sulphadiazine, pyrimethamine, and folinic acid. Depending on the severity of the disease, intravitreal injections of clindamycin may be added; systemic steroids may also be employed. Treatment is for six weeks, followed by secondary prophylaxis with co-trimoxazole; in HIV patients this can be discontinued once the CD4 count rises above 100 cells/ml.

33.10.2 Cytomegalovirus (CMV) retinitis

CMV reactivation occurs in those with advanced HIV infection (CD4 count < 50 cells/ml) as well as in other causes of immunosuppression—haematology patients undergoing aggressive chemotherapy and those undergoing bone marrow transplantation are at particular risk.

Diagnosis is dependent on clinical suspicion, which must be high in the immunocompromised. There is a spectrum of presentations, ranging from asymptomatic, unnoticed infection through visual disturbances to eye pain, although the latter is uncommon. The possibility of asymptomatic infection makes routine formal ophthalmological review of patients with CD4 < 50 cells/ml vital.

Formal ophthalmological assessment is essential as the diagnosis is predominantly based on the appearance of the retina along with the history of immunosuppression. As CMV infection is usually systemic, the patient should be assessed for other potential sites of end organ damage, such as colitis, hepatitis, and pneumonitis. Blood should be sent for CMV DNA quantitative PCR to help guide therapy. If there is doubt about the diagnosis, a vitreal biopsy can also be sent for PCR.

As with all CMV infection, ganciclovir is the first line therapy, with foscarnet as second line and cidofovir third. Ganciclovir and foscarnet can be delivered by intravitreal injection, which is often reserved for more severe cases. Systemic therapy is always given, as it has been shown to improve outcomes and also because intravitreal therapy will not treat disease at other sites, including the other eye. In milder cases, oral valganciclovir can be used, particularly if there is no viraemia. Duration of treatment is dictated by both clinical response and blood viral load if detectable but should not be less than two weeks. Following the active treatment phase, prophylaxis with oral valganciclovir should be continued until the immune system is restored—for example, until the CD4 count has climbed above 100 cells/ml.

33.11 Rare worm infections

Worm infections are rare in the UK. All cases should be discussed with the Hospital for Tropical Diseases.

33.11.1 Ocular larva migrans (OLM)

This mainly occurs in children, who ingest *Toxocara canis* eggs when playing in outdoor spaces contaminated by dog faeces. The larvae hatch and migrate around the body—their arrival in the eye results in decreased visual acuity. Diagnosis can be complicated by the fact that blood serology may be negative in purely ocular disease. Albendazole will kill the larvae but this will often increase inflammation and thus endanger sight. Pre-treating with steroids can prevent this, but surgery may be considered as an alternative to medical therapy.

33.11.2 Loaisis

Only seen in those who have been to West Africa, the *Loa loa* worm migrates around the body and not infrequently crosses the cornea, causing little to no damage as it does so. The best course of action is to allow it to exit the eye before treatment to avoid inflammatory damage to the eye.

33.12 Further reading

Barnes, S.D., Pavan-Langston, D., Azar, D.T., Durand, M.L., 'Section M - Eye Infections' in Mandell, G.L., Bennett, J.E., Dolin, R. 'Principles and Practice of Infectious Diseases' (7th edn, Philadelphia, 2010).

Tuft, S., Burton, M., 'Microbial keratitis' *Royal College of Ophthalmologists Focus* (2013) https://rcopth.ac.uk/wp-content/uploads/2014/08/Focus-Autumn-2013.pdf

33.13 Assessment questions

33.13.1 Question 1

A patient suffers anastomotic breakdown following a colonic resection for malignancy and is placed on empiric co-amoxiclav and metronidazole, on which she clinically stabilizes. A week later she remains well but complains of decreased visual acuity. An ophthalmologist reviews her and a diagnosis of endophthalmitis is made. He plans to perform a vitreal biopsy for culture and asks your opinion regarding her ongoing management.

What is the most important immediate course of action?
A. Broaden the antibiotic cover to meropenem.
B. Instil intravitreal amphotericin.
C. Instil intravitreal foscarnet.
D. Perform blood cultures.
E. Request an echocardiogram.

33.13.2 Question 2

A fifty-two-year-old man presents to the Emergency Department with weight loss, diarrhoea, and decreased visual acuity. A rapid HIV test is performed and found to be reactive—the patient admits being diagnosed as HIV-positive nearly a decade previously but had declined treatment. The patient is admitted and a raft of investigations requested.

What investigation is the most useful in ascertaining the cause of his visual symptoms?
A. Blood CD4 count.
B. Plasma CMV DNA load.
C. Plasma HIV RNA load.
D. Serum CMV IgG.
E. Serum Toxoplasma IgG.

33.13.3 Question 3

An eighty-four-year-old male is referred by his GP. The patient complains of a severe left-sided headache. The pain is sufficiently severe that he is struggling to sleep and he has vomited twice. On examination there are no focal neurological signs—however, a red left eye and vesicular lesions beneath the hairline on the left side of his head are noted.

What is the most appropriate therapy for this patient?
A. Intravenous aciclovir.
B. Intravenous foscarnet.
C. Oral aciclovir.
D. Oral valaciclovir.
E. Topical aciclovir.

33.14 Answers and discussion

33.14.1 Answer 1

B. Instil intravitreal amphotericin.
This patient has significant intra-abdominal pathology, presumably involving the leak of bowel contents into the peritoneum. Antibacterials have stabilized her and she remains well so broadening cover to meropenem will add little at this stage. However, in this context it is vital to be wary of fungal infection, particularly with *Candida* species. These yeasts are a common cause of endogenous endophthalmitis. The yeast will likely be present in the blood so blood cultures will be a useful investigation and an echocardiogram must be performed to exclude infective endocarditis. However, the patient is suffering from a sight-threatening condition and the priority must be to start therapy. While ophthalmology can often instil a combination of antimicrobials into the eye, amphotericin must be prioritized in this case.

33.14.2 Answer 2

B. Plasma CMV DNA load.
This patient is presenting with advanced HIV infection—the most likely cause of his visual symptoms is CMV chorioretinitis. However, the presence of CMV IgG in his serum will not prove this diagnosis—it only proves that he has been infected with the virus at some point in the past. Toxoplasma chorioretinitis is a possible diagnosis but much less likely—like CMV IgG, toxoplasma IgG in serum only proves past infection. The patient's HIV viral load is important for deciding his antiretroviral therapy but will not help in diagnosing his eye pathology. CD4 cell counts are important in assessing the risk of various opportunistic infections—however, in this case the patient is presenting with advanced HIV and is likely to have a sufficiently low CD4 count to facilitate either

CMV or toxoplasma chorioretinitis. The best option is blood CMV DNA load—the presence of CMV DNA will not only point to the diagnosis of CMV chorioretinitis but declining levels in the blood can be used to assess response to therapies such as ganciclovir.

33.14.3 Answer 3

A. Intravenous aciclovir.

The most likely diagnosis is ophthalmic shingles. Herpes zoster virus can be treated with all of these agents under different circumstances. Foscarnet is a less benign drug than aciclovir and is typically reserved for infections that develop aciclovir resistance. This infection calls for systemic therapy so topical aciclovir is insufficient. Oral aciclovir needs to be taken at high doses five times daily— valaciclovir is better absorbed and can be taken less frequently, which greatly improves compliance. However, in this case of an elderly patient with severe pain, vomiting, and possible keratitis, IV therapy is the best initial option, although stepping down to oral therapy will be appropriate once he begins to improve. In any event, he requires an urgent ophthalmological review.

Device-associated infections

Michael Millar

34.1 Understanding and recognizing device-associated infection

A great variety of biomedical devices are used in patient care. Almost all hospitalized patients will have a vascular catheter placed to support administration of drugs, fluids, electrolytes, blood products, feeding solutions, or for haemodynamic monitoring. Many will also be exposed to urinary catheters, or tracheal tubes. There is also increasing use of a variety of prosthetic devices.

34.2 Infection associated with biomedical devices

Different biomedical devices have different infection associations. Examples of associations include cardiac pacemakers with *Staphylococcus aureus* blood-stream infection, contact lenses with amoebic keratitis, tampons with toxic shock, and historically, intra-uterine devices with pelvic actinomycosis. The most common causative organisms associated with device infections are bacteria (less commonly fungi). For many devices coagulase-negative staphylococci are the most frequent cause of infection. It is important to remember that an enormous range of microbes have been reported to cause device-associated infection.

Biomedical devices predispose to infection through a wide range of mechanisms. These may include (depending on the device) traversing of anatomical barriers (such as the skin), protected niches for microbial proliferation, inappropriate immune activation, and provision of a surface(s) for biofilm formation. Few devices are completely inert. Most devices elicit an immune response, which depletes local complement levels and reduces oxidative killing by neutrophils, some directly damage tissues, and some release biologically-active products. There is much interest in the molecular mechanisms and physical interactions that underlie the formation of communal microbial structures on biomaterial surfaces. Many difference strategies have been proposed both to prevent, and to destroy microbial biofilms associated with biomedical devices.

Complications associated with devices are most likely to be mechanical or infective. It is estimated that up to 25% of patients with a central venous catheter (CVC) will suffer a serious mechanical or infection related complication. Risk factors for infection include host, device, and operator factors. Extremes of age, co-morbidities such as diabetes, active infection at the time of insertion, and loss of relevant anatomical barriers to infection are host risk factors that apply to most devices. Operator risk factors include poor compliance with insertion or post-insertion 'best practice'. Specifically, for CVCs the site of insertion (lowest for subclavian, highest for femoral), the numbers of lumens (increased number of lumens increases risk), the type of connector (decreased risk for neutral compared to positive displacement connectors), the type of CVC (port probably lower risk than tunnelled CVC, antimicrobial impregnated CVCs lower risk than non-antimicrobial, midline lower risk than central), and the use of parenteral nutrition solutions are risk factors.

Rates of infection are usually given as rate/numbers of days at risk (device days), for example, x infections/1000 CVC days. Rates of device-associated infection vary considerably depending on the risk factors prevalent in the population studied.

34.3 Diagnosing device-associated infections

The diagnosis of device-associated infection can be difficult. Infection may present non-specifically for example pain over a prosthetic joint, or confusion in an elderly patient with catheter-associated urinary tract infection, or headache in a patient with an infected ventriculo-peritoneal shunt. Microbial culture can help to support a diagnosis particularly when the device is accessible. The time to positivity of blood cultures collected through a CVC can give an indication that there a CVC-associated infection. Isolation of *Staphylococcus aureus* from a blood culture in a patient with a pacemaker should raise the suspicion of pacemaker infection. Suspect device associated infection when there is an implanted device associated with raised inflammatory markers (CRP, white cell count, procalcitonin) without other explanation. Sonication has been shown to increase the yield of microbes from colonized orthopaedic implants. There is ongoing research into the predictive value of synovial fluid biomarkers (such as interleukins) in joint implant infections.

34.4 Preventing device-associated infections

There is considerable evidence from quality improvement programmes that instigation of care bundles can prevent some types of device-associated infections. These are three to five evidence-based interventions introduced at the same time with checklists (designed to provide assurance of compliance) and regular feedback of compliance rates. Care bundles might include generic elements, such as the use of maximal sterile barrier precautions at the time of insertion, and standardization of equipment and techniques alongside device-specific measures, such as the introduction of antibiotic-impregnated devices or tunnelling for transcutaneous devices.

General principles for prevention of infection from transcutaneous devices include ensuring fixation at skin insertion site, protecting exit site, skin decontamination pre-insertion, limiting duration of placement as much as possible, and regular insertion site inspection. General principles for the prevention of implanted device infections include prophylactic antibiotics at the time of insertion, operator experience, optimizing management of co-morbidities, adequate skin decontamination, and optimizing the operating environment, including air quality.

Such interventions are best delivered through multidisciplinary teams with the ultimate outcome of improving patient care, and evidence shows care bundles are effective in the prevention of device-associated infections in intensive care settings, but less so when used in other contexts.

34.5 Treating biomedical device infections

Biofilm bacteria are relatively resistant to antimicrobials, and established device-associated infections usually involve biofilms. Also, devices do not have a vascular supply and may provide protected niches for microbial proliferation and survival. This means that effective treatment of device-associated infections often requires device removal. Some device-associated infections can be treated effectively with antibiotics, for example tunnelled CVC-associated infections with coagulase-negative staphylococci. In general device management has to be a component of effective device-associated infection treatment.

34.6 Further reading and useful resources

Loveday, H.P., Wilson, J. A., Pratt, R. J., Golsorkhi, M., Tingle, A., Bak, A., et al. Epic3: National Evidence-Based Guidelines for Preventing Healthcare-Associated Infections in NHS Hospitals in England. *Journal of Hospital Infection*, 86/Suppl 1 (2014), S1–S70.

Mermel, L. A., Allon M, Bouza E, Craven, D. E., Flynn, P., O'Grady, N. P., et al., 'Clinical Practice Guidelines for the Diagnosis and Management of Intravascular Catheter-Related Infection: 2009 Update by the Infectious Diseases Society of America', *Clinical Infectious Diseases*, 49 (2009), 1–45.

34.7 Assessment questions

34.7.1 Question 1

A six-year-old boy with short bowel syndrome receives total parenteral nutrition through a central venous catheter (CVC). The clinical team discuss with you the strategy that can be used to prevent CVC-associated infection.

Which of the following options has a *limited* role in the prevention of CVC- associated infection in this patient who requires the CVC for long-term nutrition?
A. Antibiotic-impregnated central venous catheter.
B. Antimicrobial CVC locks.
C. CVC fixation.
D. CVC hub disinfection policy.
E. CVC sub-cutaneous tunnel.

34.7.2 Question 2

A ten-year-old patient undergoing chemotherapy for malignancy presents with fever, vomiting, and diarrhoea. There is evidence of mucositis on clinical examination and of a subclavicular tunnelled central venous catheter (CVC) that has been in place for three months.

The patient is neutropenic (0.3 neutrophils $\times$ 10⁹/L), has a temperature of 39.5°C, and has a normal blood pressure. The respiratory and heart rate are only mildly elevated.

A single blood culture bottle collected in A&E from the CVC is reported as positive six hours after sample collection with gram-positive cocci.

Which of the following options is an *inappropriate* response to receiving this report?
A. Assuming that the positive blood culture reflects sample contamination.
B. Maintaining fluid balance.
C. Repeating blood cultures.
D. Sending stool samples for enteric pathogen studies.
E. Starting treatment with antibiotics.

34.7.3 Question 3

Prophylactic antibiotics are often used in clinical practice, but not always justified.

In which of the following scenarios is the prophylactic use of antibiotics *justified*?
A. Following an uncomplicated external ventricular drain insertion procedure.
B. In routine hip implantation procedures.
C. In the week following chest drain insertion.
D. Routinely in patients with a urinary catheter and associated bacteriuria.
E. When a central venous catheter is inserted.

34.8 Answers and discussion

34.8.1 Answer 1

A. Antibiotic-impregnated central venous catheter
There is evidence to support all of the options in the prevention of CVC-associated infection. However, antibiotic-impregnated catheters do not retain antimicrobial activity beyond a few weeks, so have a role in intensive care, but a limited role in prevention of infection in patients with long-term CVCs. Subcutaneous tunnelling is an effective preventive measure for any long-term CVC (oncology, long-term intravenous feeding). Antimicrobial CVC locks can be used with any long-term CVC which is not used continuously (e.g. renal dialysis). Fixation of the CVC (so that it doesn't move across the insertion site) and the hub disinfection policy are important elements in the prevention of infection with any CVC.

34.8.2 Answer 2

A. Assuming that the positive blood culture reflects sample contamination.
Fever, vomiting, and diarrhoea can be a feature of CVC-associated infection, or mucositis in children with cancer. The presence of gram-positive bacteria in a blood culture after six hours could be consistent with a diagnosis of CVC-associated infection, because the time to positivity is relatively short. It would be sensible to repeat blood cultures including samples from the CVC and peripheral vein. Sepsis can be rapidly fatal in patients with neutropenia so starting treatment with antibiotics, including an antibiotic active against Gram positives such as vancomycin, is appropriate. Assuming blood culture contamination would be a high-risk strategy in this scenario. This patient may have several potential causes for fever, vomiting, and diarrhoea, but may also have an enteric infection, so it is worth sending samples to check for enteric pathogens.

34.8.3 Answer 3

B. In routine hip implantation procedures.
Antibiotics do not generally have a role in in the prevention of device-associated infection after placement, or when a CVC is inserted. There is strong evidence that antibiotics given immediately before a hip device procedure do reduce the risk of infection. Bacteriuria is common in patients with a urethral catheter and is not an indication for antibiotics.

CHAPTER 35

Zoonotic infections

Marta Gonzalez Sanz and Caoimhe Nic Fhogartaigh

35.1 Definition of zoonosis

The term zoonosis comes from the Greek: ζῷον (*zoon*) 'animal' and νόσος (*nosos*) 'sickness', and means an infection transmissible from animals to humans (Table 35.1). Infected animals can be symptomatic or asymptomatic, and humans usually become accidental hosts through close contact with the reservoir animal. Six out of ten infections in humans globally are spread from animals, and 75% of emerging infections are zoonotic. Some occur worldwide e.g. *E. coli* O157:H7, whereas some are more restricted geographically, e.g. Ebola virus. The highest burden is in developing countries.

35.2 Classifying zoonoses

There are various classifications of zoonoses.

- **Causative pathogen:** bacterial (anthrax, non-typhoidal Salmonelloses); viral (rabies, Yellow Fever, hantaviruses); parasitic (hookworm, Giardia, toxoplasmosis); fungal (dermatophytes, histoplasmosis); or prion (new-variant Creutzfeldt-Jakob disease).
- **Mode of transmission** (see Section 35.3 and Table 35.1 below)
- **Distribution**: *endemic* zoonoses are continually present in a population (e.g. leptospirosis, brucellosis); *epidemic* zoonoses occur intermittently (e.g. anthrax, Rift Valley Fever); *emerging* zoonoses are new infections, or existing infections that are increasing in incidence or geographical range (e.g. Nipah virus, Middle East Respiratory Syndrome coronavirus).

35.3 Modes of transmission from animals to humans

- **Direct contact**: infectious particles are present on an infected animal, in its body fluids, and in its excreta. Q fever, caused by *Coxiella burnetii*, and brucellosis may be acquired by direct

Table 35.1 Common zoonoses, reservoir animal hosts, and modes of transmission.

Disease	Main reservoirs	Usual mode of transmission to humans
Anthrax	livestock, wild animals, environment	direct contact, ingestion
Animal influenza	livestock, humans	may be reverse zoonosis
Avian influenza	poultry, ducks	direct contact
Bovine tuberculosis	cattle	milk
Brucellosis	cattle, goats, sheep, pigs	dairy products, milk
Cat scratch fever (*Bartonella henselae*)	cats	bite, scratch
Cysticercosis	cattle, pigs	meat
Cryptosporidiosis	cattle, sheep, pets	water, direct contact
Mycobacterium marinum ('fish tank granuloma')	fish	direct contact, water
Campylobacter	poultry, farm animals	raw meat, milk
Salmonella	poultry, cattle, sheep, pigs	foodborne
Giardiasis	humans, wildlife	waterborne, person to person
Glanders (*Burkholderia mallei*)	horse, donkey, mule	direct contact
E. coli O157:H7	ruminants	direct contact (and foodborne)
Hantavirus syndromes	rodents	aerosol
Hepatitis E	not yet known	not yet known
Hydatid disease	dogs, sheep	ingestion of eggs excreted by dog
Leptospirosis	rodents, ruminants	infected urine, water
Listeriosis	cattle, sheep, soil	dairy produce, meat products
Louping ill	sheep, grouse	direct contact, tick bite
Lyme disease	ticks, rodents, sheep, deer, small mammals	tick bite
Lymphocytic choriomeningitis	rodents	direct contact
Orf	sheep	direct contact
Pasteurellosis	dogs, cats, many mammals	bite/scratch, direct contact
Plague (*Yersinia pestis*)	rats and their fleas	flea bite
Psittacosis	birds, poultry, ducks	aerosol, direct contact
Q fever (*Coxiella burnettii*)	cattle, sheep, goats, cats	aerosol, direct contact, milk, fomites
Rabies	dogs, foxes, bats, cats animal	bite
Rat bite fever/'Haverhill fever' (*Streptobacillus moniliformis*)	rats	bite/scratch, milk, water
Rift Valley fever	cattle, goats, sheep	direct contact, mosquito bite
Ringworm	cats, dogs, cattle, many animal species	direct contact
Tickborne encephalitis	rodents, small mammals, livestock	tick-bite, unpasteurized milk products
Toxocariasis	dogs, cats	direct contact
Toxoplasmosis	cats, ruminants	ingestion of faecal oocysts, meat
Trichinellosis	pigs, wild boar	pork products
Tularemia	rabbits, wild animals, environment, ticks	direct contact, aerosol, ticks, inoculation
Ebola, Crimean-Congo HF, Lassa and Marburg viruses	variously: rodents, ticks, livestock, primates, bats	direct contact, inoculation, ticks
West Nile fever	wild birds, mosquitoes	mosquito bite

Reproduced with permission from Public Health England.

contact with infected animals, particularly during parturition; cat-scratch disease caused by *Bartonella henselae*, and *Pasteurella spp.* may be acquired by bites or scratches from cats, and rabies from canine bites. Many zoonoses are also transmitted via indirect animal contact through exposure to soil or water contaminated by infectious material, e.g. leptospirosis may be acquired when water contaminated with infected rats' urine comes into contact with broken skin or mucous membranes.

- **Ingestion**: infection occurs by ingesting contaminated food or water, e.g. unpasteurized milk, poorly processed or undercooked meat, or by eating/drinking after handling animals without handwashing. Listeria, bovine tuberculosis, and brucellosis may be transmitted by unpasteurized milk and dairy produce; Hepatitis E through processed pork, and Ebola and Marburg through bushmeat.

- **Vector-borne:** infection is transmitted through a biting arthropod vector. Examples include West Nile Virus and Japanese encephalitis from mosquitoes, Lyme disease, tick-borne encephalitis, and Rocky Mountain Spotted Fever from ticks, and *Rickettsia typhi* from rat fleas.

- **Aerosolization:** infection is transmitted via inhalation of infectious aerosolized particles from an infected animal or contaminated environment. Most exposure occurs when aerosols are created during birthing, or generated from dust or soil contaminated with faeces, urine, or bacterial spores during adverse weather events or as a result of bomb blasts. Examples include Q fever and hantaviruses.

- **Fomites:** infection may occur via indirect transmission through contact with contaminated objects or surfaces, such as feeding bowls and straw bedding. Examples include dermatophytes, sporotrichosis, and glanders.

Many zoonotic infections use more than one route for transmission, and may result in different clinical syndromes, e.g. cutaneous versus inhalational anthrax. Occupations involving close contact with animals and the environment increase the risk of zoonotic infection, e.g. farming, veterinary work, animal slaughter, forestry, mining, military work. Recreational activities have also been linked to outbreaks of zoonotic disease e.g. leptospirosis following watersports.

35.4 Factors leading to the emergence of zoonotic diseases

The emergence or re-emergence of a zoonotic disease requires a variation in the pathogen (e.g. virulence mutation) or its introduction into a new host population (a new host species or the same host in a new geographical region), followed by establishment and further dissemination within the population. These occurrences are a result of the following, often in combination:

- Ecological changes, such as those due to agricultural or economic development, or climate change;
- Technology and industry;
- Human demographic changes, including urbanization;
- Breakdown of public health measures;
- Travel and commerce;
- Human behaviour, including social and cultural factors such as food habits, religious practice, conflict;
- Microbial adaptation and change.

As the human population increases, demands for food and fuel have increased dramatically. This has led to 'high density farming', closer contact between man and farm animals, and trade of livestock across international borders promoting spread of zoonotic infection. Live animal markets in Asia create a melting pot for interspecies transmission, and the emergence of pandemic influenza viruses due to reassortment of genes from pig and duck influenza strains. Globalization of food production and processing has enabled contaminated food produce to be transported across large distances causing global outbreaks.

In order to meet increased global energy demands expanding deforestation and mineral extraction industries have disrupted natural ecosystems leading to the emergence of zoonoses such as Nipah virus in Malaysia and Mayaro virus in Brazil. Global warming has enabled the geographical spread of Lyme disease and tick-borne encephalitis into new regions due to spread of the tick vector.

Uncontrolled urbanization and mass migration of refugees has increased population density and overwhelmed public health control measures leading to rapid transmission of zoonotic diseases, e.g. dengue, chikungunya, and epidemic typhus.

Ease of international travel has led to global pandemics such as Severe Acute Respiratory Syndrome (SARS), and international ecotourism and volunteer work exposes travellers to a range of endemic zoonoses. Increasing popularity of exotic pets such as reptiles has resulted in unusual nontyphoidal salmonellae in humans. Occasionally, zoonotic agents have been used for the purposes of bioterrorism.

35.5 The most common UK and worldwide zoonotic infections

Foodborne zoonoses, e.g. campylobacter and salmonellosis, are the most common zoonoses in the UK. In 2015, Public Health England also received reports of the following zoonoses: Lyme disease (n = 872), hepatitis E (n = 848), *Pasteurella multocida* (n = 641), toxoplasmosis (n = 337), leptospirosis (n = 71), Hydatid disease (n = 23), Q fever (n = 19), and brucellosis (n = 11). Only three cases of rabies (all imported) have been reported in the last decade.

According to the International Livestock Research Institute, the most common zoonoses worldwide are also foodborne, followed by cysticercosis, Q fever, toxoplasmosis, leishmaniasis, leptospirosis, zoonotic tuberculosis, brucellosis, hydatid disease, and rabies. The foodborne zoonoses are responsible for the greatest morbidity and mortality, and the greatest burden of zoonotic disease is in developing regions.

35.6 Zoonoses transmitted through animal bites

Thousands of hospital attendances occur annually in the UK as a result of animal bites. Up to 30% of dog bites may become infected, and an even higher proportion of cat bites (up to 80%). Wound infections are usually polymicrobial and include *Pasteurella spp.*, staphylococci, streptococci, anaerobes, and the fastidious gram-negative rod *Capnocytophaga canimorsus*, which is part of the normal flora in dogs but can cause severe infection with abscess formation, pneumonia, meningitis, and severe sepsis in immunosuppressed patients, particularly asplenics. Other bite-related infections include cat-scratch disease (*Bartonella spp.*), rat-bite fever (*Streptobacillus moniliformis*), rabies, simian herpesvirus B, and monkeypox. A risk assessment for rabies and other potentially life-threatening viral infections should be carried out where bites have occurred abroad.

35.7 Presentation

Zoonoses have a wide range of clinical presentations depending on the pathogen, including diarrhoeal illness, hepatitis, skin lesions (e.g. erythema migrans in Lyme disease), non-specific febrile illness (e.g. leptospirosis), atypical pneumonia, arthritis, endocarditis, meningitis, and other neurological symptoms, as well as pyrexia of unknown origin.

35.8 Diagnosing zoonoses

Zoonoses must be considered if the patient has risk factors such as occupation, recreation, travel, and animal exposure. Most of the foodborne zoonotic infections may be diagnosed by faecal microscopy and culture in microbiology laboratories. PCR methods have been developed which are more sensitive for gastro-intestinal pathogens but require local validation and careful interpretation. Some of the bacterial zoonoses require higher levels of containment, e.g. Anthrax and Brucella, and should be handled in containment Level 3, or referred to the relevant reference laboratory. For diagnosis of the more fastidious bacterial zoonoses, e.g. *Coxiella burnettii*, Lyme, and leptospirosis, serum must be sent to reference laboratories for specialized diagnostic testing and interpretation, although advances are being made in molecular diagnostics. Erythema migrans of early Lyme is a clinical diagnosis—serology is often negative at this time and is not recommended. Many of the viral and parasitic zoonoses will also require specialist reference laboratory testing.

35.9 Treating zoonoses

Many of the foodborne zoonoses will be self-limiting and do not require treatment in immunocompetent individuals. For other bacterial zoonoses, treatment is directed against the suspected pathogen, but a combination of a beta-lactam and doxycycline would be a reasonable empirical regimen until results are available. Appropriate isolation precautions are important to prevent onward transmission of gastro-intestinal pathogens, severe respiratory illness, and suspected viral haemorrhagic fevers.

Management of viral zoonoses is largely supportive, however, there may be a role for ribavirin if administered in the early phase of hantavirus pulmonary syndromes and Lassa fever. Rabies is universally fatal.

Animal bites may require surgical debridement in addition to antibiotics to prevent deeper infection. Antibiotic prophylaxis, tetanus vaccination, and, in high-risk cases, rabies vaccination and post-exposure prophylaxis with immunoglobulin are required to prevent infections.

35.10 Preventing zoonoses

In order to prevent the emergence of zoonoses it is mandatory to risk assess and control animal-associated infections that pose a threat to public health. Increasing awareness of zoonotic infections in high-risk occupations and ensuring adequate training in personal protective measures is imperative. A number of vaccinations are available for animal use and a limited number for human use, e.g. anthrax vaccine in military recruits. The following surveillance tools are in place in the UK to monitor zoonoses: statutory notifiable disease reports and laboratory notifications (animal diseases are reported to the Animal Health and Veterinary Laboratories Agency), screening of imported animals and annual screening in farm animals for certain diseases, horizon-scanning surveillance, and international web-based surveillance systems. Successful zoonoses control requires the collaboration of human, animal and environmental health experts, such as that represented in the 'One Health' concept.

35.11 Further reading and useful resources

Grace, D., Mutua F., Ochungo, P., Kruska, R., Jones, K., Brierley, L., et al., 'Mapping of poverty and likely zoonoses hotspots', *Zoonoses Project 4, Report to Department for International Development* (ILRI Nairobi, 2012).

Jones, K. E., Patel, N. G., Levy, M. A., Storeygard, A., Balk, D., Gittleman, J. L., et al., 'Global Trends in Emerging Infectious Diseases', *Nature*, 451 (2008), 990–993.

Morse, S. S., 'Factors in the Emergence of Infectious Diseases', Emerging Infectious Diseases, 1/ 1 (1995), 7–15.

35.12 Assessment questions

35.12.1 Question 1

A 77-year-old lady attended A&E following a bite from her neighbour's dog. The wound was not deep, and there were no local signs of infection.

Which of the following conditions does *not* require antibiotic prophylaxis?
A. The patient has a prosthetic heart valve.
B. The patient has diabetes.
C. The wound is localized to the hand.
D. The wound is more than forty-eight hours old.
E. There is devitalized tissue at the wound site.

35.12.2 Question 2

A 30-year-old man, usually fit and well, has been hiking in the New Forest over the weekend and discovers a tick in his groin area on Monday morning. He has removed it carefully with tweezers and attended his GP.

Which of the following do you advise?
A. No action required.
B. Reassurance and counselling on signs and symptoms of Lyme disease to facilitate early treatment.
C. Request Lyme serology.
D. Single dose Doxycycline 200mg prophylaxis and counselling.
E. Two week course of Doxycycline 100mg twice daily and counselling.

35.12.3 Question 3

A 42-year-old sheep farmer in southwest England presents in April with three weeks of fever, myalgia, dry cough, and fatigue. Physical examination was unremarkable, although laboratory investigations showed a transaminitis and mild thrombocytopenia.

What is the most likely cause of his illness?
A. Anaplasmosis.
B. *Bartonella henselae*.
C. Brucellosis.
D. Leptospirosis.
E. Q fever.

35.13 Answers and discussion

35.13.1 Answer 1

D. The wound is more than forty-eight hours old

Antibiotic prophylaxis is recommended in all cat bites, but for other animals will depend on the timing, depth, location of bite and initial management. Wounds presenting more than six hours after the bite without being cleaned are at high risk of becoming infected, although cleaned wounds with no signs of infection forty-eight hours later are unlikely to become infected and do not require prophylaxis. Patient conditions that would indicate antibiotic prophylaxis are immunosuppression (including diabetes, cirrhosis, and asplenia), prosthetic valves, and prosthetic joints. See https://cks.nice.org.uk/bites-human-and-animal#!topicsummary.

35.13.2 Answer 2

B. Reassurance and counselling on signs and symptoms of Lyme disease to facilitate early treatment

Lyme post-exposure prophylaxis is not routinely recommended in Europe but single dose doxycycline 200mg may be considered in immunosuppressed cases (amoxicillin if pregnant but the optimal dose and duration is unknown). In the United States however, single-dose doxycycline is recommended for adults and children over eight years in areas where tick infection prevalence > 20%, the tick has been present > 36 hours, and patients present within seventy-two hours of tick removal. According to a US study transmission is unlikely to take place within the first thirty-six hours of tick attachment.

35.13.3 Answer 3

E. Q fever

Lambing season takes place in spring, and these clinical and laboratory features in a sheep farmer at this time of year would be most suggestive of acute Q fever. Diagnosis is made on acute and convalescent serology and PCR, but work up would also include chest X-ray and echocardiogram. Brucella and leptospirosis are important differentials and blood cultures, serology, and PCR testing should be performed. Anaplasmosis could present similarly and is diagnosed on blood film showing neutrophil intracytoplasmic inclusions, but prevalence of *A. phagocytophilum* in UK ticks is low with only occasional cases reported in Scotland. *B. henselae* is more common in children and presents with an inoculation lesion and self-limiting regional lymphadenopathy. In immunosuppressed individuals it may cause more disseminated infections including bacillary angiomatosis and peliosis hepatis.

Exanthemata

C. Y. William Tong

36.1 What are exanthemata?

An exanthem (or exanthema) is a widespread skin rash accompanying a disease or fever. It usually occurs in children as part of a common systemic childhood viral infection, but can also occur in adults and can be caused by bacterial infections, toxin or drug reactions. An enanthem (or enanthema) is a rash that occurs in the mucous membrane, typically in the mouth, as the result of the same disease process of an exanthema.

Because the presence of a rash is a very striking feature, historically, several of the commonly seen febrile illnesses associated with rash have been recognized and named in numerical order (see Table 36.1).

36.2 Assessing a patient with exanthema

There are various things to look out for when assessing a patient with exanthema. These can include the type and evolution of the rash, as well as contact, vaccine, drug, sexual, and travel history.

- Type of rash:
    - maculopapular;
    - vesicular;
    - petechial.
- Evolution of the rash:
    - prodrome, if any;
    - date of onset of fever;
    - date of onset of the rash;
    - progression of the rash (e.g. starting location and spread);
    - other associated features (e.g. conjunctivitis, lymphadenopathy, hepatosplenomegaly).

Table 36.1 Historical naming of rashes.

Historical name	Current commonly used name	Causative micro-organisms
First disease	Measles	Measles virus
Second disease	Scarlet fever	*Streptococcus pyogenes*
Third disease	Rubella	Rubella virus
Fourth disease	Scalded skin syndrome (previously called Duke's disease which is no longer recognized as an entity)	*Staphylococcus aureus*
Fifth disease	Erythema infectiosum/slapped cheek syndrome	Erythrovirus (parvovirus) B19
Sixth disease	Exanthem subitum/roseola infantum	Human herpes virus 6 (or 7)

- Contact history:
  - history of contact with anyone with febrile or rash illness;
  - recent local outbreaks, if any;
  - contact with other vulnerable individuals before and after onset of illness (for infection control purposes).
- Vaccine history:
  - recent history of any vaccination;
  - previous vaccination history (particularly MMR and varicella);
  - timing of these vaccines and number of doses.
- Drug history:
  - including antibiotics given for the illness.
- Sexual history:
  - always consider this in any patient.
- Recent travel history:
  - record timing and location;
  - history of insect bites.

36.3 Different types of rash

A good description of the rash can help in narrowing down the possible causes. The commonly seen rashes can be maculopapular, vesicular, or petechial.

Maculopapular rash can be further categorized into subtypes. These include:

- morbilliform—a red rash which is measles-like, two to ten mm in diameter, and which merge to form confluent patches. Experienced clinicians can diagnose measles clinically, usually in conjunction with other signs and symptoms such as concurrent conjunctivitis, coryzal symptoms, and cough, presence of Koplik spot (an enaxthem associated with the early stage of measles) and a typically miserable child. However, other conditions could present in a similar way, e.g. Kawasaki disease.
- rubelliform—fine, pale pink, relatively flat maculopapular rash resembling rubella. However, many viral (e.g. enteroviruses, glandular fever) and non-viral rashes (e.g. drug rash) could present as rubelliform. Posterior cervical lymphadenopathy, notably occipital nodes, is said to be a common feature in rubella.
- roseoliform—a transient red rash that appears at the time of defervescence of fever commonly associated with primary HHV6 or 7 infection. Unlike measles, the child is typically relatively well, though the high fever may be associated with febrile seizures.

- scarlatiniform—a rash with a sandpaper like texture, with tiny macules converging rapidly to form a broad red rash that is more prominent at skin creases.

Generalized vesicular rashes are usually caused by varicella-zoster virus (chickenpox or disseminated zoster). With the eradication of smallpox, there are fewer differential diagnoses. Herpes simplex viruses usually cause a localized rash, but a generalized rash could be seen in the immunocompromised and in neonatal infection. Enteroviruses can be associated with vesicular rash in hand, foot, and mouth disease. The distribution can be beyond hand, foot, and mouth, involving buttock areas, genital area, and the trunk. Herpangina can be considered as an enanthem of enterovirus with vesicular lesions in the oropharynx.

Meningococcal disease and disseminated intravascular coagulation (DIC) should be considered when petechial and purpuric rashes are seen. Rickettsial infection of the spotted fever group could also give a purpuric rash. Non-infection causes include thrombocytopenia, vasculitis (e.g. Henoch-Schonlein purpura), and nutritional deficiency (e.g. scurvy).

36.4 What investigations should be offered?

The investigations should be targeted to the possible differential diagnoses (see Table 36.2).

Table 36.2 Investigations for exanthemata.

Condition to exclude	Investigations
Enterovirus infection	Enterovirus RNA (stool, lesion swab, throat swab, blood, CSF)
Erythema infectiosum/slapped cheek syndrome	Erythrovirus (parvovirus) B19 IgG/IgM (blood) and DNA (blood)
Exanthem subitum/roseola infantum	Rarely necessary—serology not widely available Utility of HHV6/7 DNA not clear
Glandular fever-like illness (also need to exclude HIV and syphilis)	EBV VCA IgM/ EBNA IgG (blood) CMV IgM/IgG +/- IgG avidity (blood) *Toxoplasma gondii* serology (blood)
Herpesviruses infections (HSV, VZV)	HSV/VZV DNA (lesion swab)
measles	Measles RNA (oral fluid, throat swab, urine, blood); IgG/IgM (oral fluid, blood)
Primary HIV	Fourth generation HIV Ag/Ab test (blood)
Rubella	Rubella RNA (oral fluid, throat swab, urine, blood); IgG/IgM (oral fluid, blood)
Scarlet fever	Throat swab for MC&S
Secondary syphilis	*Treponema pallidum* IgG/IgM, RPR/VDRL (blood)
Travel-related infections	Serology +/- nucleic acid amplification tests (NAAT) for dengue, chikungunya, zika, rickettsia, etc. (refer to the Rare and Imported Pathogen Laboratory, RIPL)

36.5 Infectious periods

It is necessary to understand the natural history and pathogenesis of each infection in order to provide advice on infectious period for each infection (see Tables 36.3 and 36.4).

For exclusion from school, please see the UK Government website for more information (also summarized in Table 36.4).

Table 36.3 Incubation period and infectious duration of some common exanthemata.

Disease	Incubation period	First become infectious	Cease to be infectious
Chicken pox	Ten to twenty-one days	Two days before onset of rash	Cropping ceased and all lesions crusted
Erythema infectiosum/ slapped cheek syndrome	Fourteen to twenty-one days	Ten days before onset of rash	Onset of rash
Measles	Eight to fourteen days	Four days before onset of rash	Four days after onset of rash
Rubella	Fourteen to twenty-one days	Seven days before onset of rash	Ten days after onset of rash

https://assets.publishing.service.gov.uk/government/uploads/system/uploads/attachment_data/file/786356/viral_rash_in_pregnancy_guidance.pdf

36.6 Possible complications

Most viral exanthemata are self-limiting and patients generally recover without specific treatment. However, immunocompromised individuals may be severely affected and pregnant women could also have more severe illness, or result in miscarriage or foetal infection (see Table 36.5).

36.7 Preventing infection

Many of the viral infections can be avoided by appropriate vaccination. Interested readers are referred to Chapter 48, Different types of vaccines and Chapter 49, Vaccination schedules for information on the different types of vaccines and vaccination schedules, and to Chapter 51, Post-exposure prophylaxis.

Table 36.4 Suggested exclusion period from school for some common childhood exanthemata.

Examples of common exanthemata	Exclusion period
Chicken pox	Until all vesicles have crusted over.
Erythema infectiosum/slapped cheek syndrome	None once rash developed
Glandular fever	None
Hand, foot, and mouth disease	None
Measles	Four days from onset of rash
Roseola infantum	None
Rubella	Six days from onset of rash*
Scarlet fever	Twenty-four hours after starting appropriate antibiotics
Shingles	Exclude only if rash is weeping and cannot be covered

* check if female contacts are immune.

https://assets.publishing.service.gov.uk/government/uploads/system/uploads/attachment_data/file/658507/Guidance_on_infection_control_in_schools.pdf

Table 36.5 Examples of complications associated with common exanthemata.

Conditions	Complications	Additional complications in immunocompromised hosts	Complications associated with pregnancy
Chicken pox	Bacterial superinfection; viral pneumonia; acute cerebella ataxia (post-infection syndrome); encephalitis; stroke; Reye syndrome (with concurrent use of salicylates); hepatitis	Haemorrhagic varicella	More severe disease in pregnant woman; congenital varicella syndrome (1–2%); severe neonatal varicella if mother developed infection five days before to two days after delivery
Erythema infectiosum/ slapped cheek syndrome	Polyarthropathy; aplastic crisis in those with haemogobinopathy or haemolytic anaemia such as sickle cell disease; myocarditis	Chronic anaemia	Hydrop fetalis; intrauterine death (first twenty weeks)
Glandular fever (primary EBV)	Rash after treatment with ampicillin; hepatitis; respiratory obstruction; CNS (meningitis, encephalitis, myelitis, Guillain Barre syndrome); haematological (splenic rupture, mononucleosis, haemophagocytic syndrome)	Lymphoproliferative disorders	None recognized
Hand, foot, and mouth disease (HFMD)	Brain stem encephalitis; flaccid paralysis (mainly associated with HFMD caused by enterovirus A71)	/	Neonatal enterovirus infection if mother infected perinatally
Measles	Otitis media; bronchopneumonia; croup; diarrhoea; acute encephalitis (1:1000, immune mediated); subacute sclerosing panencephalitis (SSPE)	Inclusion body encephalitis	Miscarriage

(Continued)

Table 36.5 Continued

Conditions	Complications	Additional complications in immunocompromised hosts	Complications associated with pregnancy
Primary cytomegalovirus infection	Infectious mononucleosis-like syndrome; hepatitis	Pneumonitis; colitis; retinitis	Congenital cytomegalovirus syndrome (IUGR, jaundice, purpura, microcephaly, intracranial calcification); long-term hearing loss or learning disability
Roseola infantum	Febrile seizure	Encephalitis	None recognized
Rubella	Transient polyarthralgia /polyarthritis; encephalitis (1:5000); thrombocytopenia (1:3000)	/	Congenital rubella syndrome (affecting eye, heart, hearing, CNS) if pregnant women get infected before twenty weeks gestation

36.8 Other conditions like exanthemata

Drug rash is common, and in glandular fever associated with EBV rash commonly appears after treatment with ampicillin or related antibiotics.

Some conditions such as Kawasaki disease mimic infection like measles. The cause of Kawasaki disease is still uncertain. It is diagnosed clinically based on fever associated with an enanthem (strawberry tongue, cracked lip), bulbar conjunctivitis, rash (morbilliform or scarlatiniform), lymphadenopathy, and extremity changes (induration or desquamation). Many of these features are shared with measles or scarlet fever.

Erythema multiforme (the severe form being Steven Johnson syndrome) is a skin eruption characterized by target lesions and could be triggered by herpes simplex virus or *Mycoplasma pneumonia* infection. It can also be drug induced.

Adult-onset Still's disease is another condition that may present as a salmon pink maculopapular rash over trunk and limbs, and is typically associated with high spiking fevers, joint pain, and leucocytosis. It is a diagnosis of exclusion (of causes of exanthemata and pyrexia of unknown origin), though a very high level of ferritin may help in establishing the diagnosis.

Toxic shock syndrome (TSS) is a life-threatening bacterial infection caused by *Staphylococcus aureus* and *Streptococcus pyogenes* bacteria. In the former, it is caused by enterotoxin type B or TSST-1, and in the latter, streptococcal pyrogenic exotoxins. The rash may appear like sunburn, and may desquamate in later stage of the illness. The condition needs to be recognized rapidly as intensive care is often required.

36.9 Assessment questions

36.9.1 Question 1

A fourteen-month-old child presents to the emergency department with a four-day history of fever and coryzal symptoms. On examination, the child is irritable with inflamed conjunctivae.

A generalized maculopapular rash is noted. The child has not yet received the first dose of MMR. His mother is currently twelve weeks pregnant.

What is the *most* important first step in management after initial assessment?
A. Administer a dose of ceftriaxone to the child.
B. Give a dose of human normal immunoglobulin to the mother.
C. Notify the health protection team.
D. Place the child into a side room.
E. Take a sample of oral fluid to investigate for measles.

36.9.2 Question 2

A fourteen-month-old child presents to the emergency department with a four-day history of fever and coryzal symptoms. On examination, the child is irritable with inflamed conjunctivae and a red swollen tongue. A generalized maculopapular rash and cervical lymphadenopathy is noted. The child has not yet received the first dose of MMR.

What investigation is the most relevant?
A. Blood for anti-streptococcal O titre (ASOT).
B. Blood sample for measles IgG.
C. Blood sample for monospot test.
D. Echocardiogram to examine the coronary artery.
E. Oral fluid for measles RNA.

36.9.3 Question 3

A six-month-old infant presents to the emergency department with a generalized tonic-clonic seizure after a two-day history of fever and coryzal symptoms. On examination, the infant is drowsy and a generalized non-blanching maculopapular rash is noted.

What is the most appropriate immediate management?
A. Administer a dose of aciclovir after CT scan of the brain.
B. Administer a dose of ceftriaxone after blood culture.
C. Administer antipyretic after taking baseline temperature.
D. Administer anti-epileptic after baseline EEG.
E. Perform lumbar puncture after CT scan of the brain.

36.10 Answers and discussion

36.10.1 Answer 1

D. Place the child into a side room.

The clinical picture described in this case scenario is typical of that of measles, although there is room for other differential diagnoses. In the emergency department setting, the first action when a case of measles is suspected is to isolate the patient before carrying out further assessment or investigation. Measles is highly contagious and if a suspected case is allowed to stay in the main waiting or triage area for a prolonged period of time, the risk of onward transmission is high and should be avoided as much as possible. It is important to confirm the diagnosis and an oral fluid sample is recommended, but this can be done after the patient is isolated. All clinical diagnosis needs to be notified to the health protection team, and this should be done after the clinical assessment is completed. There is no need to wait for laboratory confirmation. If the pregnant mother is susceptible to measles, a dose of human normal immunoglobulin within six days of contact could be offered as post-exposure prophylaxis. However, the immune status of the mother needs to be worked up to confirm susceptibility before this action is taken, although clearly this needs to be completed within the six-day window. Unless a disseminated bacterial infection is suspected, empirical antibiotics are not recommended.

36.10.2 Answer 2

E. Oral fluid for measles RNA.

The presentation of this child is shared by a number of conditions. Some of the features of this child are compatible with measles, but they also fulfil a number of criteria for Kawasaki disease (fever, conjunctivitis, swollen tongue, rash, lymphenopathy). Scarlet fever could also be a differential diagnosis. Oral fluid for measles RNA is the recommended sample for confirming measles during the early stage of the illness. Measles RNA could also be detected in blood, urine, and respiratory secretions. If the patient presents late, RNA may not be detectable and serology becomes more important. Public Health England sends out oral fluid collection kits for suspected cases through the local health protection team that can be used to investigate for both measles RNA and IgM. Measles IgG is not present in the early stage of the illness and therefore not useful, but demonstration of sero-conversion can help. Kawasaki disease is a clinical diagnosis after exclusion of other illnesses. Coronary artery aneurysm is a late complication. However, echocardiogram is not needed in the early stage, although it may serve as a baseline for future reference when the diagnosis is eventually confirmed. Antistreptolysin O titer (ASOT) is not particularly helpful to confirm Streptococcal infection. Rather, a throat swab for culture may be more relevant. Monospot test is rarely positive in children with primary EBV infection. If primary EBV infection is suspected, EBV VCA IgM and EBNA IgG should be the tests of choice.

36.10.3 Answer 3

B. Administer a dose of ceftriaxone.

While the infant in this case shows some features of roseola or measles, the concern is the presence of a non-blanching maculopapular rash. The prodrome in this case is also shorter in that both roseola and measles have a typical prodrome of about four days. A disseminated bacterial infection such as meningococcal disease needs to be excluded. Due to the high mortality and morbidity of meningococcal disease, it is necessary to give an empirical dose of antibiotics such as ceftriaxone as soon as possible. Blood cultures are very quick and easy to do and should be done before ceftriaxone is given even if meningococcal septicaemia is suspected, especially as the organism is less likely to grow if antimicrobials have been administered, and molecular techniques often take several days to get an answer if sent to an external reference laboratory. In the GP setting, however, empirical antibiotic is often preferred. Intravenous aciclovir is often given alongside ceftriaxone in suspected cases of encephalitis. However, in this case, the suspicion of herpes simplex encephalitis is less compelling and therefore aciclovir is not the most important option. It is also not necessary for an LP to be performed after the CT scan if there is no suspicion of significant raised intracranial pressure. Other supporting measures such as antipyretics and anti-epileptics are important but probably not as immediate as antibiotics.

CHAPTER 37

Pregnancy-associated infections

Anna Riddell and Michael Millar

37.1 Differences in pregnancy in relation to infection

An important consideration in pregnancy is the relationship between infection in the mother and the developing foetus (Figure 37.1). Infections can indirectly impact the foetus through effects on the mother, for example, maternal urinary tract infection is associated with preterm birth, or can infect the foetus. Routes of infection can be ascending from the birth canal through the cervical os, transplacentally, or rarely, contiguously.

The effect on the mother is also important: pregnancy is considered an immunosuppressive state and the growing foetus causes significant mechanical and physiological changes. Although the first trimester is the key developmental phase for the growing foetus, during the third trimester the mother is more susceptible to severe respiratory infection and some viral infections such as varicella zoster virus (VZV), due to the mechanical changes produced by the growing foetus.

37.2 General principles on treating infection during pregnancy

There is a paucity of evidence supporting the safety of drugs in pregnancy. Use of any medicinal drug in pregnancy, including antibiotics, requires good reasons. The optimum choice of antibiotics depends on the trimester of the pregnancy. In general, beta-lactams are safe and tetracyclines should be avoided throughout pregnancy. Nitrofurantoin is safe until after thirty-five weeks gestation and trimethoprim should be avoided in the first trimester but is safe otherwise (perhaps with folic acid supplementation if < 20 weeks).

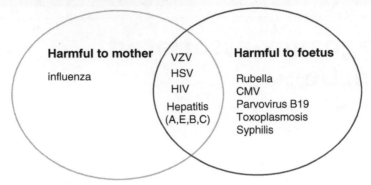

Figure 37.1 A Venn diagram showing the differential effect of some infections on mother and foetus.

37.3 The relationship between patterns of genitourinary colonization and pregnancy outcome

Specific patterns of colonization and infection of the genitourinary tract can be associated with an increased risk of an adverse pregnancy outcome, particularly preterm birth. Sexually transmitted diseases such as gonorrhoea and chlamydia are associated with an increased risk of spontaneous preterm birth, which may extend to infection in the pre-conception period. Bacterial vaginosis is an abnormal pattern of vaginal colonization and is also linked with an increased risk of preterm birth. The US Center for Disease Control recommends screening all pregnant women for chlamydia, gonorrhoea, syphilis, HIV, and hepatitis B, symptomatic women for trichomonas and genital herpes, women considered at high risk of preterm birth for bacterial vaginosis, and women at high risk of blood-borne virus infection for hepatitis C. Treatment is administered to reduce the risk of an adverse pregnancy outcome (syphilis, gonorrhoea, chlamydia, trichomonas, and bacterial vaginosis) or to prevent transmission to the infant (herpes, HIV, hepatitis B, and C).

37.4 Preventing group B streptococcal infection

Group B streptococci (GBS) colonize the vagina and rectum of up to 30% of pregnant women. Approximately 1% of pregnant women colonized with GBS will give birth to a baby infected with GBS (usually presenting with pneumonia and septicaemia).

Many countries have national policies designed to control the risk of GBS infection of the newborn infant. These policies may be based on screening pregnant women for GBS (usually at thirty-five to thirty-seven weeks gestation) or on the identification of women with risk factors for neonatal infection, such as previous delivery of an infant with GBS, GBS bacteriuria during pregnancy, preterm delivery, prolonged rupture of membranes (greater than eighteen hours), or maternal pyrexia during labour. If the pregnant woman screens positive or has risk factors, then GBS infection of the infant can be prevented by the administration of antibiotics (usually penicillin) pre-delivery.

37.5 Urinary tract infections

Asymptomatic bacteriuria is common in pregnancy (up to 15%) and is a risk factor for preterm birth and pyelonephritis. Therefore, pregnant women are screened and those who are positive should be treated (See NICE and SIGN guidelines).

37.6 Infections during pregnancy adversely impacting the foetus

The infections acquired congenitally which have significant adverse outcomes in the foetuses were traditionally known as TORCH infections. This term was first proposed in 1971 due to the similar ways in which toxoplasma, rubella, cytomegalovirus (CMV), and herpes simplex virus (HSV) infections present. However it was soon realized that congenital infections are more than the four TORCH agents.

37.6.1 Toxoplasmosis

Toxoplasmosis is caused by the parasite *Toxoplasma gondii*. Cats are the natural hosts. An infected cat excretes oocysts in their faeces for between one and three weeks after primary infection. Humans then ingest these oocysts either via direct contact with cat faeces (gardening, unwashed vegetables, handling cat litter) or indirectly through eating infected meat.

Once a human has ingested oocysts they may have a low-grade fever and lymphadenopathy, although a significant proportion of infection is asymptomatic. About 40% adults are seropositive for toxoplasma in the UK. It is higher in other European countries depending on the diet of the indigenous population.

In pregnant women, the main concern is primary acquisition of the parasite during pregnancy. Congenital toxoplasmosis is most significant to the foetus during the first trimester of pregnancy, although it is most commonly transmitted during the third trimester.

The diagnosis is complex and the test results can be difficult to interpret. Toxoplasma IgG persists for life and IgM can persist for years making the timing of infection difficult to assess. The gold standard serology test is the dye test (Sabin-Feldman). Antibody avidity testing may be of help. Other tests available include an immunosorbent agglutination assay (ISAGA) for Toxoplasma IgM and PCR (which can be performed on amniotic fluid). A combination of these tests is normally required to determine if a foetus has been infected and the timing of infection which will in turn inform treatment.

Toxoplasma has a tropism for certain tissues: brain, eyes, and muscle (skeletal and cardiac) and tends to cause problems in these tissues for the foetus, e.g. intrauterine growth restriction (IUGR), hydrocephalus, cerebral calcifications, hepatosplenomegaly.

If acute toxoplasmosis infection is suspected during early pregnancy (i.e. before eighteen weeks), foetal ultrasound should be performed and treatment with spiramycin is recommended to reduce the risk of transmission to the foetus. After eighteen weeks, amniotic fluid PCR should be performed to determine further management. If the amniotic fluid PCR is positive and/or ultrasound is positive, treatment should be switched to pyrimethamine, sulfadiazine, and folinic acid, as spiramycin does not cross the placenta and so cannot be used to treat foetal infection. Cases with confirmed congenital toxoplasmosis should be managed in a specialist unit.

37.6.2 Rubella

Rubella is a self-limiting illness and is rare in the UK after the introduction of the MMR (Measles, Mumps and Rubella) vaccine in 1998. Congenital rubella, is a serious consequence of rubella infection. If a woman has primary rubella infection during the first trimester of pregnancy, there is a 90% risk of the foetus being affected. This risk falls with progression of the pregnancy.

Congenital rubella can be a devastating disease with multi system effects:

- Cataracts and other ocular sequelae leading to blindness;
- Micrognathia;
- Hepatosplenomegaly;
- Hearing loss;
- Congenital heart disease; and
- Neurodevelopmental delay.

Rubella serology was a part of the UK antenatal screening. Due to the lack of endemic circulation of rubella virus and high degree of herd immunity, antenatal screening was stopped in April 2016.

37.6.3 Cytomegalovirus (CMV)

CMV is an extremely common virus of the family Herpesviridae. Approximately 60% adults are CMV IgG positive, i.e. have evidence of past exposure to CMV. A large majority of infections are asymptomatic.

CMV remains latent after primary infection and reactivation is common throughout a person's lifetime. However, it is maternal primary CMV infection that carries the greatest risk for congenital CMV infection in the foetus, particularly acquisition during the first trimester.

The prevalence of congenital CMV is seven per one thousand births, although only 12% of babies with congenital CMV are symptomatic at birth. The symptoms of congenital CMV include jaundice, hepato-splenomegaly, microcephaly, and cerebral calcification. There is some evidence that ganciclovir therapy in symptomatic congenital CMV disease prevents hearing deterioration in these neonates. The duration of treatment is controversial (six weeks of IV ganciclovir vs six months of oral valganciclovir) although a study suggested that prolonged treatment may modestly improve hearing and developmental outcomes. These benefits have to be considered against the side effects of neutropenia during therapy.

The more significant *sequelae* of congenital CMV is sensorineural hearing loss (SNHL). Approximately 10% of asymptomatic congenitally infected children are diagnosed with SNHL in the first five to seven years of life. However, screening of children only normally continues for the first two years of life, and therefore up to 50% children may be missed with the current screening programme. Retrospective testing to establish congenital infection relies on CMV DNA PCR of the Guthrie card which is limited in its sensitivity (due to the low volume of blood available).

37.6.4 Syphilis

Syphilis is caused by the spirochete *Treponema pallidum subspecies pallidum*, not to be confused with the other treponemes—yaws (*subsp pertenue*) and pinta (*subsp endemicum*).

The risk of congenital syphilis is dependent on the stage of syphilis the mother has: the highest risk is associated with primary and secondary infection during pregnancy, 40% in latent infection, and 10% in tertiary syphilis probably related to the high bacterial load in primary and secondary infection.

Syphilis antibody testing is currently part of the UK antenatal screening programme. Individuals with positive screening test serology should be further tested with additional treponemal-specific (e.g. TPPA) and non-treponemal-specific serology test (e.g. RPR/VDRL). Pregnant women with no previous adequate treatment should be treated as soon as possible, with long-acting penicillins the treatment of choice.

37.6.5 Parvovirus B19 (erythrovirus B19)

Parvovirus B19 is usually a self-limiting infection. Approximately 60% of UK adults have serological evidence of past infection.

The cellular target of parvovirus B19 is erythroblasts and other cell lines with the P antigen receptor.

In those patients with a high red blood cell turnover, dramatic falls in haemoglobin can occur (as in the foetus) due to the destruction of infected red cells.

Foetal infection can be fatal (9%) and the biggest risk to the foetus is acquisition during the first twenty weeks of pregnancy. Non-immune hydrops fetalis is the consequence of red cell aplasia secondary to parvovirus B19 infection and diagnosis of parvovirus during pregnancy warrants enhanced ultrasound surveillance; intra-uterine cord blood transfusions can be given.

37.6.6 Herpes simplex virus (HSV)

HSV infection in humans can be due to HSV type 1 (HSV 1) or type 2 (HSV 2). HSV 1 is ubiquitous (> 90% seropositivity in those above forty years old). HSV 2 seroprevalence is related to sexual activity and is higher in developing countries. HSV is responsible for a wide spectrum of disease, and the classical clinical syndrome associated with HSV 1 is oral ulceration in children and adults; HSV 2 is commonly associated with genital ulceration, although there is considerable crossover between HSV 1 and HSV 2. HSV infection can cause other more serious complications such as encephalitis, oesophagitis, hepatitis, or disseminated infection, particularly in the immunocompromised. More than 80% of primary infections are asymptomatic. In the UK 50% of neonatal HSV infection is due to HSV 1.

Primary HSV in pregnancy can have significant consequences for the foetus if the primary infection is within six weeks of birth. This is due to persistent viral shedding and limited passive transfer of maternal antibodies. The majority of neonates acquire HSV perinatally due to direct contact with lesions in the birth canal, although up to 25% may be due to close contact with a relative with active oral herpetic lesions. If the mother has a symptomatic infection within six weeks of birth, Caesarean section is recommended as well as aciclovir treatment for the mother. Instrumentation during a vaginal delivery can also increase the risk of HSV transmission.

Maternal primary HSV infection should be treated with aciclovir and then maintained on daily suppressive aciclovir from thirty-six weeks gestation.

Neonatal herpes (due to primary maternal HSV infection) can cause localized infection (skin/eye/mouth), local central nervous system (CNS) infection, and disseminated infection. Nearly all neonates who are exposed to HSV perinatally manifest the disease, with 70% cases being disseminated. Mortality in these cases is high without treatment (30%) and neurological morbidity can be lifelong. Delays in diagnosis are thought to be responsible for the poor outcome of these neonates.

37.6.7 Zika virus

Zika virus is a mosquito-borne flavivirus which is usually mild/asymptomatic or can present with similar clinical features to dengue and chikungunya, which are transmitted by the same species of A. aegypti mosquito. In the recent large-scale outbreaks in South America, it is recognized that it can be a cause of congenital infection if acquired by pregnant women during the early part of gestation. Manifestations in infected foetuses include microcephaly, craniofacial disproportion, spasticity, seizures, irritability, and brainstem dysfunction, including feeding difficulties and ocular abnormalities. Neuroimaging shows calcifications, cortical disorders, and ventriculomegaly. It is also recognized that Zika virus can be sexually transmitted and can persist in semen for up to six months.

37.6.8 Human immunodeficiency virus (HIV)

The most recent British HIV Association Guidelines (2015) recommend starting antiretroviral therapy (ART) independent of CD4 and HIV viral load and this includes pregnancy. The goals of treatment of an HIV positive woman are to 1) prevent progression of HIV and deterioration in the mother's health, and 2) to prevent transmission of HIV to the newborn.

In the UK, antenatal screening of HIV (along with HBV and HCV) is now 'opt out' (since 2000) which in itself has led to a reduction in mother-to-child transmission.

HIV transmission from mother to child most commonly happens during labour/delivery via maternal secretions (35–40%), but other factors which also increase risk are prolonged rupture of membranes and instrumentation during labour, presumably due to increased risk of contact with maternal blood or fluids. In-utero transmission of HIV accounts for 10–25% neonatal infection and the risk increases from early to late pregnancy. After birth, breastfeeding is also a risk factor for HIV transmission (between 35–40%) and is therefore not recommended in developed countries if the mother has a detectable HIV viral load. With optimal intervention however, the risk of transmission is reduced to 1 in 1000.

The aim of diagnosis of HIV in pregnancy is to allow for early combination ART; the product of early treatment being an undetectable plasma viral load. Ideally once ART is started, these women should remain on treatment lifelong especially now due to the demonstrated benefits on morbidity and mortality.

There is good evidence that higher plasma HIV-1 viral loads in a mother are associated with perinatal transmission of HIV. Although ARTs are not licenced for use in pregnancy, there is worldwide experience with their use in pregnancy and the US Antiretroviral Pregnancy Registry has not reported an increase in congenital anomaly rates above background rates (i.e. > 2–3%). However, there is less experience with newer drugs and potentially an increased risk of congenital anomalies with dolutegravir.

A further benefit of ART and reduction in the plasma HIV viral load to undetectable levels is that it is possible in this case to have a normal vaginal delivery. However, if the pregnant mother does have a detectable viral load at thirty-six to forty weeks, an elective Caesarean section at between thirty-eight and forty weeks is recommended to reduce the risk of HIV transmission; the benefit of this intervention can be demonstrated even at very low viral loads.

Treatment of neonates after delivery with ART is only recommended if the mother has a viral load > 1000 copies/ml and should be started in conjunction with a specialist experienced in managing HIV in pregnancy as this may involve combination therapy. In an unbooked mother with a new diagnosis of HIV or in an untreated mother, ART treatment will be offered to the mother and given to the neonate and will likely mean combination ART after/at delivery if viral load > 50 copies/ml.

37.7 Further reading and useful resources

BASHH and RCOG. Management of Genital Herpes in Pregnancy, October 2014. https://www.rcog.org.uk/globalassets/documents/guidelines/management-genital-herpes.pdf
British HIV Association Guidelines for the Management of HIV Infection in Pregnant Women 2012. http://www.bhiva.org/documents/Guidelines/Pregnancy/2012/BHIVA-Pregnancy-guidelines-update-2014.pdf
Kimberlin, D. W., Jester, P. M., Sánchez, P. J., Ahmed, A., Arav-Boger, R., Michaels, M. G., et al. 'Valganciclovir for Symptomatic Congenital Cytomegalovirus Disease', New England Journal of Medicine, 372/10 (2015), 933–943.
Liu, B., Roberts, C. L., Clarke, M., Jorm, L., Hunt, J., Ward, J., 'Chlamydia and Gonorrhoea Infections and the Risk of Adverse Obstetric Outcomes: A Retrospective Cohort Study', Sexually Transmitted Infections, 89/8 (2013), 672–678.
NICE. Urinary tract infection (lower)—women. July 2015. http://cks.nice.org.uk/urinary-tract-infection-lower-women
Scottish Intercollegiate Guidelines Network. Management of Suspected Bacterial Urinary Tract Infection in Adults. (Edinburgh, 2012). http://www.sign.ac.uk/assets/sign88.pdf

37.8 Assessment questions

37.8.1 Question 1

A lady who is sixteen weeks pregnant and originally from Bangladesh but living in the UK for the past five years is reported to have been exposed to a child with chicken pox.

What is the most important next step in management?
A. Arrange urgent VZIG (Varicella Zoster Immunoglobulin) for the pregnant lady.

B. Ask the lab to perform a VZV IgG on the pregnant woman's booking bloods.

C. Ask the pregnant lady to re-present if she develops chicken pox.

D. Clarify the nature of the exposure and when it occurred.

E. Immunize the pregnant lady against VZV.

37.8.2 Question 2

A lady who is twenty weeks pregnant has her routine twenty-week ultrasound scan and the foetus is reported as 'small for dates'. The serology results of a contemporaneous blood sample show the following results:

- CMV IgG detected
- CMV IgM detected
- Parvovirus (erythrovirus) B19 IgG detected
- Parvovirus (erythrovirus) B19 IgM not detected
- Rubella IgG detected
- Syphilis total antibody not detected
- Toxoplasma IgM/IgG not detected

What is the most appropriate next step in investigation?

A. Nothing further need to be done.

B. Request CMV DNA PCR on a plasma sample.

C. Request CMV avidity on this sample.

D. Request CMV IgG and IgM on the booking bloods.

E. Request foetal ultrasound scan to look for hydrops fetalis.

37.8.3 Question 3

A twenty-five-year-old woman, recently migrated to the UK, presents at twenty-five weeks gestation with fever and abdominal pain. She has a C-reactive protein measured at 210 mg/L at the time of presentation. She gives birth within six hours of admission.

Blood cultures taken at admission show a positive result twelve hours after incubation. A faintly haemolytic growth of a gram-positive bacillus is noted the following day on a blood agar plate that had been inoculated from the blood culture bottle and left on the bench.

What is the most likely organism?

A. *Bacillus cereus.*

B. *Corynebacterium diphtheriae.*

C. *Listeria monocytogenes.*

D. *Propionibacterium acnes.*

E. *Streptobacillus moniliformus.*

37.9 Answers and discussion

37.9.1 Answer 1

D. Clarify the nature of the exposure and when it occurred.

The single best response in this case is to clarify the nature of the exposure and when it occurred as this will dictate what to do next. The lady is from Bangladesh but has lived in the UK for five years. This is of interest as in temperate climates chicken pox exposure tends to be as a child with a 90% seropositive rate in adults, whereas in the tropics/subtropics exposure tends to be later and so a higher proportion of adults will be non-immune to chickenpox.

Chickenpox is infectious two days before the onset of the rash and until the lesions are crusted. After establishing the nature and the timing of the contact, the next stage is to arrange for an urgent

VZV IgG to be performed, either on the pregnant lady's booking bloods (usually taken after twelve weeks) or on another sample if not available. If the pregnant lady is immune no further action is required. If the pregnant woman is non-immune and the exposure to the child with chicken pox (i.e. not all the lesions had crusted) was within the last ten days, the next stage is to arrange urgent VZIG. VZV vaccine is a live attenuated vaccine and therefore is not safe during pregnancy. If the pregnant woman is both non-immune and within the ten days from exposure, as in this case, VZIG is indicated. However, if the exposure occurred more than ten days before presentation, the pregnant woman should be advised to present to a healthcare provider if she develops a rash/clinical features of chicken pox and aciclovir should be given. Although aciclovir is not licenced for pregnancy, experience has shown that it is safe in pregnancy and early use is recommended to reduce the severity of chicken pox and to prevent complications, e.g. pneumonitis which is more common later in pregnancy due to the growing size of the foetus and the anatomical splinting of the diaphragm.

37.9.2 Answer 2

D. Request CMV IgG and IgM on the booking bloods.
Although the CMV serology may be consistent with acute infection (IgM and IgG positive), IgM can persist for long period post-initial infection and also can be detected in reactivation of CMV. As the timing of primary infection is the main concern regarding congenital CMV infection, this needs to be chased down further. By reviewing the booking bloods and requesting a CMV IgG and IgM, this allows better interpretation of the recent serological results and if similar in detection, an avidity should also be added to the booking blood sample. CMV avidity is more useful on the booking blood sample than on the sample taken at twenty weeks. If a high avidity was detected on the earlier booking sample, the likely infection is outside of pregnancy thus reducing the concern regarding congenital infection. There is no suspicion of parvovirus B19 infection here, and hence the ultrasound scan feature of hydrops fetalis is not expected.

37.9.3 Answer 3

C. *Listeria monocytogenes.*
The correct answer is *Listeria monocytogenes* given the clinical scenario—Listeria can be a cause of premature labour. The other organisms are all gram-positive rods, although with different haemolytic properties in blood agar. The key microbiological feature here is the beta-haemolytic growth on blood agar of a gram-positive rod after overnight incubation on the bench, i.e. room temperature—characteristic of *Listeria monocytogenes*.

Listeria is a cause of severe and sometimes fatal neonatal infection (20–30% of cases) and can present as sepsis, pneumonia, and meningitis. The most appropriate treatment for this is IV amoxicillin and gentamicin.

Many foods are contaminated with Listeria including raw vegetables, meats, cheese, and ingestion is common. Listeria can survive the cool environment of the fridge and multiply, thus increasing the potential inoculating dose of bacterium and increasing the risk of listeria infection. Listeria is a notifiable disease in the UK and tracing of cases to identify an infected food source is undertaken due to the significant risks of Listeria infection to neonates and immunosuppressed patients.

CHAPTER 38

Infections in neonates and young children

Michael Millar and Steve Kempley

CONTENTS

38.1 The scope of the chapter

This chapter covers infections in neonates and young children. In this chapter the term 'young children' indicates children under two years of age. For information on congenital infections interested readers are referred to Chapter 37.

38.2 Infections during the first week of life

Early neonatal infection is variably defined as infection presenting up to a week after birth, but most infections present in the first seventy-two hours. Microbial invasion of the chorio-amniotic membranes or uterine cavity occur in a significant proportion of pregnancies before rupture of membranes (> 50% with preterm birth before thirty weeks gestation, 10% with term delivery), and in the majority of those with prolonged rupture of membranes (> 24 hours). It is likely that the majority of cases of early sepsis arise through ascending infection of the uterus (through the cervical canal). Ascending infection may be important in the pathogenesis of preterm birth and is more common in infants born preterm. Group B Streptococci (GBS) (*Streptococcus agalactiae*) and *Escherichia coli* are the most common agents of early neonatal infection. Infection with *Listeria monocytogenes* probably arises following ingestion of contaminated food by the mother, blood stream infection, and transplacental spread. Early infection with GBS usually presents with respiratory distress and can be difficult to differentiate from respiratory distress associated with other causes, particularly prematurity. The incidence of GBS blood stream infection in England and Wales has been 0.3–0.45/1000 live births over the last five years.

Maternal genital herpes simplex infection can spread to the newborn infant and cause a wide range of serious clinical presentations, with skin, systemic, and central nervous system involvement. Maternal infection with *Neisseria gonorrhoea* or *Chlamydia trachomatis* can also infect the infant. Either can cause conjunctivitis which can sometimes be of sufficient severity to cause substantial damage to the eyes. Gonococcal conjunctivitis usually presents in the first few days of life. Infection with *Chlamydia trachomatis* (conjunctivitis or pneumonitis) tends to present later.

38.3 Treating and preventing early neonatal infection

Traditionally, penicillin and an aminoglycoside have been used to treat infants with suspected early sepsis (to cover GBS and *Escherichia coli*). Newborn infants are often empirically treated because it can be difficult to differentiate early bacterial sepsis from respiratory distress associated with prematurity, and death may ensue rapidly if the infection is not treated. As gestational age decreases so an increasing proportion of infants are treated with penicillin and gentamicin. Herpes simplex infection may require the use of aciclovir.

Early GBS disease can be prevented if antibiotics are given to the mother intrapartum. In the UK the current recommendations from the Royal College of Obstetrics and Gynaecology and from NICE is to base the use of prophylactic antibiotics on risk factors. In many other countries in the developed world the decision to use prophylactic antibiotics is based on screening pregnant women for vaginal or rectal colonization with GBS.

38.4 Infections after the first seven days of life

Late neonatal infection is usually defined as infection that presents after the first seven days of life. Newborn infants are vulnerable to the wide range of infections prevalent in the community (see Infections in infants and young children). Some early infections can present late and this probably includes GBS disease, which has an estimated incidence of late infection of 0.2/1000 live births. Infants born preterm are the most vulnerable to late neonatal sepsis, often acquired from carers and environmental sources in hospital.

38.5 Infection and adverse outcome in preterm infants

The incidence of preterm birth has not changed substantially over the last thirty years. Approximately 8% of births are before thirty-seven weeks gestational age and 1% are very preterm (< 32 weeks gestational age). As other outcomes have improved, infection is accounting for an increasing proportion of deaths and adverse outcomes amongst infants born too early. Risk factors for infection include increasing prematurity, intensity of care, use of biomedical devices particularly intravascular cannulae, and necrotizing enterocolitis (NEC). Exposure to antibiotics is itself a risk factor for infection and NEC. One of the commoner hospital infections in preterm infants undergoing neonatal intensive care is staphylococcal infection associated with vascular catheters (caused by coagulase-negative staphylococci or *Staphylococcus aureus*). It is important to remember that infants nursed in intensive care are still at risk of viral infections acquired from breast milk, visitors, and staff.

38.6 Treating late neonatal infection and nosocomial infection

The choice of antimicrobial depends on the source of infection and aetiological agent. Source control is essential, especially central venous and umbilical vessel catheters. NICE provides guidelines on the management and treatment of neonatal infection.

Many hospital-acquired neonatal infections can be prevented. A particular focus is on the use of care bundles, which are defined as three to five evidence-based interventions introduced contemporaneously, combined with feedback on compliance.

38.7 Infections in infants and young children

Infectious disease is one of the most common reasons for admission of infants to hospital. The aetiology is usually viral. Common presentations in the first year of life include fever and rash, e.g. roseola infantum, erythema infectiosum (see Chapter 36), and respiratory tract infection. Clinical syndromes associated with viral respiratory infection include bronchiolitis (RSV), croup (parainfluenza type 3), and pneumonia. Bacterial infection most commonly arises secondary to viral infection (particularly respiratory).

For vaccine-preventable diseases, please refer to Chapter 15 and the Green Book.

38.8 Treating common respiratory tract infections in young children

Respiratory tract infection presenting in infancy is usually caused by viruses, and these infections account for > 20% of admissions of infants to hospital in the UK and > 50% of general practice consultations.

Clinical syndromes associated with viral respiratory infection include bronchiolitis (RSV), croup (parainfluenza type 3), and pneumonia. RSV is probably the most common cause of infection and cause outbreaks annually during winter. Rhinovirus, parainfluenza virus, adenovirus, human metapneumovirus, coronavirus, and influenza virus all also contribute. Bacterial infection most commonly arises secondary to viral infection.

If influenza is diagnosed in infants older than three months of age, neuraminidase inhibitors (oseltamivir and zanamivir) can be used for treatment within thirty-six hours of symptom onset. Neuraminidase inhibitors can also be used for prophylaxis but must be given within forty-eight hours of exposure. Data on dose, efficacy, and safety is lacking in infants younger than three months of age.

Palivizumab is used for the prophylaxis of RSV in high-risk groups including preterm infants, those with chronic lung disease, and congenital heart disease. The role of ribavirin in the treatment of RSV remains controversial.

Bronchodilators, steroids, and antibiotics all have a role in the treatment of viral lower respiratory tract infection.

38.9 Urinary tract infection in young children

Since the introduction of effective vaccines for *Haemophilus influenza* type B and *Streptococcus pneumonia* infection, urinary tract infection (UTI) has accounted for an increasingly substantial proportion of serious bacterial infections in infants. The prevalence of urinary tract infection in children presenting with fever in the first two years of life probably exceeds 5%. Current NICE guidelines advocate testing for UTI in those children presenting with unexplained fever in addition to those with relevant signs or symptoms (such as pain on micturition). The urine sample can be a clean catch, supra-pubic aspirate, catheter sample, or from a urine collection pad. Samples should be tested for pyuria and bacteriuria. The bedside strip tests for leucocytes esterase and nitrite are useful in identifying children requiring further investigation and treatment. Evidence of bacteriuria (positive nitrite test or culture of > 10^4 bacteria/ml of urine) is an indication for treatment. Negative test results for nitrites and leucocyte esterase indicate that UTI is unlikely.

Infants younger than three months of age with suspected UTI should be referred to a paediatrician for assessment and treatment (often requiring systemic antibiotics). Duration of antibiotic treatment depends on the extent to which there is renal involvement. Cystitis can be treated with three days of appropriate oral antibiotics whereas pyelonephritis requires ten to fourteen days.

There are various imaging modalities, including ultrasound, radio-isotope MAG3 (mercapto acetyl tri-glycine) or DMSA (dimercaptosuccinic acid) scans, and a micturating cystogram. The role of imaging modalities is discussed in the relevant NICE guidelines.

Prophylactic antibiotics may be considered for children with recurrent episodes of UTI, but in this era of burgeoning antibiotic resistance this may simply select for infections that are more difficult to treat.

38.10 Further reading and useful resources

NICE. Neonatal Infection: Antibiotics for Prevention and Treatment. Clinical Guidance CG149 (London, 2012). https://www.nice.org.uk/Guidance/cg149

NICE. Neonatal Infection Quality Standard. Quality Standard QS75 (London, 2014). https://www.nice.org.uk/guidance/qs75

NICE. Bronchiolitis in Children: Diagnosis and Management. NICE Guideline NG9 (London, 2015). https://www.nice.org.uk/guidance/ng9

NICE. Fever in Under 5s. Quality Standard QS64 (London, 2014). https://www.nice.org.uk/guidance/qs64

38.11 Assessment questions

38.11.1 Question 1

An infant presents at three days of life with a history of irritability and poor feeding. The infant was born by vaginal delivery at thirty-six weeks gestational age and is breast-fed. There is a history of maternal diabetes, prolonged rupture of membranes, and maternal pyrexia pre-delivery. Antibiotics have not been administered. Following a lumbar puncture *E. coli* is isolated from the CSF of the infant.

What is the most significant risk factor for infection in this infant?
A. Failure to use antibiotics in the peripartum period.
B. Maternal diabetes.
C. Prolonged rupture of membranes.
D. Poor infant feeding.
E. Prematurity.

38.11.2 Question 2

A six-month-old previously healthy infant with no comorbidities is admitted to a paediatric ward with acute onset respiratory distress just before Christmas.

What is the most likely cause of this infant's illness?
A. Cytomegalovirus.
B. *Kingella kingiae.*
C. *Mycoplasma pneumoniae.*
D. Respiratory syncytial virus.
E. *Staphylococcus aureus.*

38.11.3 Question 3

A ten-month-old infant presents with fever and has stopped crawling over the last two days. The infant cries when the left leg is moved. There is evidence of an effusion in the left hip which is purulent when aspirated.

What bacterial species is a common cause of the illness in this infant but less common in older children or adults?

A. *Streptococcus pyogenes.*

B. *Haemophilus influenza* type B.

C. *Kingella kingiae.*

D. *Staphylococcus aureus.*

E. *Streptococcus pneumoniae.*

38.11.4 Question 4

A fourteen-month-old child presents to the GP with vesicular lesions on the trunk. The mother is 20 weeks pregnant and has a clear documented history of chicken pox infection in the past. The mother regularly attends antenatal classes and brings her child with her.

What action should the GP prioritize?

A. Administration of varicella-zoster immunoglobulin to the mother.

B. Advising the mother not to attend antenatal classes for three weeks.

C. Determining whether other pregnant women have been exposed to the child.

D. Notifying public health authorities.

E. Prescribing aciclovir to the child.

38.12 Answers and discussion

38.12.1 Answer 1

C. Prolonged rupture of membranes.

Prolonged rupture of membranes is defined as rupture of the membranes more than twenty-four hours preceding the onset of labour. Prolonged rupture of membranes is probably the substantive risk factor in this case. The risk of ascending infection in association with prolonged rupture of membranes rises with decreasing gestational maturity but is substantial even at term. Suspicion of maternal chorio-amnionitis is an indication for the administration of antibiotics to the mother and use of antibiotics may have reduced the risk of neonatal meningitis. The degree of prematurity is insufficient by itself to increase the risks of infection. Maternal diabetes is a risk factor for infection but again not as substantial as prolonged rupture of membranes.

38.12.2 Answer 2

D. Respiratory syncytial virus.

Viral infection is the most common cause of respiratory illness in infancy and RSV is most commonly implicated in the winter. The incidence of *Mycoplasma pneumoniae* infection varies considerably from year to year and older children and young adults are more frequently infected than infants. *Kingella kingiae* and *Staphylococcus aureus* can both cause serious invasive disease but are a much less common cause of a primary respiratory infection.

38.12.3 Answer 3

C. Kingella kingiae.

Staphylococcus aureus is a common cause of bone and joint infection in all age groups. *Streptococcus pyogenes* and *Streptococcus pneumoniae* are less common causes in age group. *Haemophilus influenza* type B infection is uncommon in countries that have introduced vaccination. *Kingella kingiae* is a gram-negative rod which is found in the oropharynx of children. Bone or joint infection often follows an upper respiratory tract infection. Bone and joint infection with *Kingella kingiae* is uncommon after the age of two years.

38.12.4 Answer 4

C. Determining whether other pregnant women have been exposed to the child.

This mother has a history of chicken pox. If in doubt then chicken pox immunity can be checked. While the child is infectious with new crops of vesicles, then the child should not attend antenatal classes. The public health authorities should be notified. The child does not normally require treatment unless there is an underlying condition which increases the risks associated with chicken pox infection, such as immunosuppression. The priority is to identify contacts who are vulnerable to severe forms of chicken pox (such as pregnant women) so that appropriate prophylaxis can be offered.

CHAPTER 39

Infections in the immunocompromised host

Anna Riddell, Marta Gonzalez Sanz, and Jonathan Lambourne

39.1 Caring for an immunocompromised patient

An understanding of the main aspects and functions of the immune system is important, i.e. physical barriers, innate, humoral, and cell-mediated immunity (see Chapter 6, Basic Immunology), when caring for the immunocompromised patient. In adults, secondary immunodeficiency is much more common than primary, and is most often due to iatrogenic immunosuppression with drugs, e.g. corticosteroids, chemotherapy agents, immunosuppressive agents, 'biological' therapies. For example, treatment with corticosteroids for more than one month is enough to increase the risk of some fungal infections such as Candida and *Pneumocystis jirovecii*, such that PCP prophylaxis should be considered in patients receiving $\leq$ 20mg/day prednisolone for four or more weeks. Chemotherapy and immunosuppressive agents may cause profound immunosuppression. The degree and duration of immunosuppression following a transplant, and the conditioning regimen used before the transplant varies with respect to the type of transplant: heart and lung transplant recipients typically receive more significant immunosuppression, and so are at increased risk of opportunistic infection compared to other solid-organ transplant recipients.

Infections (e.g. HIV), cancer, and autoimmune disorders and the treatment of these conditions can also affect the immune system. Other diseases are also considered immunosuppressive although the exact nature of this is less well defined, for example, poorly controlled diabetes mellitus increases the risk of candidal infections and common bacterial infections. Cirrhosis is also considered to be a relatively immunosuppressed state.

Understanding the nature of immune defects in both primary and secondary immunodeficiency allows more accurate prediction of overall infection risk and risk of specific pathogens, allowing a rational approach to infection prevention and investigation when patients become unwell. The initial assessment of the immunocompromised host should be to identify why the patient is immunocompromised, how long they have been immunocompromised (is it a congenital or acquired immunodeficiency?), and whether there is potential for immune recovery. Clearly, a person with a congenital immunodeficiency will have lifelong susceptibility to specific infections, unlike an acquired deficiency due to chemotherapy or transplantation which may be transient. If the immunosuppression is due to a drug, is it possible to reduce or change the immunosuppression? If an infection is suspected, pre-immunosuppression infection screening results can help identify whether the current presentation represents reactivation of a latent infection or primary infection.

39.2 Bacterial infections in the immunocompromised host

One approach to considering which bacterial infections affect immunocompromised patients is to consider the different mechanisms of immunocompromise.

When *physical barriers* to infection, e.g. skin, mucosa, are broken either through intravenous cannulae, mucositis (e.g. secondary to chemotherapy,) and surgery, infection is often due to endogenous flora of the skin and/or gastro-intestinal tract.

The innate immune system acts as the second line of defence against invading organisms and includes the complement cascade and phagocytes. Deficiencies in complement function render individuals uniquely susceptible to infection with Neisseria species. Complement defects may be inherited or acquired, for example, following use of Eculizumab, a monoclonal antibody directed against C5, and used to treat paroxysmal nocturnal haemoglobinuria and acute renal transplant rejection. Defects in neutrophil number and/or function may also be primary, for example, in chronic granulomatous disease, or secondary, for example, neutropaenia following chemotherapy. Pseudomonas infections are of particular concern in neutropaenic patients and may cause an array of problems that range from fever and sinus infection to necrotizing skin and soft tissue infections such as ecthyma gangrenosum. For this reason, empiric antimicrobial therapy for neutropaenic patients typically includes an anti-pseudomonal agent.

Impaired humoral immunity, with impaired antibody production and/or function, predisposes to recurrent sinopulmonary infection and invasive infection due to encapsulated organisms such as *Streptococcus pneumonia, Haemophilus influenzae*, and *Neisseria meningitidis*. Patients with an absent or dysfunctional spleen are also susceptible to infection with these encapsulated organisms. Immunoglobulin replacement, immunization, and prophylactic antibiotics may prevent infections, with the ideal approach varying on the nature of the immune defect and infections the patient has had.

Impaired cell mediated immunity (e.g. post chemotherapy, HIV infection) leads to problems controlling intracellular bacteria, including *Mycobacterium, Salmonella,* and *Listeria* species. *Mycobacterium avium* is significantly more common in patients with advanced HIV infection, i.e. with a CD4 cell count $<50 \times 10^6/L$.

39.3 Viral infections in the immunocompromised host

Both the innate and adaptive immune system are important for control and elimination of viral infections, but the failure of the adaptive immune system (either congenital or acquired) is responsible for the majority of significant presentations of viral infections in the immunocompromised host.

Impaired humoral immunity is associated with increased susceptibility to enterovirus infections, a failure to control Hepatitis B virus replication, and protracted infection with norovirus and rhinovirus. Enteroviral infections in the immunocompromised may cause chronic meningoencephalitis, hepatitis, and dermatitis. Examples of primary immunodeficiencies associated with hypogammaglobulinaemia include X-linked agammaglobulinaemia (due to a failure of B cell development) and Common Variable Immunodeficiency. Immunoglobulin replacement may be considered to control other viral infections, for example, chronic parvovirus B19 infection.

Table 39.1 Risk of post-transplant CMV infection in relation to donor and recipient serostatus.

Donor	Recipient	Solid organ transplant	Stem cell transplant
+	−	High risk, primary infection	Medium risk, protected by host T cells
+	+	Medium risk, reactivation, or reinfection	Medium risk, reactivation, or reinfection
−	+	Medium risk, reactivation	High risk, uncontrolled reactivation
−	−	Low risk	Low risk

For the majority of viral infections, virus eradication or control is determined by the cell-mediated immune response. Diminished T cell responses to varicella zoster virus are seen in older populations and correlate with increased frequency and severity of herpes zoster. Reactivation in significantly immunocompromised patients can lead to multidermatomal or disseminated, infection, which is associated with a high mortality. A young person presenting with shingles should always have an HIV test. Cytomegalovirus (CMV) and Epstein-Barr virus (EBV) infection can have devastating effect in post-transplant patients. The severity and risk of reactivation differs depending on type of transplant (Table 39.1), and this determines when and how to give prophylaxis or pre-emptive therapy. CMV also seems to have an immunomodulatory affect leading to increased prevalence of acute and chronic transplant rejection, bacterial and fungal infections, and EBV-driven post-transplant lymphoproliferative disease (PTLD). EBV is an oncogenic herpes virus and EBV viraemia in a transplant patient raises the possibility of PTLD as well as other EBV-associated non-Hodgkin's lymphomas. PTLD has a mortality of up to 40% and is most common in the first year post transplant.

Polyoma viruses are also important in the context of transplantation and HIV. Similar to herpesviruses they are near ubiquitous in the adult population. BK virus is a major cause of loss of renal graft due to BK nephropathy. Viraemia typically predates and is predictive of nephropathy and should prompt consideration of reducing immunosuppression. BK viruria and the presence of decoy cells are less specific. JC virus is the causative agent of progressive multifocal leukoencephalopathy (PML), which may complicate advanced HIV and therapy with agents impeding lymphocyte migration into the CNS, such as natalizumab, which is used to treat multiple sclerosis.

39.4 Fungal infections in the immunocompromised host

The risks and types of fungal infection to which immunocompromised patients are susceptible vary with the nature of the immune defect.

Patients with impaired physical barriers, e.g. mucositis, most commonly develop infections due to endogenous, colonizing fungi, for example, Candida sp. Due to its association with mucositis, invasive candidiasis is often seen at an early stage of immunosuppression; 90% of invasive disease is caused by C. albicans, C. glabrata, C. tropicalis, C. parapsilosis, and C. krusei. Whether fluconazole or an echinocandin is used first line depends in part on the local prevalence of non-albicans Candida species, and the focus and severity of infection. If Candidal infection is IV catheter-related, the catheter should ideally be removed and clearance blood cultures taken. Due to the risk of endocarditis and endophthalmitis associated with candidaemia, an echocardiogram and an ophthalmology review are recommended.

Infections due to environmental, saprophytic moulds such as Aspergillus and the Mucorales species are seen in patients both with profoundly impaired phagocyte number/function and/ or impaired T cell function, such as that seen in patients receiving immunosuppression for Graft vs host disease. Invasive aspergillosis most commonly manifests as pulmonary disease although other sites can be affected, causing CNS infection, sinusitis, or endocarditis. Diagnosis of invasive aspergillosis is based on combination of histology, culture, antigen detection, and radiology. Serum and BAL galactomannan measurements are recommended in haematological patients; PCR testing can be useful but it is not yet widely available. CT scanning is a useful imaging modality and is more sensitive than plain X-rays. The treatment of choice for invasive aspergillosis is a triazole, e.g. voriconazole, posaconazole, isavuconazole, and itraconazole, although liposomal amphotericin B and echinocandins can be used as alternatives.

Impaired cell-mediated immunity is also associated with infections due to *Pneumocystis jiroveci* and *Cryptococcus neoformans*, described in more detail in Chapter 55, Opportunistic infections in HIV patients. Another group of pathogens to consider in patients with impaired cell-mediated immunity includes the intracellular endemic fungi such as *Histoplasma, Coccidioidomycosis,* and *Paracoccidioidomycosis*. Diagnosing endemic fungal infection requires taking a good travel history and having a high degree of suspicion. Diagnosis is made by demonstration of the fungus in tissue, serology, and PCR. Prolonged treatment with antifungals such as amphotericin B or itraconazole is usually required.

39.5 Parasitic infections in the immunocompromised host

Parasitic infections associated with impaired humoral immunity are mainly gastro-intestinal protozoa, which often cause chronic diarrhoea and non-specific gastro-intestinal symptoms. Intestinal protozoa affecting immunocompromised patients include *Giardia lamblia, Cryptosporidium parvum, Cyclospora cayetanensis, Microsporidia species,* and *Isospora belli.* Intestinal parasites can be diagnosed by microscopy or enteric PCR. Protozoal infections associated with impaired cell-mediated immunity are usually due to reactivation of quiescent infection as opposed to *de novo* infection and includes infection with *Toxoplasma gondii* and *Leishmania donovani.* Toxoplasma and leishmania are usually diagnosed by histology, serology, and/or PCR. The treatment of protozoal infections in the immunocompromised should be tailored to each parasitic disease. Immunocompromised hosts typically require longer treatment courses as they are more prone to treatment failure and relapse.

Patients with impaired cell-mediated immunity are more susceptible to infection with specific helminths. *Strongyloides stercoralis* can complete its life cycle in the human being, and immunocompromised patients are at greater risk of hyperinfection and disseminated infection, presenting with nausea, vomiting, diarrhoea, abdominal pain, gastrointestinal haemorrhage, cough and fever, gram-negative meningitis, renal failure, respiratory failure, and death. Screening for *Strongyloides* with serology should be considered in patients who have travelled and/or who were born in endemic areas when the diagnosis of immunosuppression is made, and/or prior to receiving immunosuppressive treatment. *Strongyloides stercoralis* infection is usually treated with ivermectin.

39.6 Assessment questions

39.6.1 Question 1

A twenty-seven-year-old Caribbean woman with systemic lupus erythematosus treated with rituximab reports chronic diarrhoea.

Which of the following parasites is most likely to be causing her symptoms?

A. *Cryptosporidium parvum.*

B. *Cyclospora cayetanensis.*

C. *Giardia lamblia.*

D. *Isospora bella.*

E. *Strongyloides stercoralis.*

39.6.2 Question 2

A thirty-five-year-old patient receiving renal replacement therapy is being worked up for renal transplant. She is CMV IgG negative. A potential living donor has been found who is CMV IgG positive.

What is the most important next step in management?
A. Do not go ahead with the transplant.
B. Go ahead with the transplant and give IVIG post-operatively.
C. Go ahead with the transplant and give valganciclovir prophylaxis for ninety days.
D. Go ahead with the transplant and monitor CMV DNA monthly.
E. Go ahead with the transplant and no prophylaxis or monitoring is required.

39.6.3 Question 3

A fifty-seven-year-old woman with severe rheumatoid arthritis is being worked up pre-rituximab. Her hepatitis B serology is as follows:
  Hepatitis B surface antigen negative
  Hepatitis B core antibody positive
  Hepatitis B surface antibody 10 mIU/ml
  Hepatitis B DNA < 20 IU/ml

What is the most appropriate next step in the management of this patient?
A. Do not do anything—this patient has evidence of past exposure to hepatitis B.
B. Monitor HBV DNA and LFTs weekly after commencing rituximab.
C. Offer a booster dose of hepatitis B vaccination prior to starting rituximab.
D. Start entecavir prophylaxis and continue until end of the course of rituximab.
E. Start prophylaxis with lamivudine before starting rituximab and continue until eighteen months after cessation of immunosuppression.

39.7 Answers and discussion

39.7.1 Answer 1

C. *Giardia lamblia*.
Giardia lamblia, also known as *Giardia intestinalis*, is the most common cause of diarrhoea secondary to parasites in immunocompromised. *Cryptosporidium parvum, Cyclospora cayetanensis, Isospora bella*, and *Strongyloides stercoralis* can also cause diarrhoea. Chronic giardiasis is associated with reduced mucosal IgA and may be a problem for patients with IgA deficiency and other forms of hypogammaglobulinaemia. Rituximab is a monoclonal antibody is a monoclonal antibody directed against CD20, expressed on all mature B cells except plasma cells and may cause hypogammaglobulinaemia.

While *Giardia lamblia* and *Cryptosporidium parvum* are usually seen in the UK, *Cyclospora cayetanensis, Isospora bella*, and *Strongyloides stercoralis* are usually linked to travel. The symptoms of giardiasis include diarrhoea, abdominal cramps, bloating, flatulence, and nausea. Cysts of *Giardia lamblia* can be seen in stool microscopy, and stool PCR is also available for diagnosis. The treatment is usually based on metronidazole, tinidazole, or nitazoxanide. Immunocompromised patients are more likely to fail treatment than immunocompetent host and might require combination therapy to treat giardiasis.

39.7.2 Answer 2

C. Go ahead with the transplant and give valganciclovir prophylaxis for ninety days.
This a D+/R- solid organ transplant which carries the highest risk of primary CMV infection in the transplant recipient. Prophylactic rather than pre-emptive therapy with valganciclovir is recommended in this patient group.

39.7.3 Answer 3

E. Start prophylaxis with lamivudine before starting rituximab and continue until 18 months after cessation of immunosuppression.

This lady is at risk of reactivation of hepatitis B virus after commencing rituximab. As per NICE and EASL guidelines regarding hepatitis B, any person who is surface antigen negative but anti-hepatitis B core antibody positive (irrespective of the anti-hepatitis B surface antibody status) commencing rituximab or other B cell depleting therapy should be offered lamivudine prophylaxis. This should be continued for at least 18 months after cessation of immunosuppressive therapy in this case and monitoring should continue for a further 12 months. However, as generic versions of entecavir and tenofovir become available it is likely that these second-generation nucleotide reverse transcriptase inhibitors will become used in preference to lamivudine in most healthcare settings due to their higher genetic barrier to resistance development. Lamivudine can be used in this setting although HBV exacerbation due to lamivudine resistance has been reported.

CHAPTER 40

Post-infection syndrome

Sherine Thomas

CONTENTS

40.1 Defining post-infection syndrome (PIS/CFS)

Post-infection syndrome (PIS) or chronic fatigue syndrome (CFS) is a complex debilitating disorder. It is usually characterized by fatigue that is worsened by physical activity or mental exertion, and is experienced in the aftermath, or with ongoing concurrent infections. Other symptoms may also be present including myalgia, impaired concentration, impaired memory, insomnia, and post-exertion malaise that can last for more than twenty-four hours after exertion.

40.2 Causes of PIS/CFS

PIS/CFS is a complex disorder with symptoms related to cognitive, autonomous, and immune dysfunction. No single causal factor has been identified, but there is some evidence that indicates that immunological dysfunction and infections interacting with genetic and psychosocial factors probably contribute to the development of PIS/CFS.

40.3 Diagnosing PIS/CFS

There are no tests to diagnose PIS/CFS. There are many conditions where the symptoms of PIS/CFS can appear, and therefore diagnosing PIS/CFS may rely on ruling out other conditions.

There are published guidelines that are available in order to help with diagnosing these conditions. The most frequently used ones are from the CDC (the 1994 Fukuda criteria) and the 1991 Oxford criteria. The CDC case definition for CFS requires individuals to meet three criteria before receiving this diagnosis. These are:

1. Severe chronic fatigue which must have been present for six or more consecutive months, and not as a result of other medical conditions associated with fatigue.

2. Fatigue that interferes significantly with activities of daily life.
3. Four or more of the following symptoms are present:
   a. Post-exertion malaise that lasts for longer than twenty-four hours.
   b. Impairment of short-term memory.
   c. Myalgia.
   d. Unrefreshed sleep.
   e. Headache (of new type or severity).
   f. Arthralgia (without swelling or erythema around the joints).
   g. A frequent or recurring sore throat.
   h. Tender lymphadenopathy.

However, the Oxford criteria differentiates CFS of unknown aetiology and CFS related to PIS, which is CFS that either follows an infection or is associated with an ongoing current infection. These guidelines suggest that in order to diagnose CFS, individuals must meet the following criteria:

1. The principle symptom experienced by patients should be fatigue that affects physical and mental functioning, and should have been present for at least six months.
2. The presence of other symptoms, including myalgia and sleep disturbances.
3. The symptoms must not have been lifelong, but have had a definite onset.
4. Patients with established medical conditions known to produce chronic fatigue, including mental health disorders or proven organic brain diseases, are precluded from the diagnosis.

PIS is then further subcategorized in this criteria and can be diagnosed based on the following:

1. The criteria for CFS as defined by the Oxford definition must be met.
2. In addition, the following should be fulfilled:
   a. Definite evidence of an infection at the onset of symptoms.
   b. Symptoms are present for at least six months after the onset of infection.
   c. Laboratory evidence of infection.

However, in 2011, a panel of researchers, clinicians, and patient advocates have challenged these diagnostic criteria and have suggested altering some of the criteria to no longer include requiring the six-month symptomatic period before diagnosis, having less emphasis on fatigue, and focusing on symptom clusters instead.

40.4 Risk factors for developing PIS/CFS

Ongoing research has failed to identify a single causative factor for developing PIS/CFS. Potential triggers for the condition include infections. The different types of infections studied to date include the Epstein-Barr virus (EBV), human herpes-virus 6 (HHV-6), and enterovirus infections, and although no one infection has been found to cause PIS/CFS, the syndrome can be triggered by an infection.

Other potential triggers could include immune dysfunction, with groups of CFS patients having been found to have different T cell activation markers compared to healthy controls. Trauma and toxins as well as stress are also possible risk factors and it is likely that this condition has multiple risk factors. Research is ongoing.

40.5 Managing PIS/CFS

There are no drugs that can cure this condition. Management of PIS/CFS can be complicated and requires a multidisciplinary team approach. PIS/CFS can affect patients differently and therefore an individualized management plan is often needed in order to reach the best possible outcomes for each patient. Recent randomized controlled trails have suggested that graded therapy programmes and clinical psychology input, including cognitive behavioural therapy regarding activity management and thought processes around behaviour, may be key factors in improving outcomes from this debilitating condition.

40.6 The prognosis regarding PIS/CFS

In general, prognosis regarding this condition can be difficult to predict, but it is thought that outcomes are better in those that have not had the condition for long periods of time and seek early help from an experienced multidisciplinary team, including clinical psychologists.

Relapses can be common in PIS/CFS and can be triggered by numerous factors including further infections and unplanned activity. Relapses should be handled in the same way as the original condition, with individualized management plans according to the patient's main symptoms and complaints.

40.7 Further reading and useful resources

CDC. *Myalgic Encephalomyelitis/Chronic Fatigue Syndrome* (Atlanta, GA, 2018). http://www.cdc.gov/cfs/index.html

Fukuda, K., Straus, S. E. , Hickie, I., Sharpe, M. C., Dobbins, J. G., Komaroff, A., et al. 'The Chronic Fatigue Syndrome: A Comprehensive Approach to its Definition and Study', *Annals of Internal Medicine*, 121 (1994), 953–959.

http://bestpractice.bmj.com/best-practice/monograph/277/diagnosis/criteria.html

40.8 Assessment questions

40.8.1 Question 1

A twenty-six-year-old woman presents with significant fatigue, myalgia, and arthralgia for a period of over six months. Preceding the onset of symptoms is a glandular, fever-like illness which she feels she never recovered from. She has a background history of mental health problems and struggles with a bipolar disorder.

Which of her clinical features is against the diagnosis of post-infection fatigue?
A. Evidence of infection at onset of symptoms.
B. History of mental health problems.
C. Ongoing myalgia and arthralgia.
D. Significant fatigue.
E. Symptoms being present for at least six months.

40.8.2 Question 2

There are a number of treatment modalities suggested for the management of chronic fatigue/post-infection syndrome.

Based on current evidence, what is the *most* effective approach in management?
A. Activity management.
B. Cognitive behavioural therapy.
C. Graded therapy programmes.
D. Individualized programmes.
E. Reducing overall activity levels.

40.9 Answers and discussion

40.9.1 Answer 1

B. History of mental health problems.

A history of mental health problems precludes the diagnosis of PIS/CFS according the CDC and Oxford diagnostic criteria. A history of or evidence of infection at the onset of symptoms is one of the main diagnostic criteria for PIS, and at present these symptoms should have been present for at least six months. Although this is contentious, it is still part of the diagnostic criteria for PIS/CFS. People commonly complain of fatigue, myalgia, arthralgia, and impaired short-term memory.

40.9.2 Answer 2

D. Individual programmes.

More research needs to be done looking into the management of this condition, but recent randomized controlled trials suggest that individualized programmes (including a combination of graded therapy programmes) and clinical psychology input (including cognitive behavioural therapy regarding activity management and thought processes around behaviour) may be key factors in improving outcomes after PIS/CFS.

PART SEVEN

UNDERSTANDING USE OF ANTIMICROBIAL AGENTS

CHAPTER 41

Mechanism of action of antimicrobial agents

Ruaridh Buchanan and Armine Sefton

CONTENTS

41.1 Selective toxicity

Antibacterial and antifungal agents aim to kill pathogens, or at the very least incapacitate them. To achieve this aim these agents must have a reasonable degree of toxicity at the cellular level. If this toxicity was equally manifest against all cell types then the drugs would be unusable in patients as the side effect profile would be unacceptably severe. Selective toxicity, whereby the agents are orders of magnitude more toxic to bacteria or fungi than human cells, allows for the safe and effective administration of these agents to patients.

There are a number of different mechanisms by which an antimicrobial agent can yield selective toxicity:

- Target a cellular structure that exists only in bacteria/fungi—e.g. the cell wall;
- Target a cellular structure that has a significantly different structure in bacteria/fungi—e.g. the ribosome; the fungal cell membrane;
- Target cellular enzymes that are significantly different in bacteria/fungi e.g. topoisomerase;
- Target a synthetic pathway that exists only in bacteria e.g. folate synthesis.

41.2 Antibacterial targets

Broadly, antibacterial drugs can be divided into the following categories:

- Agents that target the cell wall;
- Agents that target the cell membrane;

- Agents that inhibit protein synthesis;
- Agents that inhibit DNA replication/transcription of RNA;
- Agents that target folate synthesis;
- Agents that directly damage intracellular structures.

41.3 Drugs targeting the bacterial cell wall

The cell wall is unique to bacteria, and therefore an ideal target. Disrupting the complex cross-linking process required to produce the cell wall leads to loss of bacterial cell integrity and therefore to cell death. The following classes of antibiotics target the cell wall:

41.3.1 Beta-lactams

The first class to be discovered, and still in many cases the most effective, incorporates the four-membered beta-lactam ring—its homology to d-alanyl-d-alanine allows beta-lactam-containing compounds to bind to cell wall peptidoglycans and act as chain terminators.

41.3.1.1 Penicillins

The beta-lactam ring is fused to a five-membered sulphur-containing ring. Variations in side chains account for the differing pharmacokinetics and spectra of action of the different compounds—for example, the addition of an amino group to benzylpenicillin produces ampicillin. Antipseudomonal activity can be produced by replacing the amino group with a cyclic urea group (ureidopenicillin—piperacillin).

41.3.1.2 Cephalosporins

The beta-lactam ring is fused to a six-membered sulphur-containing ring. Once again, variations in side chains differentiate the compounds; the extra carbon atom in the ring allows for a greater variety of modifications and thus a large number of different cephalosporins are available. Adaptations allow for antipseudomonal compounds (ceftazidime) and for compounds with action against MRSA (ceftaroline).

41.3.1.3 Carbapenems

The beta-lactam ring is fused to a five-membered carbon-only ring. The differing structure renders these compounds resistant to the majority of beta-lactamase enzymes produced in bacterial defence. Additionally, side chains confer a broad spectrum of activity, although some, e.g. ertapenem, do not possess antipseudomonal activity.

41.3.1.4 Monobactams

The beta-lactam ring stands alone in these compounds, active only against Gram negative organisms—aztreonam is the only one in clinical use.

41.3.2 Glycopeptides

Vancomycin and teicoplanin are the two glycopeptides used routinely in British practice, although new compounds are coming on market. Comprised of a polypeptide chain with sugar moieties incorporated into it, they act by binding to nascent peptidoglycan molecules and preventing addition of further subunits. Their large size means that they cannot traverse the outer membrane of Gram negative bacteria and consequently are used solely against Gram positive bacteria; it also means they are very poorly absorbed from the gut and are thus given parentally, except when prescribed for C. difficile treatment.

41.3.3 Fosfomycin

Fosfomycin, an older and little-utilized drug in the UK, is finding a new role in treating resistant Gram negative infections, predominantly simple UTIs. However, it is now licensed for a wider variety of infections. It inhibits the enzyme pyruvyl transferase and thus an early stage in the peptidoglycan synthesis process.

41.4 Drugs targeting the bacterial cell membrane

The difference in structure between the bacterial and human cell membranes is much smaller than with the other structures used as drug targets. These agents thus come associated with a more significant risk of toxicity and tend to be used only when other options are unavailable.

41.4.1 Daptomycin

Only available as an IV preparation, daptomycin is a lipopeptide that is incorporated into the cell membrane, resulting in physical disruption and a breakdown in membrane integrity. The subsequent leakage of intracellular ions results in the loss of membrane potential which has knock-on effects on essential cellular activity. Active mainly against Gram positive organisms, it is used for resistant staphylococcal and enterococcal infections.

41.4.2 Polymyxins

A variety of different compounds exist in this class—the combination of polymyxin A and B, known as colistin, is finding increasing usage in the treatment of multi-drug resistant Gram negative infections. Polypeptides with attached fatty acids, they incorporate into the cell membrane where they act as a detergent and cause loss of membrane integrity.

41.5 Drugs inhibiting protein synthesis

Protein synthesis is mediated by ribosomes. The bacterial ribosome is significantly different from those found in human cells. It is comprised of the 30S subunit (including 16S RNA) and the 50S subunit (including 23S RNA). Several classes of antibacterial agent inhibit protein synthesis by targeting various parts of the ribosome complex.

41.5.1 Aminoglycosides

These agents bind to the 30S ribosomal subunit, preventing peptide elongation and thus protein synthesis. The first in this class was streptomycin, though gentamicin and amikacin are the most commonly used today. Tobramycin is sometimes used in pseudomonal infections, and paromomycin is used as an antiprotozoal agent. Available only as parenteral preparations, they are mainly used for their activity against Gram negative organisms, though they retain a degree of activity against Gram positives as well.

41.5.2 Tetracyclines

So named because of their four-ringed structure, these compounds also bind to the 30S ribosomal subunit, although at a different site to aminoglycosides. They prevent the binding of t-RNA/amino acyl complexes to the ribosome, thus preventing peptide formation. The parent compound tetracycline is still used, though doxycycline is more common in routine practice. Tigecycline, a newer intravenous compound, was briefly in vogue but studies showing excess all-cause mortality have lessened its appeal; it remains a drug of last resort for multi-drug resistant Gram negatives. Tetracyclines have a broad spectrum of action, including against spirochaetes and rickettsial species.

41.5.3 Macrolides

Like aminoglycosides, these agents also prevent peptide elongation, although they differ in that they bind to the 23S RNA portion of the 50S ribosomal subunit, physically blocking the process. Clarithromycin, erythromycin, and azithromycin are the most commonly used. Clarithromycin has good Gram positive activity and also covers respiratory tract Gram negatives; azithromycin has much broader Gram negative cover but at the expense of a degree of its Gram positive cover. Spiramycin, used to treat toxoplasmosis in pregnancy, also belongs to this class.

41.5.4 Lincosamides

Clindamycin is the only drug in this class in common usage. Similarly to macrolides, it binds to 23S RNA, again inhibiting peptide elongation. It covers Gram positive organisms as well as anaerobes but has no meaningful Gram negative action.

41.5.5 Oxazolidinones

Currently linezolid is the only member of this class available. It inhibits protein synthesis, probably by preventing initiation of translation, but the mechanism is not clearly defined. It is likely due to interactions with 23S RNA as resistant strains of *Staphylococcus aureus* often show mutations in this region. Activity is limited to Gram positive organisms as the drug is actively pumped out of Gram negative bacteria.

41.5.6 Streptogramins

These compounds come in two varieties—A and B. Both are capable of binding to the 50S subunit, preventing peptide elongation and causing release of incomplete chains. However, the binding of streptogramin A causes a conformational change in the ribosome which increases its affinity for streptogramin B by up to 100 times—using the two compounds in combination is therefore much more effective. Synercid®, an IV formulation, is no longer available; pristinamycin, available orally, is used occasionally for non-life threatening, resistant, Gram positive infections.

41.5.7 Chloramphenicol

Less commonly used in the UK than previously due to concerns about its side effect profile, chloramphenicol retains a broad spectrum of activity. It also binds to 23S RNA to inhibit peptide elongation. It remains the drug of choice for community-acquired bacterial meningitis in individuals with severe penicillin allergy.

41.5.8 Fusidic acid

Used either topically for infections such as impetigo, or orally to treat staphylococcal infections in conjunction with a beta-lactam, fusidic acid does not target the ribosome directly. Rather, it acts by inhibiting elongation factor, resulting in reduced efficiency of the peptide elongation process.

41.6 Drugs targeting DNA replication/RNA transcription

41.6.1 Fluoroquinolones

This family of compounds targets topoisomerase enzymes involved in the uncoiling of DNA prior to replication or transcription. The result is nuclear fragmentation and subsequent breakdown in cellular activity. Different compounds have stronger affinity for different subclasses of topoisomerase, resulting in differing spectra of activity. Anti-topoisomerase II (also known as DNA gyrase) activity results in broader Gram negative cover (ciprofloxacin) while anti-topoisomerase IV activity results in improved Gram positive cover (moxifloxacin, levofloxacin).

41.6.2 Rifamycins

Rifamycins bind to and inhibit the action of bacterial DNA-dependent RNA polymerase, thus inhibiting transcription from DNA. Rifampicin is the most commonly used, mainly for treating mycobacterial infections and as an adjunct in the treatment of staphylococcal infections; it also has good activity against *Legionella* species.

41.7 Drugs targeting folate synthesis

While humans utilize dietary folic acid, bacteria synthesize their own—this pathway is therefore an ideal target for antimicrobial agents as actively dividing bacteria require a large supply of folic acid. Drugs acting on this pathway can broadly be subdivided into sulphonamides and diaminopyridines—the two classes act synergistically and are frequently used in combination.

41.7.1 Sulphonamides

These compounds competitively inhibit the enzyme dihydropteroate synthase (DHPS), a catalyst early in the folate synthesis pathway. Members include sulphadiazine, used against toxoplasmosis, and sulphamethoxazole, used in combination with trimethoprim as co-trimoxazole.

41.7.2 Diaminopyridines

Dihydrofolate is converted to tetrahydrofolate by the enzyme dihydrofolate reductase (DHFR)—inhibition of this enzyme prevents the final step in the synthesis pathway. Trimethoprim, commonly used to treat urinary tract infections, is a DHFR inhibitor, as is pyrimethamine, used in the treatment of toxoplasmosis.

41.8 Drugs that directly damage intracellular components

As with agents acting on the cell membrane, these drugs are less selective in their toxicity—prolonged courses should therefore be avoided if at all possible.

41.8.1 Nitrofurantoin

Very commonly used in the community for urinary tract infections as it concentrates within the urine, it is of no utility in systemic infection. It accumulates within cells where it is reduced by bacterial flavoproteins to produce a number of reactive species which cause damage to DNA, proteins, and other cellular components.

41.8.2 Nitroimidazoles

Metronidazole is by far the most commonly used example of this class. The molecule is reduced intracellularly by enzymes such as nitroreductase, generating damaging reactive species. This process only occurs within anaerobic bacteria, thus antimicrobial activity is limited to these organisms. Some protozoa, such as *Giardia* and *Entamoeba*, are also susceptible to its actions.

41.9 Antifungal targets

Although the structure of fungi is distinct to that of bacteria, the same principles apply—areas where the cellular biology differs from that of the human host are the best targets for antimicrobial drugs. In practice, commonly used agents target either the fungal cell wall or fungal cell membrane, though agents that directly damage intracellular structures also exist.

41.10 Drugs targeting the fungal cell wall

Unlike the wide variety of drugs targeting the bacterial cell wall, only one class currently exists that specifically targets the fungal cell wall:

41.10.1 Echinocandins

The major component of the fungal cell wall is beta-D-glucan, synthesized within the cell by the enzyme beta-1, 3-glucan synthase. Echinocandins inhibit this enzyme in a non-competitive fashion, decreasing cell wall integrity and causing breakdown of cellular processes. Commonly used drugs in this class are caspofungin and micafungin, both covering a wide variety of *Candida* and *Aspergillus* species.

41.11 Drugs targeting the fungal cell membrane

The fungal cell membrane is structurally quite distinct from that of the human cell, incorporating ergosterol rather than cholesterol as its major component. Drugs that target the fungal cell membrane are thus less toxic to human cells than those that target the bacterial cell membrane and form the mainstay of antifungal therapy.

41.11.1 Triazoles

Ergosterol is produced from lanosterol by the enzyme 14α-demethylase—triazoles act by inhibiting this enzyme. There are a variety of different agents available, the newer agents having a broader spectrum of activity. Fluconazole is effective against dermatophytes and most yeasts, including *Candida* and *Cryptococcus sp*. Voriconazole maintains this spectrum with additional activity against *Aspergillus sp.* and various endemic mycoses; posaconazole is additionally effective against mucormycoses. Ketoconazole is available as a topical solution and can be used for scalp infections; clotrimazole is a useful topical agent against intertrigo and vaginal candidiasis.

41.11.2 Polyenes

These agents directly attack the fungal membrane by binding to ergosterol and causing structural changes that result in membrane leakage, cell depolarization, and disruption of cellular functions. The most well known is amphotericin B, available as a variety of lipid preparations (Ambisome® is the most commonly used in the UK). This is given parenterally for a wide variety of invasive fungal infections, although it is no longer considered first-line therapy with the exception of cryptococcal meningitis. Another commonly used member of this family is nystatin, used topically for oral candidiasis.

41.11.3 Allylamines

This family of compounds again inhibit the ergosterol synthesis process, this time by inhibiting the formation of lanosterol by the enzyme squalene epoxidase. The most commonly used member of this family is terbinafine, applied topically or taken orally for dermatophyte infections.

41.12 Drugs that directly damage fungal intracellular structures

41.12.1 Flucytosine

This acts as a prodrug and it is converted to 5-fluorouracil within fungal cells, where it directly interferes with RNA synthesis; other products interfere directly with DNA replication. Its only mainstream use at present is in combination therapy with amphotericin B in the treatment of invasive cryptococcal infection.

41.12.2 Griseofulvin

Active only against dermatophytes, griseofulvin binds to fungal microtubules, inhibiting mitosis and thus cell division. It is given systemically for severe dermatophyte infections.

44.13 Further reading

Finch, R., Davey, P., Wilcox, M., Irving, W., *Antimicrobial Chemotherapy* (6th edn, Oxford, 2012).

Finch, R., Greenwood, D., Ragnar Norrby, S., Whitley, R. J., *Antibiotic and Chemotherapy: anti-infective agents and their use in therapy* (9th edn, Edinburgh, 2010).

Kapoor, G., Saigal, S., Elongavan, A., 'Action and resistance mechanisms of antibiotics: a guide for clinicians', *Journal of Anaesthesiology and Clinical Pharmacology*, 33/3 (2017), 300–305.

41.14 Assessment questions

41.14.1 Question 1

A 53-year-old woman on warfarin for deep vein thrombosis presents with a cough productive of green sputum, fever, and breathlessness. A chest x-ray shows right middle lobe consolidation. She is treated empirically with amoxicillin but while her symptoms improve she develops diarrhoea. Her stool tests negative for *C. difficile* glutamate dehydrogenase.

Blood cultures are negative. A sputum culture grows *Streptococcus pneumoniae* with the following sensitivity pattern:

Amoxicillin—sensitive

Erythromycin—sensitive

Tetracycline—resistant

Vancomycin—sensitive

The patient improves and is to be discharged after two days in hospital. She refuses to continue taking amoxicillin due to the diarrhoea.

Which antibiotic should she be prescribed orally at discharge?
A. Clarithromycin.
B. Doxycycline.
C. Linezolid.
D. Temocillin.
E. Vancomycin.

41.14.2 Question 2

An 82-year-old man presents with a several-week history of fevers and malaise. Multiple sets of blood cultures grow Vancomycin-resistant *Enterococcus faecium*. His medical history is notable for a history of depression, for which he is taking phenelzine, and an endovascular aortic aneurysm repair graft some six months previously. A CT aortogram is suggestive of a collection surrounding the graft.

While awaiting surgery, which antibiotic should he be treated with?
A. Amoxicillin.
B. Ceftriaxone.
C. Daptomycin.
D. Linezolid.
E. Metronidazole.

41.14.3 Question 3

A 43-year-old deteriorates on the Haematology unit three weeks after completing his most recent course of chemotherapy. He has previously suffered from a *Candida glabrata* Hickman line infection—during his therapy he developed a widespread rash following administration of caspofungin.

He is noted to be breathless and has oxygen saturations of 90% on air; his temperature is 39.1°C. Blood tests reveal a neutrophil count of 0.3 x10⁹ /L—review of his previous results shows it has been at this level for several weeks. He is commenced on piperacillin/tazobactam but fails to improve over the next few days. A chest CT scan shows widespread ground glass change and the presence of halo sign is noted in the report. His condition deteriorates and he is transferred to the Intensive Care Unit.

Which antimicrobial agent is the most appropriate at this stage?
A. Fluconazole.
B. Flucytosine.
C. Micafungin.
D. Terbinafine.
E. Voriconazole.

41.15 Answers and discussion

41.15.1 Answer 1

C. Linezolid.
The patient has pneumococcal pneumonia. The bacterium is resistant to tetracycline so doxycycline, a related compound, is unlikely to be effective. Vancomycin, while effective in vitro, is not absorbed from the gut when taken orally and will thus not be an effective therapy in this case. Temocillin only has activity against Gram negative bacteria—*S. pneumoniae* is Gram positive; additionally, temocillin is only currently available as an IV formulation. Clarithromycin, while effective, will interact with the warfarin the patient takes, increasing her INR markedly, and should therefore be avoided unless there are no other options. In this case there is another option linezolid. Although sensitivity testing has not been performed, the rates of resistance to linezolid in pneumococci are so small as to be clinically irrelevant, especially in patients without bacteraemia, as is the case here.

41.15.2 Answer 2

C. Daptomycin.
Enterococcus faecium is intrinsically resistant to amoxicillin so this should not be used. All enterococci are intrinsically resistant to cephalosporins like ceftriaxone, though there is now some evidence that they can be used as synergistic agents in *Enterococcus faecalis* endocarditis. Metronidazole is active only against true anaerobic organisms, a group to which *E. faecium* does not belong. Linezolid, while a highly effective agent against most enterococci, interacts significantly with monoamine oxidase inhibitors such as phenelzine, and is therefore contraindicated in this patient. Daptomycin, though not used first line when treating enterococcal infections, is the best choice in this situation.

41.15.3 Answer 3

E. Voriconazole.
Although the patient has suffered from candidaemia in the past, the most likely fungal pathogen at this stage is *Aspergillus fumigatus*—prolonged neutropaenia is a risk factor and his CT scan is suggestive of invasive aspergillosis. Empirical antifungal therapy must therefore target this pathogen. Fluconazole does not cover *Aspergillus*, nor does terbinafine. Flucytosine does have activity against *Aspergillus* but would always be used as part of a combination therapy, not as a single agent. Both voriconazole and micafungin cover *Aspergillus*. In this case the patient has previously had an allergic reaction to caspofungin, an echinocandin, the class to which micafungin also belongs, so voriconazole is the best choice.

CHAPTER 42

Use of antimicrobials and toxicity

Armine Sefton

CONTENTS

42.1 Defining and using narrow- or broad-spectrum antimicrobials

Broad-spectrum antibacterial agents kill most bacteria including gram-positive rods and cocci, gram-negative rods and cocci, and often anaerobes too. Narrow-spectrum agents kill a narrow range of microbes, e.g. benzylpenicillin is mainly active against gram- positive cocci.

By and large a narrow-spectrum antimicrobial is less likely to disrupt a patient's normal flora than a broad-spectrum agent. Hence, if the likely organism is causing an infection it is best to give a narrow-spectrum antimicrobial to treat that specific organism. If a patient presents 'septic' and the source of infection is unknown, relevant cultures should be taken followed by broad-spectrum antimicrobial cover. This can later be modified either when the source of infection is found or as a result of microbiology culture results.

- Agents mostly active against gram-positive bacteria include:
    - Penicillin (Also active against *Neisseria spp.*).
    - Fusidic acid.
    - Macrolides (Also active against *Legionella, Campylobacter, Bordetella spp.*).
    - Clindamycin.
    - Glycopeptides.
    - Oxazolidinones.
    - Streptogramins.
- Agents mainly active against gram-negative bacteria include:
    - Polymyxin.
    - Trimethoprim.

- Aminoglycosides (also active against staphylococci and show synergy when combined with beta-lactams against/glycopeptides against streptococci).
- Monobactams.
- Temocillin.
- Broad-spectrum antimicrobials include:
  - Beta-lactam plus beta-lactamase inhibitor combinations.
  - Cephalosporins.
  - Carbapenems.
  - Chloramphenicol, Tetracyclines/Glycyclines.

42.2 Bacteriostatic and bactericidal compounds and their use

A bactericidal agent is a compound that actively kills multiplying bacteria. A bacteriostatic compound inhibits the growth of bacteria. Whether or not an antimicrobial is bactericidal or bacteriostatic depends on a variety of things, including the type of agent, its concentration, and the organism it is being used to treat. It is especially important to try and use a bactericidal agent if the patient's immune system is impaired or the infection is at a site where it is difficult for the immune system to access, e.g. the heart valves in bacterial endocarditis, the meninges in meningitis. Examples of each are given here:

- Bactericidal agents include beta-lactams, glycopeptides, fluoroquinolones, and aminoglycosides.
- Bacteriostatic agents include macrolides, clindamycin, tetracyclines, trimethoprim, and sulphonamides.

42.3 The therapeutic index

The therapeutic index of a drug is the ration of the concentration of drug likely to be toxic to the patient divided by the concentration of drug likely to be clinically effective (Figure 42.1). Generally speaking, drugs with a high therapeutic index, e.g. beta-lactams are likely to be safer to use and less likely to need monitoring than drugs with a lower therapeutic index, e.g. aminoglycosides. For treating relatively trivial infections it is important to always try and use an antibiotic with a high

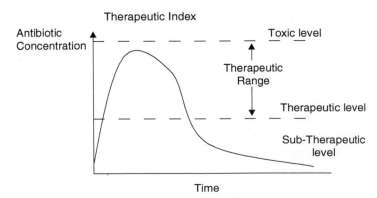

Figure 42.1 The relationship between therapeutic level and toxic level.

therapeutic index whereas for treating serious infections it is important to use the antibiotic likely to be most effective.

Some examples of side-effects/ toxicity of some antimicrobials (NB this is NOT a comprehensive list) include:

- Aminoglycosides: Ototoxicity and renal toxicity especially in the elderly or in patients with renal failure. Can impair neuromuscular transmission and should not be given to patients with myasthenia gravis
- Beta-lactams: Hypersensitivity reactions (see above). Can cause encephalopathy in very high doses, especially in patients with renal failure.
- Chloramphenicol: Bone marrow suppression. Usually dose related but occasionally idiosyncratic.
- Glycopeptides: Vancomycin is nephrotoxic and requires monitoring. If infused rapidly can frequently lead to 'Red Man syndrome' with hypotension, bronchospasm, and urticaria.
- Linezolid: Bone marrow suppression.
- Macrolides: Frequently cause gastro-intestinal side effects but otherwise generally very safe. Should be used with caution in people with a predisposition to an increased QT interval. Can cause hepatoxicity and occasionally hearing loss if used in very high doses.
- Metronidazole: Disulfiram-like reactions with alcohol.
- Quinolones: Should be used in caution in people with a predisposition to seizures. Can prolong the QT interval. Use in children is generally not advised as can cause arthropathies in joints of young animals.
- Sulphonamides: Skin reactions, including Stevens Johnson syndrome. Occasional bone marrow suppression.
- Tetracyclines: May increase muscle weakness in myasthenia gravis. Should not be given to children under the age of twelve years as can get deposited in growing bones and teeth. Their absorption is decreased by antacids and milk.

42.4 Considerations for combination therapy

Combination therapy should be considered in the following situations:

- For empirical therapy of serious sepsis likely to be due to mixed infections or where likely focus of infection and thus likely organisms causing it is unknown.
- Avoidance of resistance, e.g. TB.
- Synergy: e.g. penicillins and aminoglycosides in the treatment of streptococcal endocarditis.
- Toxicity sparing: when by using two potentially toxic drugs together you can use each in a lower concentration than if using alone and hence may reduce toxicity, e.g. amphotericin B and 5-flucytosine.

42.5 Considerations for chemoprophylaxis

Chemoprophylaxis means the prevention of infection by giving antimicrobials. Examples include;

- malaria prophylaxis for travellers going to areas where malaria is endemic;
- prophylaxis to patients undergoing certain surgical procedures. This may be either:

- where there is likely to be a high likelihood of bacterial contamination during surgery, e.g. surgery on the large bowel;
- if the likelihood of bacterial contamination of surgical site is low but the consequences of this occurring are potentially severe, as in joint replacement surgery or heart valve replacement surgery;
- prophylaxis against *Pneumocystis jirovecii* in AIDS patients with low CD4 counts.

42.6 Things to know about antimicrobial agents

- Class of antimicrobial, e.g. beta-lactam, macrolide, etc.;
- Site of action;
- Spectrum of activity;
- Mechanisms of resistance;
- Mode of administration;
- Pharmacology, including absorption, penetration into various sites, and routes of administration;
- Clinical uses;
- Drug interactions and contraindications;
- Side-effects;
- Toxicity and need to monitor; and
- Approximate cost (cheap or expensive).

Each clinician must know these facts about all the main antimicrobials (active against bacteria, fungi, viruses, and protozoa) as they are likely to be used on a regular clinical basis.

42.7 Considerations before prescribing any antimicrobial

- Does the patient need an antibiotic at all?
- Does the patient have any allergies, especially to beta lactams? Remember there is some cross-sensitivity between the penicillins, cephalosporins, and carbapenems. If there is a history of allergy then *avoid* using the drug. However, it is essential to find out what the patient means when they say they are allergic to a drug; frequently the patient means side effects, rather than allergy (see Table 42.1 for different types of penicillin allergy and Table 42.2 for prescribing in penicillin allergy).
- Is therapy going to be empiric (based on likely source of infection and likely organism)?
- Is therapy going to be specific (based on laboratory report)?
- Are you going to give a broad- or narrow-spectrum agent?
- What is the likely site of infection and which antimicrobials penetrate well to that site (e.g. if treating a patient with meningitis you must use a drug that gets into the cerebrospinal fluid; for treating osteomyelitis you need one with good bone penetration, etc.)?
- Where is the patient and how sick are they?
- Does the patient have impaired metabolism (e.g. renal/liver failure, G6PD deficiency)?
- Are they a child, pregnant, breastfeeding, or immunocompromised?
- Are they on any other therapy (consider the possibility of drug interactions / contraindications)?
- What is the preferred route of administration (IV/IM/PO)?

Table 42.1 Types of penicillin allergy.

	Immediate Type 1	Delayed
Timing of onset	Usually one to four hours from onset (rarely up to seventy-two hours)	More than seventy-two hours from exposure
Severe	Anaphylaxis, laryngeal oedema, wheezing/ bronchospasm, angioedema, generalized urticaria, diffuse erythema	Steven Johnson syndrome Toxic Epidermal Necrolysis
Mild	Minor rash	Minor rash, contact dermatitis, maculopapular rash, morbilliform rash, drug fever

Table 42.2 Prescribing in patients with a history of penicillin allergy.

RED! -- DO NOT USE:
Antibiotics contra-indicated in all __true__ penicillin allergic patients: amoxicillin, ampicillin, benzylpenicillin (Penicillin G), co-amoxiclav (Augmentin®), flucloxacillin, phenoxymethylpenicillin (Penicillin V), piperacillin/tazobactam (Tazocin®), temocillin, and ticarcillin/clavulanic acid (Timentin®)

AMBER -- SHOULD BE AVOIDED WHEREVER POSSIBLE:
Antibiotics which should be avoided in patients with history of severe penicillin allergy: cefalexin, ceftazidime, cefixime, ceftriaxone, cefotaxime, cefuroxime, ertapenem, meropenem, imipenem, and aztreonam. NB: In patients with a vague or non-severe history of penicillin allergy, cephalosporins and carbapenems may be used with caution

GREEN -- CONSIDERED SAFE TO USE:
Antibiotics considered safe in penicillin allergic patients:
amikacin, azithromycin, ciprofloxacin, clarithromycin, clindamycin, cotrimoxazole, doxycycline, erythromycin, gentamicin, levofloxacin, linezolid, metronidazole, moxifloxacin, nitrofurantoin, rifampicin, sodium fusidate, Synercid^d, teicoplanin, tetracycline, tigecycline, trimethoprim, tobramycin, and vancomycin

It is vital that IV antibiotics should only be initiated in patients with severe symptoms, where no equivalent oral antibiotics are available, or where the oral administration is contra-indicated/ compromised. IV-to-oral switch should be considered in a patient who has shown clear evidence of improvement with the following features:

- Resolution of fever for more than twenty-four hours;
- Absence of hypoxia;
- Pulse rate < 100 beats/min (WCC);
- Resolution of tachypnoea;
- Resolution of hypotension;
- Clinically hydrated and taking oral fluids;
- No concerns over gastro-intestinal absorption;
- Improving white cell count;
- Non-bacteraemic infection:
  - How often does the drug need to be given?
  - How safe is the drug? Is there specific toxicity to the liver, kidney, bone marrow? Is there a need to either monitor drug levels for achievement of safe/effective levels or toxicity or the patient for potential abnormalities in haematological or biochemical parameters?

- What are its likely side-effects?
- How cost-effective is it likely to be?
- Is there likely to be resistance to the drug/ is resistance likely to develop during treatment?
- How long will you need to give it?

42.8 Accessing national and local guidelines

National guidelines on toxicity, interaction, and contra-indication, where applicable, are available from websites such as the British Society of Antimicrobial Chemotherapy, The British Infection Association, the Hospital Infection Society, the British Thoracic Society, etc. Additionally, each hospital department may also hold copies of these.

Most trusts have their own guidelines, which are generally based on national guidelines, if available, but may be modified slightly dependent on local susceptibility/ resistance patterns, etc. Local guidelines may via the hospital's intranet, a mobile app, or paper versions. It is important to verify that the most up-to-date version of local guidelines are checked in each case. Most trusts will have a restricted antimicrobials list. The agents on this list can only be prescribed under the direction of Medical Microbiology unless these are used as part of a departmental protocol/guideline

The British National Formulary (BNF) is generally good for doses, contraindications, drug interactions, and chemoprophylaxis. It comes in both an electronic and paper version and there is also a paediatric version. Pharmacy may also be able to provide advice as might a more senior member of your department. Drug companies will also have a medical information unit that you can contact.

42.9 Assessment questions

42.9.1 Question 1

When treating patients with an infection, it is often desirable to use an antimicrobial drug with a high therapeutic index.

What is the most likely benefit of using a high therapeutic index agent?
A. Cheaper.
B. Easier to monitor.
C. Lower dose.
D. More effective.
E. Safer.

42.9.2 Question 2

A patient comes into hospital hypotensive and febrile and requires ITU admission. He has no significant past medical history. He is thought to be septic but has no obvious focus of infection.

What is the most appropriate management after taking appropriate cultures and checking for drug allergy?
A. Await culture results before giving any antimicrobial.
B. Give (a) broad-spectrum bactericidal antimicrobial(s).
C. Give (a) broad-spectrum bacteriostatic antimicrobial(s).
D. Give both a broad-spectrum bactericidal antimicrobial and an anti-fungal agent.
E. Give a narrow-spectrum antimicrobial to minimize the risk of the patient developing *Clostridium difficile* diarrhoea.

42.9.3 Question 3

A patient presents with septic shock of unclear source and is known to have a past history of anaphylaxis to penicillins.

Which of the following options is the most appropriate to be given before culture and sensitivity results are available?
A. Ciprofloxacin and metronidazole.
B. Co-amoxiclav.
C. Meropenem.
D. Vancomycin, amikacin, and metronidazole.
E. Vancomycin, aztreonam, and metronidazole.

42.10 Answers and discussion

42.10.1 Answer 1

E. Safer.
When using a drug with a high therapeutic index there is a large margin between what constitutes a therapeutic level compared to a toxic level in a patient. Hence it is much easier to ensure that the patient has an adequate dose of the drug for treating their infection as there is then no worry (within reason) about giving them too high a dose of the drug. Drug levels do not normally have to be monitored if using an antimicrobial with a high therapeutic index. As always, it is important to check for possible allergy before prescribing any antimicrobial. For instance, beta-lactam agents are antimicrobials with a high therapeutic index, whereas aminoglycosides are drugs with a low therapeutic index, but allergy to beta-lactams is much more common than allergy to aminoglycosides.

There is a danger when using drugs with a low therapeutic index that patients are underdosed because the doctors treating them are worried about causing toxicity. If treating a fairly trivial infection it is important to try and use a drug with a high therapeutic index, but when treating a life-threatening infection the antimicrobial(s) most likely to be effective for treating the sepsis should be used, even if it does not have a high therapeutic index, e.g. a single dose of an aminoglycoside is commonly given in combination with a beta-lactam antibiotic in this situation.

42.10.2 Answer 2

B. Give (a) broad spectrum bactericidal antimicrobial(s).
If a patient is admitted to hospital septic but with no obvious source of infection relevant cultures should be taken to try and help find the source and then start the patient on broad-spectrum antimicrobials. Always culture the blood and urine and then other sites as appropriate. Ideally where possible use bactericidal rather than bacteriostatic antimicrobials, as these actively kill the microbes, unlike bacteriostatic agents, which prevent their multiplication and require the host to have a reasonable immune system for them to be really effective.

In a patient thought to have life-threatening sepsis do not wait for the culture results before starting the antimicrobials, as the prognosis is improved if treatment is started immediately. Once any positive culture results are obtained it is possible to modify treatment; e.g. change to a narrower-spectrum agent to treat a specific organism if one is cultured and this should be less likely to cause antibiotic-associated diarrhoea. Some trusts will use one broad-spectrum antimicrobial but others will use combination therapy of two or three antimicrobials, which together will have broad-spectrum activity against both gram-positive and gram-negative organisms and also anaerobes. In a patient with no significant past medical history it is unlikely that an invasive fungal infection would be the cause of his/her sepsis and so normally such a patient would not be started on antifungals as well as antimicrobials on their admission.

42.10.3 Answer 3

D. Vancomycin, amikacin, and metronidazole.

Always check for a history of allergy before prescribing any antimicrobial. Although beta-lactam drugs are generally very safe, a considerable amount of people claim to be allergic to penicillin. If a patient says that they are allergic to a drug it is very import to ascertain what they mean by this as sometimes it means that the drug has given them diarrhoea or indigestion. However, if someone is truly allergic to penicillin there may be some cross-sensitivity to cephalosporins and carbapenems as well (between 1–10%). Therefore, if a patient has had a severe reaction to a penicillin they should not be prescribed any beta-lactam (although some people feel that aztreonam is the exception to this rule as there is very little cross-sensitivity with this).

In a patient presenting with septic shock and with no obvious focus coverage for infections due to both gram-positive and gram-negative bacteria is necessary, and probably anaerobes as well. Vancomycin, amikacin, and metronidazole are all non-beta-lactam drugs and do this, although the combination is relatively nephrotoxic. Amikacin is also effective against most ESBL-producing coliforms. The combination of ciprofloxacin and metronidazole provides good cover against most gram-negative bacteria and anaerobes, but relatively poor cover against gram-positive bacteria such as streptococci and staphylococci. In addition, many of the ESBL producing gram-negative bacteria are ciprofloxacin resistant and fluoroquinolones have been implicated as one of the common causes of *Clostridium difficile* diarrhoea.

CHAPTER 43

Mechanisms of antibiotic resistance

Ruaridh Buchanan and David Wareham

CONTENTS

43.1 Is antibiotic resistance a new problem?

Although antibiotic resistance has come to the fore in the media and clinical practice relatively recently, it is by no means a new issue; Alexander Fleming discussed the risks of penicillin resistance more than sixty years ago, but even he was behind the times. Bacteria have been competing with each other for millions of years, producing compounds which kill or inhibit other species—it is not surprising that bacteria have evolved defence mechanisms. Current major concerns are the rise of pan-drug resistant gram-negative organisms and the spread of multi-drug resistant TB.

43.2 How antibiotic resistance arises

Bacterial cells turn over rapidly—this rate of reproduction leads to many errors in DNA replication. Many of these mutations are deleterious to the organism, but others confer new properties, such as changing the structure of an enzyme. The application of selection pressure in the form of antimicrobial therapy leads to the survival of mutants that have randomly acquired resistance mechanisms.

43.3 Categorizing antibiotic resistance mechanisms

There are two useful ways to categorize resistance mechanisms: by how bacterial cells acquire them and by the physical mechanism of action. The types of acquisition have important infection control ramifications.

Resistance can be subdivided into three separate categories:

- Intrinsic resistance—mechanisms hard coded into all members of a bacterial species at the chromosomal level. If an organism's antibiogram suggests susceptibility to an agent to which it should be intrinsically resistant, further work should be done to check that the identification is correct. Examples include gram-negative bacteria being resistant to glycopeptides due to the outer cell membrane, anaerobes being resistant to aminoglycosides due to lack of an uptake mechanism, and amoxicillin resistance in *Klebsiella* due to beta-lactamase production.
- Mutational resistance—resistance that arises randomly due to DNA replication errors in conjunction with selection pressure applied by antimicrobial agents. This is the basis of the majority of the mechanisms detailed in this chapter.
- Transferrable resistance—mutational resistance that is passed horizontally from the bacterium in which it arose to another cell, possibly of a different species entirely. This happens through either transposons (DNA that incorporates into the bacterial chromosome) or plasmids (rings of DNA that replicate independent of the main chromosome). Often multiple genes conferring resistance to multiple classes of antimicrobial are linked on one plasmid.

Mechanisms of resistance are best thought of logically as follows:

- Preventing a drug from reaching its target:
  - The drug is prevented from entering the cell due to decreased membrane or wall permeability;
  - The drug enters the cell as normal but is then actively pumped out; or
  - The drug is enzymatically destroyed, either inside or outside the cell.
- The drug target is modified such that the drug can no longer bind to it;
- Alteration of metabolic pathways such that:
  - The step targeted by the drug is bypassed; or
  - The prodrug is no longer metabolized to its active form.

43.4 Examples of decreased membrane permeability

Decreased membrane permeability is a relatively uncommon cause of resistance, being generally confined to gram-negative bacteria, particularly *Pseudomonas* and *Stenotrophomonas* species. Hydrophobic drugs, such as fluoroquinolones, can pass through relatively freely; however, the majority of drugs are hydrophilic and thus cannot pass directly through the lipid bilayer. They must therefore either be actively transported by carrier proteins (e.g. aminoglycosides, macrolides) or travel through porin structures which contain water (e.g. beta-lactams). Mutations causing porin loss are a common cause of beta-lactam resistance in *Pseudomonas* species; carrier protein mutations are a common cause of aminoglycoside resistance in a number of gram-negative bacteria.

43.5 Examples of increased drug efflux

Bacterial cells often actively pump antimicrobial compounds out through their membranes. Mutations can increase the rate of this in one of three ways:

1. Increased efficiency of an existing efflux mechanism;
2. Increased expression of an existing efflux mechanism, i.e. more individual units;
3. Acquisition of an efflux mechanism from another bacterium.

The majority of efflux pumps are proton linked. Although some are specific to individual drugs, many have a broad range of substrates and can thus give rise to multidrug resistance. Horizontal transmission of genes for these pumps can cause resistance to jump between bacterial species when they co-exist in the same host.

Examples in gram positive organisms include the *mefA* transporters that extrude macrolides from *Streptococcus* species and the *tetK* transporters that extrude tetracyclines.

Examples in gram-negative organisms include the *Mex* family in *Pseudomonas* species, capable of extruding beta-lactams, fluoroquinolones, and aminoglycosides, amongst others; the *Acr* family in *E. coli* which extrude beta-lactams, fluoroquinolones, and trimethoprim, and a wide variety of tetracycline-extruding *tet* pumps.

43.6 Examples of enzymatic drug destruction

43.6.1 Beta-lactams

The most clinically relevant enzymes are the beta-lactamases, a broad family with varying spectra of action. They are responsible for the vast majority of beta-lactam resistance, stretching from the relatively common enzymes giving rise to amoxicillin resistance, through to the emerging threat of carbapenem resistance.

The Ambler classification divides beta-lactamases structurally into four sub-groups. However, this classification, while simple, gives no real clues as to the spectra of action.

A: the families TEM, SHV, CTX-M and KPC.

B: the metallo-beta-lactamases IMP, VIM, and NDM.

C: the AmpC enzymes.

D: the OXA family.

The Bush criteria form a more functional framework. Some of more relevant categories are described here.

- **Class 1**—the AmpC enzymes: this family can hydrolyse cephalosporins and penicillins and are not inhibited by the beta-lactamase inhibitor clavulanic acid. This means that they can cause resistance to combination drugs such as co-amoxiclav and piperacillin-tazobactam. Though some are constitutively active (derepressed AmpC) others are inducible, thus bacteria may initially appear susceptible only to develop resistance during treatment. Cefoxitin rapidly induces the expression of the gene and thus *in vitro* cefoxitin resistance may herald the presence of AmpC genes. The so-called ESCHAPPM organisms—*Enterobacter cloacae, Serratia marcescens, Citrobacter freundii, Hafnia alvei, Acinetobacter baumanni, Proteus vulgaris, Providencia* species, and *Morganella morganii*—have these enzymes. They are predominantly chromosomal and thus not easily passed to other bacteria.
- **Class 2**—subdivided into:
  - 2a—simple penicillinases.
  - 2b—hydrolysers of simple penicillins and cephalosporins: the cause of amoxicillin resistance in many *Enterobacteriaceae*. The first identified was TEM-1; others include TEM-2 and SHV-1.
  - 2be—extended spectrum beta-lactamases (ESBLs): These enzymes are able to hydrolyse a broader range of beta-lactams, including modified penicillins, such as piperacillin, and third-generation cephalosporins, such as cefotaxime. Though many are susceptible in vitro to beta-lactam/beta-lactamase inhibitor combinations (e.g. amoxicillin/clavulanic acid), clinically it is generally advisable to choose either a carbapenem, temocillin, or non-beta-lactam antimicrobial for therapy, especially in severe infections. Examples include TEM-3, SHV-2, and the CTX-M family. They are plasmid borne and thus relatively easily transferred between bacteria.
  - 2d—oxacillinases: enzymes preferentially targeting flucloxacillin, e.g. OXA-1.
  - 2de—ESBL oxacillinases, e.g. OXA-15.

- 2df—carbapenemase oxacillinases: These enzymes are capable of hydrolysing drugs such as meropenem, providing resistance to all beta-lactams except the monobactam aztreonam. OXA-48-like enzymes are the most prevalent in UK isolates and phenotypic detection can be difficult due to the lack of a specific enzyme inhibitor.
- 2f—carbapenemases, including the KPC family: These enzymes provide resistance to all beta-lactams including aztreonam. They can be distinguished phenotypically as their activity is inhibited in vitro by boronic acid. They are mainly found in *Klebsiella pneumoniae* (hence KPC) but are plasmid borne and can be transferred to other *Enterobacteriaceae*.

- **Class 3**—the metallo-beta-lactamases, including the carbapenemase families VIM, IMP, and NDM. VIM enzymes are more commonly found in *Pseudomonas* species, whereas NDM is predominantly found in *Enterobacteriaceae*; IMP enzymes can be found in both. The distinguishing phenotypic feature is their inhibition *in vitro* by EDTA and dipicolinic acid; they also do not confer resistance to aztreonam.

The biggest challenge facing infection specialists over the coming years will doubtless be the increase in prevalence of carbapenemase-producing organisms, particularly *Enterobacteriaceae*. Patients with nearly untreatable infections are already seen in the UK, particularly within London and Manchester, and much research is being undertaken as to the optimal treatment strategies for affected patients.

43.6.2 Aminoglycosides

Enzymatic modification is the commonest mechanism of aminoglycoside resistance, often conferring high-level resistance. The enzymes can be found in many bacterial species and are subdivided into acetyltransferases, phosphotransferases, and nucleotidyltransferases. Some confer resistance to a specific drug while others are broad in their range of action, sometimes giving rise to resistance to other classes of antibiotics. There is a great geographic variation in distribution and thus each local area has to examine their resistance patterns and determine which aminoglycoside is the most suitable for use in their patients.

43.7 Examples of target modification

Target modifications only persist if the mutation is not in itself lethal to the bacterial cell. Some of these mutations are thus quite subtle and involve only single nucleotide changes—they can thus arise quite rapidly within a population of bacteria but tend not to spread as they are chromosomal rather than plasmid borne.

43.7.1 Cell Surface

Altered penicillin-binding proteins with decreased affinity for penicillins account for resistant strains of *Streptococcus pneumoniae*. These changes are often acquired in a stepwise fashion, with each individual mutation increasing resistance further. Knowing the organism's minimum inhibitory concentration (MIC) is helpful as lower-level resistance can be overcome with increased penicillin dosing. This mechanism can also be found in other *Streptococci* and the gram-negative *Haemophilus* and *Neisseria*.

MRSA (meticillin-resistant *Staphylococcus aureus*) acquires its resistance to flucloxacillin by the acquisition of a gene from the *mec* family. This encodes a modified penicillin-binding protein, PBP 2a, with vastly reduced affinity for the drug. Generally speaking this resistance cannot be overcome with dose increases, and alternative drugs should be used.

Glycopeptide resistance can arise due to changes in peptidoglycan precursor structure, usually with the exchange of d-alanyl-d-alanine termination for either d-alanyl-d-lactate or d-alanyl-d-serine—these changes prevent glycopeptides from binding. They are encoded by the *Van* family of genes: the most important are *VanA*, which confers high-level resistance to vancomycin and teicoplanin, and *VanB*, which confers lower-level resistance to vancomycin only. These genes are mainly found in the *Enterococci* termed vancomycin- or glycopeptide-resistant (VRE/GRE) though they can transfer to other gram-positive organisms, including *Staphylococcus aureus*.

True resistance to glycopeptides in *Staphylococcus aureus* is thus far a rare entity, but strains termed vancomycin intermediate (VISA) are increasingly common. The mechanisms for this are complex and polygenetic, resulting in a number of phenotypic changes in the cell wall, including increased thickness and reduced peptidoglycan cross-linking.

43.7.2 Ribosome

The major target modification at the ribosome is methylation of the 23S RNA in the 50S subunit. This is mediated by a family of enzymes encoded by the *erm* family of genes. These genes generate resistance to the so-called MLS$_B$ group of antimicrobials—macrolides, lincosamides (clindamycin), and streptogramin B. These enzymes can be constitutively active or inducible, with erythromycin the most potent inducer. This mechanism is usually seen in gram-positive cocci.

Resistance to the oxazolidinone, linezolid, arises either due to direct mutation of 23S RNA or by methylation of the binding site. The former is more commonly seen in *Enterococcus* species, while the latter is more common in *Staphylococcus* species, encoded by the *cfr* gene which also confers resistance to streptogramin A and clindamycin. The gene is plasmid borne and can therefore transfer between bacterial species.

43.7.3 Topoisomerase enzymes

These are targeted by the fluoroquinolone family of antimicrobials, including ciprofloxacin, levofloxacin, and moxifloxacin. Topoisomerase II (DNA gyrase) is responsible for the majority of activity against gram-negative bacteria—a single mutation in the *GyrA* gene encoding one of its subunits can render the organism resistant. This can arise rapidly and causes significant problems in the treatment of pseudomonal infections, where ciprofloxacin is the only active oral agent. Mutations in the Topoisomerase IV gene confer resistance in gram-positive bacteria, though the genetic barrier to resistance is higher.

43.8 Examples of metabolic pathway modification

Metabolic pathway modification can occur either by the alteration of a pathway to circumvent a bottleneck caused by antibacterial enzyme inhibition, or by the loss of an enzyme critical to modifying a prodrug to its active form.

The bacterial folate synthesis pathway is targeted by trimethoprim and the sulphonamide family of antibacterials. These agents act as enzyme inhibitors, preventing the bacteria from producing the folic acid they require for normal cellular function. Genes encoding altered forms of the target enzymes can be carried on plasmids between bacterial species. In the presence of the antibacterial compound the new enzyme can retain sufficient synthetic activity to compensate for the reduced activity of the native form of the enzyme.

Metronidazole, used against anaerobic infections, is inactive until chemically reduced. The reduced form is cytotoxic, damaging DNA and other structures. The *nim* family of genes, most clinically relevant in *Bacteroides* species, encodes an alternative enzyme which can process metronidazole into a far less cytotoxic form, rendering it ineffective as an antibacterial agent. A similar process is responsible for generating resistance to nitrofurantoin in *E. coli*.

43.9 Further reading

Finch, R., Davey, P., Wilcox, M., Irving, W., *Antimicrobial Chemotherapy* (6th edn, Oxford, 2012).
Finch, R., Greenwood, D., Ragnar Norrby, S., Whitley, R. J., *Antibiotic and Chemotherapy: anti-infective agents and their use in therapy* (9th edn, Edinburgh, 2010).

Holmes, A. H. et al., 'Understanding the mechanisms and drivers of antimicrobial resistance', Lancet, 387 (2016), 176–187.

Kapoor, G., Saigal, S., Elongavan, A., 'Action and resistance mechanisms of antibiotics: a guide for clinicians', Journal of Anaesthesiology Clinical Pharmacology, 33/3 (2017), 300–305.

43.10 Assessment questions

43.10.1 Question 1

A 65-year-old male undergoes an emergency colectomy for a perforated diverticulum. Intra-operative samples grow a variety of organisms including an *Enterococcus* that shows resistance to a variety of antibacterials. Sequencing of the bacterial genome reveals the presence of an *erm* gene.

Which antibacterial agent is the *most* likely to retain its activity?
A. Clarithromycin.
B. Clindamycin.
C. Erythromycin.
D. Pristinamycin.
E. Vancomycin.

43.10.2 Question 2

A 53-year-old woman presents with fevers and right upper quadrant pain. An abdominal ultrasound shows several large abscesses within her liver. She is started on empiric co-amoxiclav and her fevers began to subside.

A blood culture is positive for *Enterobacter cloacae*—susceptibility testing is performed with the following results:
Co-amoxiclav—sensitive
Cefoxitin—resistant
Ciprofloxacin—sensitive
Piperacillin/tazobactam—sensitive

Which antimicrobial is the *most* appropriate for ongoing therapy?
A. Aztreonam.
B. Ceftriaxone.
C. Ciprofloxacin.
D. Co-amoxiclav.
E. Piperacillin/tazobactam.

43.10.3 Question 3

An 82-year-old Greek woman presents to her GP with dysuria and urinary frequency. She has recently returned from a lengthy trip to Athens, during which she spent a week in hospital following a non-ST elevation myocardial infarction. Her GP sends a urine sample which yields the following results:
Organism—*Klebsiella pneumoniae*
Amoxicillin—resistant
Aztreonam—resistant
Gentamicin—resistant
Meropenem—resistant
Meropenem + boronic acid—sensitive
Meropenem + EDTA—resistant

Which carbapenemase is *most* likely to be present?
A. IMP.
B. KPC.

C. NDM-1.
D. OXA-48.
E. VIM.

43.11 Answers and discussion

43.11.1 Answer 1

E. Vancomycin.

The *erm* gene is found in a number of organisms, coding for a methylase enzyme. It targets the ribosome, altering the binding site for the MLS$_B$ antibiotics—macrolides, lincosamides, and streptogramins. Erythromycin and clarithromycin are macrolides, clindamycin is a lincosamide, and pristinamycin belongs to the streptogramin family. Vancomycin is thus the only antibiotic listed which will definitely be unaffected by the presence of this gene.

43.11.2 Answer 2

C. Ciprofloxacin.

This patient is suffering from a deep-seated *Enterobacter cloacae* infection. *E. cloacae* possesses a chromosomal AmpC beta-lactamase enzyme which is more frequently expressed in the presence of beta-lactam antibiotics. The gene is also found in *Serratia, Citrobacter, Hafnia alvei, Acinetobacter, Proteus vulgaris, Providencia,* and *Morganella.* It is most rapidly induced by cefoxitin, which is also the beta-lactam compound most rapidly affected by the enzyme. In this case, *in vitro* resistance to cefoxitin is an indicator of the presence of the AmpC gene, despite the apparent susceptibility to co-amoxiclav and piperacillin/tazobactam. While the patient has exhibited an initial favourable response to co-amoxiclav, it is likely that this response will arrest as the AmpC gene becomes switched on in the majority of the bacteria.

In this situation, co-amoxiclav, ceftriaxone, and piperacillin/tazobactam are not suitable long-term therapies. AmpC additionally causes resistance to the monobactam aztreonam—however, it has no impact on fluoroquinolones such as ciprofloxacin, which is therefore the best option here.

43.11.3 Answer 3

B. KPC.

Hospitalization in a country with a high prevalence of carbapenemase-producing organisms is a major risk factor for becoming colonized with such an organism. Key to the identity of the carbapenemase are the organism present, aztreonam susceptibility, and the effect of various inhibitor agents.

- *Klebsiella pneumoniae* most commonly possess KPC but can possess a variety of carbapenemases.
- This isolate is aztreonam resistant—KPC causes resistance to aztreonam whereas OXA-48-like enzymes and the metallo-beta-lactamases do not. However, organisms with these enzymes can gain aztreonam resistance through other mechanisms, so alone this is insufficient for identification.
- This isolate remains resistant to meropenem in the presence of EDTA making it highly unlikely that a metallo-beta-lactamase (VIM, IMP, NDM-1) is present. The key in this instance is the reversion to meropenem susceptibility in the presence of boronic acid—this is the hallmark of the KPC family of enzymes.

CHAPTER 44

Detecting antimicrobial resistance

Lynette Phee and David Wareham

CONTENTS

44.1 Looking for resistance

- To optimize antimicrobial therapy for the management of individual patient's infection.
- For surveillance purposes, which in turn inform local/national/international clinical guidelines.
- For the management of infection control and prevention.

44.2 Detecting resistance in the laboratory

Broadly speaking, resistance is detected by observing its phenotypic expression (activity of the candidate drug(s) against the target bacterium) or detecting the underlying genotypic determinant (resistance genes).

Commonly used methods in clinical diagnostic laboratories generally fall under the 'phenotypic' category. These share similar traits—ease of use, reproducibility, scalability, quick turnaround of results and relative low cost of materials/reagents required. Moreover, decades of experience and fine-tuning have seen them established as methods of choice in most microbiology laboratories.

Most phenotypic test methods are reliant on the use of clinical breakpoints set by national and international bodies (e.g. EUCAST and CLSI) to determine susceptibility/resistance. These guidelines are regularly subject to updates with input from leading experts and latest research findings. It is important for clinical diagnostic laboratories to adhere to best practice guidance set out by these bodies and keep up-to-date with the latest guidelines.

Growth characteristics (on artificial media) of the bacterium of interest are extremely important in conventional phenotypic methods. As this presents a big obstacle for slow growers and 'unculturable' pathogens (e.g. *Mycobacterium tuberculosis, Mycoplasma spp.*) it has led to the introduction of genotypic methods of resistance detection in the clinical diagnostic laboratory. Rapid improvements in range/reliability/cost and expertise in genotypic methods precipitated their meteoric rise in the world of microbiology. Compared with conventional phenotypic methods, molecular genotypic-based tests are better suited for automation and reduce dependence on skilled workers for result interpretation. They therefore deliver the rapid turnaround demanded by modern medicine.

44.3 Antimicrobial susceptibility tests

Antimicrobial susceptibility tests (ASTs) is a term used to describe a range of phenotypic methods that employ direct observation of the action of antimicrobials against a target microorganism. This is the most commonly used method in clinical diagnostic laboratories for detecting resistance in bacteria.

A. Disc diffusion (Figure 44.1)

Growth medium: Standardized agar plates (usually unsupplemented, but addition(s) may be necessary for bacteria with specific growth requirements).

Antibacterial component: Fixed dose in standard size circular paper discs or tablets.

Bacterial component: Bacterial suspension at standardized turbidity.

Equipment required: Appropriate incubator.

Determination of susceptibility: Zone diameter inferring susceptibility/resistance based on guidelines (e.g. EUCAST, CLSI)

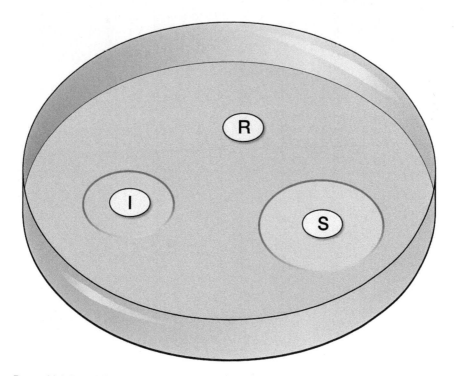

Figure 44.1 Disc diffusion assay.
S—susceptible; I—intermediate; R—resistant.

Features: Cheap, scalable, has the flexibility to incorporate multiple antibacterials onto the same
plate, easy to make changes to the antibacterials selected for each series, robust, specialist
equipment outside of a conventional microbiology laboratory not required.

B. Gradient strips (e.g. Etest®—Figure 44.2)

Set-up is similar to disc diffusion, with the following differences:

Antibacterial component: Range of doses across a plastic strip, allowing a specific minimum
inhibitory concentration (MIC) to be determined for each agent/bacterium combination.

MIC methods are superior to disc diffusion mainly due to the fact that the degree of in vitro
susceptibility or resistance can be observed, thus allowing the clinician to make better therapeutic
choices based on the understanding of pharmacokinetic and pharmacodynamic parameters

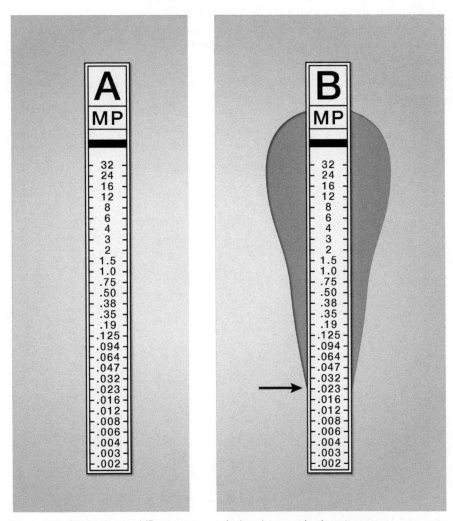

Figure 44.2 Gradient strips. MP—meropenem. Isolate A is completely resistant to meropenem,
MIC > 32 mg/L. Isolate B is susceptible to meropenem, MIC 0.023 mg/L.

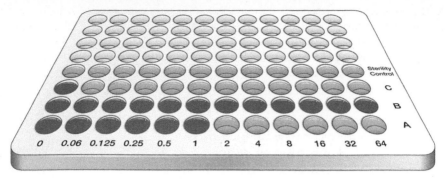

Figure 44.3 Broth microtitre dilution. Clear—no growth; Black—bacterial growth. Range of concentrations across rows (0, 0.06 mg/L to 64 mg/L). A: MIC 2 mg/L; B: > 64 mg/L; C: < 0.06 mg/L.

(PK/PD) of each agent and the primary source of infection. Due to the simplicity of set-up and interpretation, this is usually the MIC method of choice in conventional microbiology laboratories.

Gradient strips are more expensive than discs and, as the strips themselves are larger, impractical to set up more than one per plate.

C. Agar dilution and Broth microtitre dilution (Figure 44.3)

Growth medium: Standardized agar plates (agar dilution) or standardized broth aliquots in microplates (broth microtitre dilution).

Antibacterial component: Incorporated into growth medium across a range of concentrations.

Bacterial component: Standardized turbidity of bacterial suspension in fixed volume aliquots.

Equipment required: (optional) Multi-point inoculator (agar dilution), multi-channel pipette (broth microtitre dilution), appropriate incubator.

Determination of susceptibility: MIC based on lowest inhibitory concentration. Susceptibility/ resistance inferred from guidelines.

Features: Similar to gradient strips, with the additional ability to individualize the range of concentrations and repertoire of antibacterials tested makes it more flexible. It is, however, more time consuming, labour-intensive, and expensive to perform. As a result, these methods tend to be used in reference laboratories, but are generally accepted as gold standard antimicrobial susceptibility testing methodologies.

In resource-poor settings, a modification of agar dilution known as 'breakpoint plates', where two to three concentrations around the susceptible breakpoint of key antimicrobials are chosen, may be performed to provide information about resistance.

D. Commercial automated susceptibility systems

The common platforms available utilize similar principles to broth microtitre dilution, often in a multiplexed format with a smaller range of concentrations per antibacterial (around the susceptibility breakpoint). These automated systems have contributed to the modernization and efficiency of conventional microbiology laboratories.

44.4 Other types of phenotypic tests

Other phenotypic tests have been developed to allow for faster turnaround of result or more accurately detect resistance, which may otherwise be missed on AST.

The following are some examples:

A. Other susceptibility methods:
- Not commonly utilized outside of research settings.
- Examples include:
  a) Time-kill assays.
  b) Population analysis profile.
B. Specific antibacterial/inhibitor tests:
- Can be either agar or broth based.
- Common examples include:
  a) Double disc diffusion tests for ESBL detection.
  b) AmpC/ESBL combination disc diffusion test kits.
  c) Inducible MLS$_b$ resistance.
  d) Disc diffusion sets or gradient strips for detection of various beta-lactamases (e.g. metallo-beta-lactamases).
C. Detection of enzymes/binding proteins:
- Enzymatic reactions. Examples include:
  a) Nitrocefin for beta-lactamase production.
  b) pH indicators to detect acidic by-products of beta-lactam (e.g. imipenem) hydrolysis.
  c) Use of MALDI-TOF to detect by-products of beta-lactam catalytic reactions (e.g. ertapenem).
  d) Modified Hodge test for carbapenemase production (Figure 44.4**).**

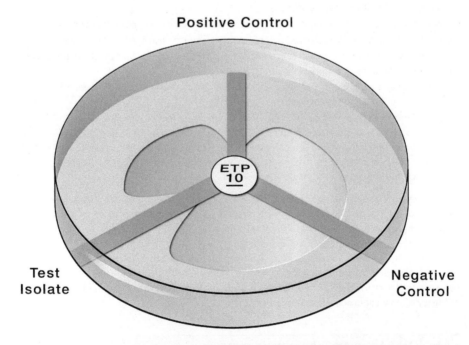

Positive Control

ETP 10

Test Isolate

Negative Control

Figure 44.4 Modified Hodge test. For detection of carbapenemases. A carbapenem disc is placed in the centre of an evenly applied lawn of a suitable antibiotic-susceptible type strain. A sterile 1 µL loop is used to create a thick streak of test isolate as well as positive (known carbapenemase-producing type strain) and negative (known carbapenemase-negative strain) controls preferably utilizing similar species.

e) PBP mutants indicating resistance to various penicillins (e.g. PBP2' for methicillin-resistance in *Staphylococcus aureus*).
- Lateral flow devices.
- Others (usually in research settings): Western blot, utilizing MALDI-TOF to detect specific enzymes.

D. Identification of species (species-specific antimicrobial resistance).
- Examples include:
  a) e.g. *Morganella morgannii*—imipenem and colistin.
  b) e.g. chromosomal inducible AmpC—e.g. *Enterobacter spp.*

44.5 Molecular methods for detecting antibacterial resistance

The blueprints to antibacterial resistance (e.g. β-lactamases, efflux pumps, porin changes) are encoded on DNA (chromosomal or mobile elements). Once known, these resistance determinants can be detected using myriad of methods. Most require a two-step process of amplification of the target determinant (e.g. polymerase-chain reaction or PCR) and an identification process (e.g. probes, gel electrophoresis, sequencing).

As they are not dependent on bacterial growth (unlike most phenotypic methods), molecular methods tend to turn around results in a shorter timeframe. Rapid development continues to further shorten this time to result; there has been a significant rise in commercially available point-of-care systems. Consequently, the relative predominance of phenotypic over genotypic detection methods has narrowed.

Most molecular platforms require specialist equipment and dedicated facilities, which may be cost prohibitive. In addition, skills necessary for performing molecular techniques may be lacking in conventional microbiology laboratories. When performed and maintained correctly, however, there is far less subjectivity when interpreting results compared with traditional phenotypic techniques. Molecular methods of resistance detection are well suited for automation and round-the-clock services, with the expressed aim of providing timely results at the frontline.

Caution, however, should be taken when interpreting molecular resistance profiles as organisms may harbour resistance determinants that are quiescent and not phenotypically expressed. This may lead to falsely positive results. Likewise, falsely negative results may arise from previously unknown (or undetectable by commonly available multiplex resistance panels) resistance determinants.

44.6 Further reading

Clinical and Laboratory Standards Institute. *Performance Standards for Antimicrobial Susceptibility Testing; Eighteenth Informational Supplement.* CLSI document M100-26 (Wayne, PA, 2016).

European Committee on Antimicrobial Susceptibility Testing (EUCAST). Breakpoint tables for interpretation of MICs and zone diameters. Version 6.0 (Sweden, 2016). http://www.eucast.org/fileadmin/src/media/PDFs/EUCAST_files/Breakpoint_tables/v_6.0_Breakpoint_table.pdf

Fluit, A. C., et al., 'Molecular Detection of Antimicrobial Resistance', Clinical Microbiology Review, 14/4 (2001), 836–871.

Jorgensen, J. H., Ferraro, M. J., 'Antimicrobial Susceptibility Testing: A Review of General Principles and Contemporary Practices', *Clinical Infectious Diseases*, 49/11 (2009), 1749–1755.

44.7 Assessment questions

44.7.1 Question 1

Which of the following methods is *best* suited for confirming the presence of extended-spectrum beta-lactamases?
A. Broth microtitre dilution.
B. Disc diffusion.
C. Gradient strip.
D. Plating on ESBL selective agar.
E. Real-time PCR.

44.7.2 Question 2

Blood culture taken from an elderly patient transferred from a psychiatric ward has grown methicillin-resistant *Staphylococcus aureus* (MRSA). Despite treatment with vancomycin, he continues to deteriorate clinically. Careful investigation for other sources of infection (apart from the previously identified and removed central venous catheter) does not yield any results. Further sets of blood cultures taken while on vancomycin reveal growth of MRSA. Serum vancomycin levels remain within the therapeutic window. The vancomycin disc diffusion test is reported as being susceptible.

What is the *most* appropriate next diagnostic laboratory test?
A. Repeat the vancomycin disc diffusion test to confirm the zone size.
B. PCR for *mecA* and *mecC* genes.
C. PCR for *vanA* and *vanB* genes.
D. Teicoplanin Etest®.
E. Vancomycin Etest®.

44.7.3 Question 3

Figure 44.5 shows a pure growth of *Enterobacter cloacae*, cultured from a sample of cerebrospinal fluid.

What is the *most* appropriate next diagnostic laboratory test?
A. Cefepime/clavulanic acid double disc diffusion test.
B. Ceftriaxone Etest®.
C. Nitrocefin beta-lactamase test.
D. None required. Report the final result as ESBL negative.
E. None required. Report the final result as ESBL negative, AmpC positive.

44.8 Answers and discussion

44.8.1 Answer 1

E. Real-time PCR.
Disc diffusion and broth microtitre dilution tests may be used for screening for extended spectrum beta-lactamases (ESBLs) by observing resistance to third- and fourth-generation cephalosporins. However, the pair-wise observation utilizing the inhibitory property of clavulanic acid on cephalosporins (i.e. increase in the antimicrobial activity of the cephalosporin with the addition of clavulanic acid) is required to confirm the presence of ESBLs. Likewise, chromogenic ESBL agar plates are screening methods requiring a further confirmation step. Real-time PCR of known ESBLs is the only option presented here which has the ability to confirm the presence of ESBLs. The main drawback of this method is the possibility of false negatives (e.g. resistance determinants not

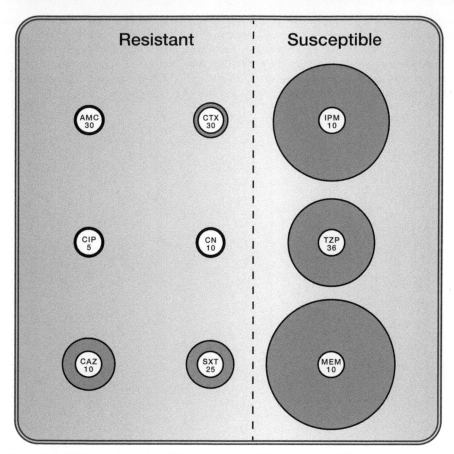

Figure 44.5 AMC—co-amoxiclav; CTX—ceftriaxone; CN—gentamicin; CIP—ciprofloxacin; IPM—imipenem; TZP—piperacillin-tazobactam; CAZ—ceftazidime; SXT—cotrimoxazole; MEM—meropenem.

included in the panel used, inhibition in the sample, mutations in the target region utilized in the chosen assay).

44.8.2 Answer 2

E. Vancomycin Etest®
Vancomycin disc diffusion is no longer recommended by most guidelines (e.g. EUCAST, CLSI), and has been replaced by the preferred MIC method. The method of choice is broth microtitre dilution, which is often not performed outside reference laboratories. *mecA* and *mecC* genes encode for resistance to methicillin, hence for MRSA. While *vanA* and *vanB* genes confer resistance to vancomycin, this is a rare cause of vancomycin resistance in *S. aureus*. Teicoplanin Etest® may be used to screen for hGISA (heterogeneous glycopeptide-intermediate *S. aureus*).

44.8.3 Answer 3

A. Cefepime/clavulanic acid double disc diffusion test.
Ceftriaxone Etest® would confirm that the isolate is resistant to ceftriaxone but will not provide further information about the presence of beta-lactamases. Nitrocefin is useful for detecting

beta-lactamases but is not selective for ESBL. Furthermore, *Enterobacter cloacae* harbours intrinsic beta-lactamases which will always yield a positive nitrocefin test regardless of the presence of ESBLs. From the given antibiogram, it is not possible to conclude that the isolate is ESBL negative. Cefepime is relatively less susceptible to hydrolysis by AmpC compared with other cephalosporins, and as *E. cloacae* carries chromosomal AmpC, cefepime +/- clavulanate double disc or combination disc diffusion tests are useful for detecting the presence of ESBL in this case.

CHAPTER 45

Immunotherapy

Jonathan Lambourne, Ruaridh Buchanan, and Emily Zinser

45.1 What is immunotherapy?

Immunotherapy implies the use of an immune-based therapy to treat infection. Broadly speaking, these therapies can be divided into antibody-based therapies (both pathogen specific and pathogen agnostic), cellular therapies (e.g. CMV-specific T cells), and immune signalling therapies (e.g. interferon-alpha in the treatment of hepatitis C infection). While agents such as corticosteroids, thalidomide, and vitamin D have profound effects on immune function and a well-established role in the treatment of some infections (e.g. corticosteroids in tuberculous and pneumococcal meningitis), in this review they are not considered as immunotherapy, as they are not directly derived from components of the immune system.

When considering immunotherapy, it is important to make a distinction between therapy and prophylaxis. There are well-established indications for using immunotherapy as prophylaxis against infection, including the use of varicella immune globulin and RSV-specific monoclonal antibodies (Palivizumab) to prevent chicken pox and RSV infection respectively. In addition, immunization is a form of immunotherapy—inducing a primary immune response and immunological memory such that on exposure to the pathogen, a secondary immune response is rapidly generated, hopefully leading to the control and eradication of the pathogen before infection occurs.

There are few immunotherapies currently in routine clinical use, and several experimental therapies under investigation (see Table 45.1).

Table 45.1 Examples of immunotherapies.

Immunotherapy	Explanation
Antibody-based immunotherapy	
Intravenous immunoglobulin (Human normal immunoglobulin—HNIg)	Polyclonal immunoglobulin, derived from blood donors. Established treatment adjunct for a number of indications (see question below) Experimental treatment of a range of infections, including Shiga toxin-mediated haemolytic uremic syndrome
Hyperimmune serum	Polyclonal immunoglobulin derived from pooled adult human plasma selected for high titres of antibody against the target organism Established treatment (and prevention) of tetanus (tetanus immune globulin) Experimental therapy for range of infections, including anthrax and CMV disease in transplant recipients
Convalescent serum	Polyclonal immunoglobulin, derived from survivors of infection, assumed to contain high titres of pathogen-specific antibodies (but antibody titres not specifically measured) Experimental therapy, investigated for a range of infections, including Ebola, MERS, 'swine 'flu', and SARS
Palivizumab	Monoclonal antibody vs RSV envelope glycoprotein Experimental for treatment of RSV. Established for prevention of RSV
Botulism immune globulin	Polyclonal, human, or equine source, specifically directed against *Clostridium botulinum* toxin type A or B. Established treatment of botulism. Human-derived used for infants younger than one year of age (BabyBIG), equine-derived for infants older than one year of age, and adults
Actoxumab and bezlotoxumab	Human monoclonal antibodies against *C. difficile* toxins A and B, respectively. Addition of Bezlotoxumab to standard antibiotic treatment is associated with a substantially lower rate of recurrent infection
HIV	Range of antibody-based immunotherapies currently under investigation for treatment/control of HIV infection, including use of anti-HIV antibodies and monoclonal antibodies against a4b7 integrin
Raxibacumab and obiltoxaximab	Monoclonal antibodies directed against protective antigen. Both approved by FDA for treatment of Anthrax
Cellular immunotherapy	
Pathogen-specific T cells	Experimental therapy, currently under investigation for specific viral infections in stem-cell transplant recipients (EBV, CMV, and adenovirus)
Granulocyte transfusion	Established treatment, but with questionable efficacy, for fungal infection in patients with prolonged neutropenia where infection is refractory to antifungal therapy
Immune signalling therapy	
Interferon-alpha	Established therapy for chronic hepatitis C and hepatitis B infection
Interferon-gamma	Established as prophylaxis in patients with Chronic Granulomatous Disease Experimental therapy for a rage of other infections, including mycobacterial (TB and non-tuberculous mycobacteria) and fungal (e.g. aspergillus and cryptococcus)
Colony-stimulating factors, e.g. G-CSF	Established treatment, but with questionable efficacy, for fungal infection in patients with prolonged neutropenia where infection is refractory to antifungal therapy
IL-2	Experimental therapy, investigated for example in treatment of HIV and TB
IL-12	Experimental therapy, investigated in treatment of fungal infection
Anti-TNF	Experimental therapy, investigated to counter some of the detrimental effects of immune overactivation thought to play a role in disease processes such a sepsis and immune reconstitution inflammatory syndrome (IRIS)
Anti-PD-1/PD-L1	Experimental therapy, investigated for example in treatment of HIV and TB

45.2 How immunotherapy works

The aim of most immunotherapy is to replicate what should happen in an effective immune response to a pathogen, but which, due to host factors, pathogen factors, or both, has failed to occur.

45.2.1 Pathogen-specific antibodies (monoclonal or polyclonal)

Antibodies exert their effect in three main ways:

1. Neutralization: Antibody binding to pathogens, or their toxins, limits the access of the pathogen or the toxin to the target cell, thereby preventing cell infection or damage. Neutralization is important for preventing viral entry into cells and preventing the actions of bacterial toxins, e.g. Staphylococcal exotoxin. Neutralization cannot prevent bacterial replication.
2. Antibody dependent cytotoxicity: Phagocytes express receptors for the Fc-portion of antibodies on their cell surface (FcRs). Ligation of phagocyte FcR with an antibody bound to a pathogen is an effective method of delivering a pathogen to a phagocyte for engulfment and destruction. Coating of pathogens with antibodies is a form of opsonization, or 'making ready to eat'.
3. Activation of the classical complement cascade: Binding of C1q to antibody-antigen immune complexes triggers the initiation of the classical pathway of the complement cascade. This leads to further opsonization and phagocytosis.

45.2.2 Intravenous immunoglobulin (IVIg)/human normal immunoglobulin (HNIg)

In treating infection, intravenous immunoglobulin may play a variety of roles. It may contain antibodies directed against the pathogen being treated, acting in the same way as pathogen-specific antibodies already discussed. For the approved indications, transfer of antibodies that neutralize microbial toxins seems to be of particular importance. In treating toxic shock syndrome (TSS), the antibodies that appear to have the greatest impact are those directed against the super-antigens, proteins which lead to indiscriminate cross-linking of MHC-II molecules with T cells, which drive the pathogenesis of TSS.

The extent to which the effect of immunoglobulin acts via pathogen-specific antibodies will depend on the amount of pathogen-specific antibody present in the immunoglobulin preparation. This may vary between preparations and will depend on the sero-prevalence within the population from which the immunoglobulin has been obtained.

In addition, immunoglobulin has a number of potential anti-inflammatory and immunomodulatory effects, including:

- Blocking of Fc receptors on phagocytic cells in the reticuloendothelial system, preventing uptake of antibody-coated pathogens;
- Inhibition of peripheral blood monocytes and tissue resident macrophages and dendritic cells through ligation of the immunomodulatory antibody receptor Fc-gamma-RIIB;
- Inducing a skew in T cell development from pro-inflammatory Th1 and Th17 responses, to an immunomodulatory response driven by regulatory T cells; and
- Inhibition of complement activation, by clearance of immune complexes.

45.2.3 Cellular therapies

Patients with impaired cell-mediated immunity, for example, due to immunosuppressive agents given to prevent transplant rejection, are at increased risk of viral infections. This may include reactivation of latent infection, infection acquired from the graft, or de novo infection. Cytotoxic T cells play a central role in the immune response to viral infection, and infusion of pathogen-specific cytotoxic T cells has been shown to be effective. Advances in understanding of interactions between viruses and T cells, and improved capacity to select and manipulate T cells ex vivo, are bringing cellular therapy closer to routine clinical use.

45.2.4 Immune signalling therapies

The common theme of virtually all immune signalling therapies is that they attempt to stimulate the immune system to a more activated phenotype, in the hope that this will encourage pathogen killing or containment. Most of these therapies drive a Th1-associated pro-inflammatory response (e.g. IL2, IL12, IFNγ), which stimulates macrophage recruitment, phagocytosis, and phagosome-lysosome fusion. It is increasingly recognized that impaired IFNγ production and/or function can arise in adulthood, for example, due to development of anticytokine antibodies, and that this may be associated with an increased susceptibility to a range of intracellular bacterial pathogens, including mycobacterial species. Administration of exogenous IFNγ may be indicated for individuals found to have impaired IFNγ production and/or function, especially if they are failing conventional therapy.

There are two types of immune signalling therapies:

A. Colony-stimulating factors: CSFs promote proliferation, differentiation, and activation of progenitor cells. For example, G-CSF increases efflux of neutrophils from the bone marrow and enhances superoxide production. CSFs act in a relatively non-specific fashion, predicated on the assumption that more activated effector cells will be more effective at controlling infection. Most clinical studies to date have not demonstrated conclusive evidence of benefit of CSFs.

B. Checkpoint inhibitor blockade: The immunological impact of chronic infection bears some resemblance to that seen in some cancers. Persistent presentation of antigen can lead to increased T cell expression of immuno-regulatory receptors, including programmed cell death protein 1 (PD-1) and cytotoxic T lymphocyte-associated protein 4 (CTLA-4). Expression of these receptors affects the balance of stimulatory and regulatory second signals and leads to reduction in pro-inflammatory effector functions, favouring a more 'tolerogenic' response towards pathogen or tumour. Use of 'immune checkpoint' inhibitors, which antagonize these regulatory second signals, is now standard of care for some malignancies, leading to activation of exhausted antigen-specific T cells, more effective tumour clearance, and tangible clinical endpoints. Trials are currently underway investigating their use in HIV and TB.

45.3 Infectious conditions needing intravenous immunoglobulin

Immunoglobulin is derived from the plasma of donors. It may be administered intravenously or subcutaneously and is used in the treatment of an array of disorders, including certain immunodeficiencies (e.g. primary and secondary hypogammaglobulinaemia), autoimmune, inflammatory, and infectious conditions. As it is a pooled blood product, its availability is limited. To address this, NHS England has established a national demand management programme for immunoglobulin, which sets out nationally agreed indications for immunoglobulin use (Table 45.2). The guideline uses colour coding to reflect the prioritization of immunoglobulin treatment, based on the availability of alternative treatments and strength of clinical evidence.

'Red' indicates conditions for which treatment is considered the highest priority, because of a risk to life without treatment. For these indications, no external authorization for immunoglobulin use is required. 'Grey' indications are those diseases for which the evidence is weak, often because the diseases are rare. Trust and Clinical Commissioning Group (CCG) approval is required for use in patients with grey indications. 'Blue' indications fall in-between red and grey, and local trust approval, via the Immunoglobulin Assessment Panel, is required prior to use.

45.4 The future of immunotherapy

As understanding of the intricacies of the host-pathogen interaction and capacity to better interrogate immune function improves, it is likely that immunotherapy will play an increasing role in the treatment

Table 45.2 NHS England-agreed indications for immunoglobulin use for infectious diseases.

Condition	Rating and dose	Selection criteria
Severe or recurrent *Clostridium difficile* colitis	Blue 0.4g/kg, one dose, consider repeating	Severe cases (WBC > 15, acute rising creatinine and/or signs /symptoms of colitis) not responding to oral vancomycin 125mg four times daily, high-dosage oral vancomycin +/- IV metronidazole 500mg thrice daily is recommended; the addition of oral rifampicin (300mg twice daily) or IVIg may be considered. If multiple recurrences, especially if evidence of malnutrition, wasting, etc., consider IVIg
Staphylococcal or streptococcal toxic shock syndrome (TSS)	Blue 2g/kg as a single dose	Diagnosis of streptococcal of staphylococcal TSS, preferably with isolation of organism; AND failure to achieve rapid improvement with antibiotic therapy and other supportive measures; AND life-threatening
Necrotizing (PVL-associated) staphylococcal sepsis	Blue 2g/kg as a single dose	As per TSS
Viral pneumonitis following heart and/or lung transplant	Blue 0.5g/kg for five days	Viruses include HSV, VZV, CMV, RSV, but excludes influenza virus

From http://www.igd.nhs.uk. Accessed 22nd May 2017.

of infection. For example, immunotherapy could be used in sepsis, to counter either the immune over activation seen in early sepsis, or the immune deficiency that frequently follows. Likewise, host tissue damage in TB infection may be pathogen driven, but in many cases, it is driven by an overexuberant immune response. Using techniques and therapeutics now available, it should be possible to use immunotherapy to tailor the immune response to one that is effective, but not pathological.

45.5 Further reading

Bollard, C. M., Heslop, H. E., 'T cells for Viral Infections after Allogeneic Hematopoietic Stem Cell Transplant', *Blood*, 127/26 (2016), 3331–3340.

UK guidelines for indications for intravenous immunoglobulin. https://www.gov.uk/government/publications/clinical-guidelines-for-immunoglobulin-use-second-edition-update

NHS England. National Demand Management Programme for Immunoglobulin. http://igd.mdsas.com/

45.6 Assessment questions

45.6.1. Question 1

A fourteen-year-old girl presents with recurrent respiratory infections. She is admitted again with viral gastroenteritis. Investigations identify common variable immune deficiency (CVID) and immunoglobulin replacement therapy is requested.

Under the NHS demand management scheme for IVIG, what indication is this under?

A. Blue indication.

B. Green indication.

C. Grey indication.
D. Not indicated.
E. Red indication.

45.6.2. Question 2

A sixty-three-year-old man sustains a cut on his hand while gardening. He presents with a lock jaw and painful spasms. He was not previously vaccinated against tetanus. He is admitted to ITU and sedated. The wound is assessed to be clean.

What is the next most effective management?
A. A stat dose of amikacin.
B. Immunization with tetanus toxoid.
C. Intravenous immunoglobulin (IVIG).
D. Intravenous vancomycin.
E. Oral metronidazole.

45.7 Answers and discussion

45.7.1 Answer 1

E. Red indication.
Immunoglobulin replacement in patients with primary or secondary immunodeficiency in which antibody deficiency is a prominent feature is an important adjunct to preventing infection in these patients and is a 'red' indication in the UK guidelines for indications for intravenous immunoglobulin.

45.7.2 Answer 2

C. Intravenous immunoglobulin (IVIG).
Antibodies binding to unbound tetanus toxin prevent further neurotransmission blockade but have no activity on toxin that is already bound. Use of tetanus immune globulin is associated with improved survival. Other key aspects of care for patients with tetanus include wound management (e.g. debridement of necrotic tissue), appropriate antibiotics (e.g. intravenous metronidazole), supportive care on ITU (in case of airway and autonomic problems), and vaccination upon recovery. In the UK, there is a shortage of tetanus immune globulin. Studies carried out by Public Health England have confirmed that commonly used immunoglobulin preparations (Subgam, Vigam, and Gammaplex) contain sufficient amounts of tetanus-specific antibody, with sufficient toxin neutralizing activity for these products to be used in place of tetanus-specific immune globulin. Interested readers are referred to the website for more information: https://www.gov.uk/government/publications/tetanus-advice-for-health-professionals

CHAPTER 46

Outpatient parenteral antimicrobial treatment (OPAT)

Mark Melzer

46.1 What is OPAT?

Outpatient parenteral antimicrobial therapy (OPAT) is the provision of intravenous (IV) antibiotics to patients in the community or an ambulatory care setting. It was first used to treat children with cystic fibrosis in the 1970s but did not become part of adult services in the UK until the 1990s. OPAT facilitates hospital admission avoidance and decreased lengths of inpatient stay. It is associated with high levels of patient satisfaction. Recent clinical guidelines on the provision of OPAT services in the UK and US have recently been published

46.2 Conditions treated with OPAT

Skin and soft tissue infections (SSTIs), in particular lower limb cellulitis, are the commonest medical conditions referred to OPAT services. Patients are typically treated for three to five days with IV antibiotics but patients with lymphoedema or underlying skin conditions typically require longer courses. Increasingly, multidrug-resistant urinary tract infections (UTIs) may be treated in the community with IV antibiotics, although oral options such as fosfomycin are now available. Patients with bone and joint infection invariably require prolonged parenteral antibiotic courses, whether this be vertebral osteomyelitis or native or prosthetic joint infection. Other less common examples, where careful patient selection is required, include infected diabetic foot ulcers (with or without osteomyelitis), infective endocarditis, empyema, liver, and tubo-ovarian and brain abscesses.

46.3 Recruiting OPAT patients

Patients are recruited on the basis of clinical syndromes (e.g. lower limb cellulitis) or laboratory referral (e.g. multidrug-resistant UTIs). Active recruitment (e.g. attendance at acute assessment unit board rounds or orthopaedic multidisciplinary teams, MDTs) compared to passive recruitment (waiting for clinical referrals) increases the yield of patients. The suitability of a patient to receive treatment out of hospital or in an ambulatory care setting needs careful assessment and is dependent upon age, comorbidities, and severity of infection. OPAT also requires patients to engage actively and reliably with therapy. Therefore, IV drug users and patients with serious mental health problems are generally not suitable.

46.4 Commonly used antibiotics

Commonly used antibiotics are those given once daily as these reduce nursing time, although some nursing teams can administer IV antibiotics up to three times per day. It is imperative to take a drug allergy history and seek an alternative class of antibiotics when a patient complains of severe penicillin allergy. When a patient describes a non-severe allergy (e.g. mild rash) it is reasonable to trial an IV cephalosporin or carbapenem. Some services insist on the first dose of antibiotic being given in hospital but many services now give the first dose of IV antibiotics in the community. Examples of commonly used antibiotics include ceftriaxone, ertapenem, amikacin, teicoplanin, and daptomycin. OPAT teams may need to monitor drug levels (e.g. pre-teicoplanin levels for efficacy or pre-amikacin levels for nephrotoxicity). For most IV antibiotics, full blood count, urea and electrolytes, C-reactive protein, and liver function tests should be monitored at least on a weekly basis.

46.5 Administering antibiotics

These can be given through a peripheral venflon, but for longer durations of treatment (for more than seven days), administration through a Hickman line or a peripherally inserted central catheter (PICC) is preferable. Insertion by a suitably trained health care professional or by an interventional radiologist reduces the risk of line-associated infection. Administration devices are available for antimicrobial administration in the community and save district nurse time.

46.6 Delivering OPAT

There are different models for delivering OPAT services. These are community based (nurses delivering treatment within the patient's home) or hospital based (patients attending hospital or an ambulatory care centre on a daily basis for IV antibiotic treatment). Ideally an OPAT team should consist of doctors, hospital-based nurses, and community nurses capable of re-siting venflons and taking blood samples from patients. Patients can also be taught to self-administer and this can be facilitated by 'antibiotic administration devices'.

46.7 Monitoring and following up OPAT patients

It is important that patients are appropriately monitored with clinical assessments, blood tests, and imaging performed at appropriate intervals. Some trusts organize patients on virtual wards which facilitates clinical ownership and follow up. Good practice includes regular MDTs (where cases are discussed with an infection specialist), taking of bloods, and organization of other investigations. While many conditions can be managed exclusively by a clinical microbiologist or infectious diseases physician, joint care is required for orthopaedic or neurosurgical cases. The treatment of lower limb cellulitis can mainly be managed by nurses and requires minimal involvement from medical staff.

46.8 Data collected for each patient

Data collection should occur locally and in the UK, data can be fed into a national database. For each patient, age, gender, comorbidities, vascular access, medical condition, antibiotic choice, duration on intravenous antibiotics, and outcomes should be recorded. Data collection is also important for the payment of national tariffs, set up at different levels depending upon admission avoidance or duration of inpatient stay. These provide a financial incentive for the further expansion of OPAT services within the UK.

46.9 OPAT-associated risks

Because of less clinical supervision there are risks associated with OPAT unless strict governance arrangements are in place. Adverse drug reactions are commonly reported and central venous access can be associated with access site infections and thrombophlebitis. Overuse of broad-spectrum IV antibiotics can be associated with *C. difficile* infection and depending upon the condition treated, relapse and hospital re-admission rates can occur. It is, therefore, important that patients are clinically supported in the community, often by nurses, and that there are formal re-admission pathways to secondary care. However, evidence suggests that OPAT is safe provided it is administered through a formal service, designed to minimize risk, which interfaces doctors and nurses working in primary and secondary care.

46.10 Key outcomes measurements

The key outcome measures are mortality, relapse, re-admission rates, adverse drug reactions, and vascular access complications. These should be periodically audited.

46.11 The future for OPAT in the UK

OPAT was recently cited as one of five antimicrobial prescribing decision options in the Department of Health guidance on antibiotic stewardship. It is likely to expand in the UK, driven by good safety and outcome data, patient choice, high levels of patient satisfaction, and health care efficiencies.

46.12 Further reading

Chapman, A. L., Seaton, R. A., Cooper, M. A., Hedderwick, S., Goodall, V., Reed, C., et al., Good Practice Recommendations for Outpatient Parenteral Antimicrobial Therapy (OPAT) in Adults in the UK: A Consensus Statement', *Journal of Antimicrobial Chemotherapy*, 67/5 (2012), 1053–1062. doi: 10.1093/jac/dks003. www.ncbi.nlm.nih.gov/pubmed/22298347

Tice, A. D., Rehm, S. J., Dalovisio, J. R., Bradley, J. S., Martinelli, L. P., Graham, D., R., et al., 'Practice Guidelines for Outpatient Parenteral Antimicrobial Therapy', *Clinical Infectious Diseases*, 38 (2004), 1651–1672. http://www.idsociety.org/uploadedFiles/IDSA/Guidelines-Patient_Care/PDF_Library/OPAT.pdf#search=%22OPAT%20guidelines%22

46.13 Assessment questions

46.13.1 Question 1

A 35-year-old man presents with a three-day history of left lower limb cellulitis. He also has lymphoedema following an inguinal node biopsy three years ago. There is no known penicillin allergy.

On examination he is alert and orientated. BP is 120/82 and he has cellulitis extending from his ankle to mid-thigh.

The patient is recruited to OPAT. What is the *most* appropriate intravenous antibiotic to administer?

A. Benzylpenicillin.
B. Ceftriaxone.
C. Daptomycin.
D. Flucloxacillin.
E. Teicoplanin.

46.13.2 Question 2

A 45-year-old woman presents with a five-day history of right upper limb cellulitis. She is known to have a severe penicillin allergy. On examination, she is alert and orientated. BP is 130/72 and she has cellulitis extending from her wrist to her shoulder.

The patient is recruited to OPAT. What is the *most* appropriate intravenous antibiotic to administer?

A. Ceftriaxone.
B. Ertapenem.
C. Flucloxacillin.
D. Teicoplanin.
E. Tigecycline.

46.13.3 Question 3

A 35-year-old woman presents with a five-day history of fever, rigors, and left-sided flank pain. On examination, she is febrile (T 38.5°C), alert, and orientated and has normal BP (135/75). She is commenced empirically on IV co-amoxiclav and amikacin and her fever settles after two days (Table 46.1).

Table 46.1

Investigations:	Creatinine	125 μmol/L
	Urea	13.2 mmol/L
	Blood culture	*E. coli* (ESBL +ve)
	Meropenem -	sensitive
	Ertapenem -	sensitive
	Amikacin -	sensitive
	USS of renal tract	Normal

The patient is recruited to OPAT. What is the *most* appropriate intravenous antibiotic to administer?

A. Amikacin.
B. Ceftriaxone.
C. Ertapenem.
D. Gentamicin.
E. Meropenem.

46.13.4 Question 4

A 35-year-old man is admitted with a three-week history of lower back pain. On examination he is alert and orientated and BP is 135/70 (Table 46.2).

Table 46.2

Investigations:	Blood culture	MSSA
	MR scan lumbar spine:	L4/5 discitis

The patient is recruited to OPAT and commences on IV ceftriaxone and oral rifampicin. What is the *likeliest* relapse rate?

A. 5%.
B. 10%.
C. 15%.
D. 20%.
E. 25%.

46.14 Answers and discussion

46.14.1 Answer 1

B. Ceftriaxone

Ceftriaxone is the most commonly used IV antibiotics to treat skin and soft tissue infection in the OPAT setting. Cohort studies demonstrate good clinical outcomes in carefully selected patients and low rates of *C. difficile* infection (< 1%). Benzylpenicillin is appropriate treatment for beta-haemolytic Streptococci, but not MSSA. Also, it is less suitable for OPAT as it needs to be given four times per day. Teicoplanin and daptomycin are generally used to treat MRSA infections or patients with severe allergy. Teicoplanin may be less effective than ceftriaxone and needs regular monitoring, including pre-teicoplanin levels and renal function.

46.14.2 Answer 2

D. Teicoplanin

As the woman has severe penicillin allergy, ceftriaxone and flucloxacillin are not suitable antibiotics. Flucloxacillin would also need to be administered four times per day. Teicoplanin is a better alternative than tigecycline and ertapenem as it has a narrower spectrum of activity and is more commonly used to treat skin and soft tissue infections.

46.14.3 Answer 3

C. Ertapenem

Ertapenem would be a better choice than meropenem as it is given once daily. Although once-daily amikacin is an alternative, this is best avoided in patients with renal impairment. Approximately

30–50% of ESBL-producing *E. coli* are resistant to gentamicin so this should be avoided unless susceptibility results are available. ESBL-producing Enterobacteriaceae are intrinsically resistant to Cephalosporins (e.g. ceftriaxone) but can be used in pyelonephritis caused by non-ESBL-producing Enterobacteriaceae.

46.14.4 Answer 4

D. 20%

The relapse rate for vertebral osteomyelitis in OPAT cohort studies, most commonly caused by MSSA, is approximately 20%. Governance arrangements should allow for appropriate clinic follow up or re-admission to hospital with early referral to appropriate teams.

Antivirals

C. Y. William Tong

47.1 The difficulty in treating viral infections

Viruses are obligate intracellular pathogens that utilize many of the host metabolic machineries for reproduction. Unlike the binary fission of bacteria, the replication process of viruses is more like a production line with a final assembly process to produce their progenies. Any agents used to prevent viral replication must be specific to the virus and cause as little problem for the host as possible.

The rate of virus replication can also cause problems. In rapidly reproducing viruses, the high replication rate generates mutants that could be selected for resistance to antivirals. On the other hand, viruses could remain latent with little metabolic activity. None of the current antivirals are effective against latent viruses.

47.2 Targets used against viruses

The life cycle of a typical virus goes through the following stages:

- Attachment;
- Entry and uncoating;
- Replication of viral nucleic acid;
- Establishing latency or persistent infection (in some viruses);
- Translation of viral protein and post-translational modifications;
- Secretion and assembly of viral particles; and
- Release from host cells.

Each of these steps can be used as antiviral targets (see Table 47.1).

Table 47.1 Steps of viral replication and some examples of currently available antivirals.

Steps	Examples of currently available antivirals
Attachment	Maraviroc – CCR5 inhibitor (HIV)
Entry and uncoating	Enfuvirtide – fusion inhibitor (HIV)
	Amantadine – M2 protein ion channel inhibitor (influenza A virus)
Nucleic acid replication	Aciclovir – nucleoside analogue (herpes simplex viruses)
	Tenofovir disoproxil fumarate – nucleotide analogue (HIV, hepatitis B virus)
	Sofosbuvir – nucleotide analogue (hepatitis C virus)
Establish persistence	Raltegravir – integrase inhibitor (HIV)
Viral protein production	Atazanavir – protease inhibitor (HIV)
	Simeprevir – protease inhibitor (hepatitis C virus)
Secretion and assembly	Ledipasvir, daclatasvir – interfere with NS5A protein which is important as a replication complex (hepatitis C virus)
Release	Oseltamivir – neuraminidase inhibitor (influenza A and B viruses)
	Zanamivir– neuraminidase inhibitor (influenza A and B viruses)

47.3 Stopping nucleic acid replication mechanism of the virus without affecting the host

The most common strategy is to use a nucleoside analogue as a false substrate. However, such a false substrate can also be taken up by host polymerase and could result in toxicity, e.g. mitochondrial toxicity in some of the earlier antiretroviral drugs. The most successful example to circumvent this problem is aciclovir, which is the prodrug of the active agent aciclovir tri-phosphate. Aciclovir is a substrate for the viral enzyme thymidine kinase carried by the herpes simplex virus (HSV) and varicella-zoster virus (VZV), which converts it into aciclovir monophosphate. As this only happens inside cells infected by HSV or VZV, it is concentrated only in infected cells. Host enzymes then add further phosphates to form the active agent aciclovir triphosphate, which has a higher affinity to viral polymerase than host polymerase. It acts as a false substrate for the viral polymerase and results in premature termination of nucleic acid replication. A similar mechanism is utilized in ganciclovir against cytomegalovirus (CMV). The viral phosphate kinase involved in the case of CMV is the UL97 protein.

Such specific activation mechanisms do not exist for other nucleoside analogues and depends on the greater effect of the agent against the viral polymerase. The reverse transcriptase of HIV and hepatitis B virus (HBV) are examples of such successful targeting. For example, lamivudine is a nucleoside analogue against both HIV and HBV. As the first phosphorylation step is often a rate limiting step, it could be more efficient to use an agent which has already had a first phosphate added, hence the development of nucleotide analogues. Some successful examples are tenofovir (HIV and HBV) and cidofovir (HSV, CMV).

An alternative approach is to use non-nucleoside analogues that can bind and inhibit viral polymerase directly. They can act very fast as there are no phosphorylation steps. Some successful examples are nevirapine and efavirenz (HIV) and foscarnet (HSV, CMV). However, such agents could have significant toxicity (e.g. nevirapine—liver toxicity, Stevens Johnson syndrome; efavirenz—CNS toxicity; foscarnet—renal toxicity).

47.4 Targeting viral proteins

Viral proteins often need modification after translation and viruses often carry a viral protease to carry out this function. Inhibition of viral protease is therefore a very attractive target. This has been used successfully in HIV (e.g. lopinavir, atazanavir, darunavir) and hepatitis C virus (e.g. telaprevir, boceprevir, simeprevir).

47.5 Preventing the entry or release of viruses from host cells

The mechanism of viral entry involves attachment of viral envelope proteins to a receptor on the target cell followed by fusion with the cell membrane, often effected through a viral fusion protein, and then an uncoating step that liberates the viral genome to allow subsequent replication.

The receptor of HIV is CD4, but it also needs to bind to a coreceptor in order to enter into cells. HIV strains could be R5 (utilise CCR5) or X4 (utilise CXCR4). In cases where R5 is utilised, a CCR5 inhibitor (maraviroc) can be used. However, it is necessary to do a tropism test prior to treatment to establish that the patient's virus is R5 tropic. Phenotypic tests are labourious and expensive. The most common method is to obtain a sequence of the envelope protein and perform a prediction algorithm to assess if the virus is likely to use CCR5 or not.

It is possible to target the fusion protein of the virus. An example is enfuvirtide, which is a peptide mimicking the fusion protein of HIV to prevent its normal action.

Influenza A and B viruses carry haemagglutinin and neuraminidase on the viral envelope. Haemagglutinin binds to sialic acid (neuraminic acid) on the cell surface of respiratory epithelium to gain entry to host cells. After completion of replication, the viral neuraminidase helps the release of the viral particles by removing its binding to the sialic acid on cell surface. Hence, it is possible to interrupt the viral life cycle by developing a neuraminidase inhibitor, e.g. oseltamivir and zanamivir.

47.6 The role for immune modulators

The human immune system is capable of clearing many viral infections without the need for antivirals. However, in some infections where the virus has persisted, it may be possible to give a helping hand to the immune system by using an immune modulator. The commonest agent used is interferon. It could be used alone (HBV) or in combination with another anti-viral, e.g. in combination with ribavirin in HCV. Ribavirin is itself a guanosine nucleoside analogue, but it probably has multiple other antiviral functions. Its most effective use is in hepatitis C as an adjunct with pegylated interferon and other direct acting agents.

In some serious infections such as post-transplant CMV pneumonitis, intravenous immunoglobulin (IVIg) is used together with ganciclovir.

47.7 Prolonging or improving antiviral biological activity

Some antivirals such as aciclovir and ganciclovir have poor bioavailability when given orally. It is possible to modify the structures of these two agents to improve their absorption in the gut by adding a valine ester to the agent (Figure 47.1). Hence, valaciclovir and valganciclovir are developed as the prodrug for aciclovir and ganciclovir, respectively. The valine ester is removed by enzymes in the gastro-intestinal (GI) tract and the liver to form the original agent. This leads to a significant improvement in drug levels of the two agents when taken orally. It has been shown that 1g thrice daily of valaciclovir achieved comparable blood level as IV aciclovir 5 mg/kg thrice daily; and 900 mg of valganciclovir provide the same drug exposure as 5mg/kg of IV ganciclovir.

It is also possible to prolong the half-life of immune modulators such as interferon by adding additional molecules to the structure. Polyethylene glycol (PEG) is added to interferon to form pegylated interferon, which lasts longer in the body. Instead of daily injection, PEG-interferon can be given once weekly.

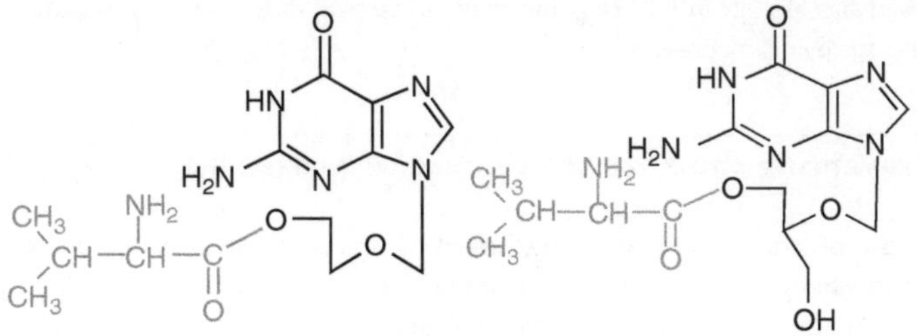

Figure 47.1 Structures of valaciclovir (left) and valganciclovir (right) with the valine ester residue in red.

Some antivirals such as protease inhibitors against HIV cannot achieve sufficient pharmacological levels when used alone. It was discovered that one of the protease inhibitors, ritonavir, while it only has modest activity against HIV, can act as a pharmacological enhancer to boost the level of other protease inhibitors. Hence, many protease inhibitors are used together with ritonavir, e.g. kaletra (a fixed-drug combination of lopinavir and ritonavir), atazanavir/ritonavir (ATV/r). Such a strategy has also been used with integrase inhibitors, e.g. boosting raltegravir with ritonavir (raltegravir/r). A newer boosting agent is cobicistat. An example of its use is in Stribild®, which is a fixed-dose combination of elvitegravir, cobicistat, emtricitabine, and tenofovir.

47.8 How viruses develop resistance to antivirals

Viral RNA polymerases, including reverse transcriptase, lack proofreading capacity. Hence, a large number of errors accumulate during the rapid viral replication process. Most of these errors lead to mutations that are either silent or lethal. However, in the presence of selection pressure such as antiviral therapy, some of these mutations that provide survival advantage will be selected. Some of these mutants are less replication-competent (also termed viral fitness) than wild type virus, but then further compensatory mutations can be selected to help maintain replicative competency of the mutated virus.

Some antivirals have a low genetic barrier for resistance. Lamivudine is an active reverse transcriptase (RT) inhibitor and binds the YMDD (tyrosine-methionine-aspartate-aspartate) domain of RT. A mutation in this domain from M to V (valine) or I (isoleucine) will result in high-level resistance to lamivudine. This same mechanism occurs in HIV (M184V/I) and HBV (M204V/I). Non-nucleoside RT inhibitors (NNRTI) also have a low genetic barrier, whereas protease inhibitors are less prone to development of resistance.

In influenza, the development of a neuraminidase mutation from histidine to tyrosine (H275Y) renders the 2009 pandemic H1N1 virus resistant to oseltamivir. However, the activity of zanamivir is not affected.

In herpesvirus, the main mechanism of resistance is through a mutation in the phosphorylation enzyme thymidine kinase in HSV/VZV or UL97 in CMV. More rarely, mutations to the viral DNA polymerase can occur which may lead to cross-resistance between different antivirals.

47.9 Antiviral strategies

The use of combination of antivirals against several targets has been successfully used in HIV, e.g. so-called highly active antiretroviral therapy (HARRT). This is now also used in the treatment of hepatitis C, which not only suppresses the virus, but could also lead to final eradication and cure. It is important to use a combination of anti-virals that complement each other and are not antagonistic or competitive. Many successful regimens use a combination against different targets, e.g. in HIV—use of two complementary nucleoside reverse transcriptase inhibitors (NRTIs) with a non-nucleoside reverse transcriptase inhibitor (NNRTI), or two complementary NRTIs with a boosted protease inhibitor (PI); in HCV— use of a nucleoside RNA polymerase inhibitor together with an NS5A inhibitor and/or a PI, with or without ribavirin. To improve compliance, the pill burden can be reduced by using fixed-dose combination pills and once daily regimen. Some examples of fixed dose combinations are:

Atripla®: efavirenz + emtricitabine + tenofovir (HIV)

Harvoni®: ledipasvir + sofosbuvir (HCV)

Kivexa®: abacavir + lamivudine (HIV)

Stribild®: cobicistat + elvitegravir + emtricitabine + tenofovir (HIV)

Triumeq®: abacavir + dolutegravir + lamivudine (HIV)

Truvada®: emtricitabine + tenofovir (HIV, HBV)

Viekira®; ombitasvir + paritaprevir + ritonavir (HCV)

47.10 Potential future targets

There are some very exciting new targets for antivirals. Some examples are:

- Brincidofovir: a prodrug of cidofovir which renders it less nephrotoxic. Active in vitro against cytomegalovirus, adenovirus, smallpox, and ebolavirus.
- Favipiravir: inhibit RNA dependent RNA polymerase and active in vitro against influenza viruses, West Nile virus, yellow fever virus, ebolavirus, and many other RNA viruses.
- Letermovir: inhibitor of CMV terminase complex.
- Pritelivir: inhibitor of HSV helicase–primase complex.
- RNA interference and gene silencing: applicable to many viruses.

47.11 Assessment questions

47.11.1 Question 1

A forty-seven-year-old man with acute myeloid leukaemia is to undergo stem cell transplantation. His pre-transplant blood test results show the following:

Hepatitis B surface antigen (HBsAg)—not detected

Hepatitis B core antibody (anti-HBc)—detected

Hepatitis B surface antibody (anti-HBs)—<10 mIU/ml

HBV DNA—340 IU/ml

What is the *most* appropriate management?
A. Give a course of accelerated hepatitis B vaccination before transplant.
B. No anti-viral required as HBsAg is negative.
C. Start adefovir.
D. Start entecavir.
E. Start lamivudine.

47.11.2 Question 2

A thirty-two-year-old man known to have HIV infection is started on combination therapy with efavirenz, emtricitabine, and tenofovir. He develops virological failure after initial successful viral control. Genotyping shows the presence of M184V and K103N mutations in the reverse transcriptase sequence.

Which of the following options is the *most* likely to be successful?
A. Intensify with maraviroc.
B. Intensify with raltegravir.
C. Switch efavirenz to ritonavir-boosted darunavir.
D. Switch emtricitabine to lamivudine.
E. Switch tenofovir to abacavir.

47.11.3 Question 3

A fifty-two-year-old man with chronic renal failure receives a cadaveric renal transplant. He is CMV seronegative and the donor is CMV seropositive. Due to HLA mismatches, he has to receive a relatively high level of immunosuppression to prevent rejection.

What strategy is the *most* likely to be effective to prevent CMV disease?
A. Intravenous ganciclovir prophylaxis for at least three months.
B. Monitor CMV viral load and offer pre-emptive therapy with IV ganciclovir when viral load is detectable.
C. Oral ganciclovir prophylaxis for at least three months.
D. Oral valaciclovir prophylaxis for at least three months.
E. Oral valganciclovir prophylaxis for at least three months.

47.12 Answers and discussion

47.12.1 Answer 1

D. Start entecavir.
Although this patient is HBsAg negative, he has positive anti-HBc and undetectable anti-HBs, suggesting previous HBV exposure and potential of reactivation. His HBV DNA result is detectable in low level, a condition recognized as occult hepatitis B. Overall, his risk of hepatitis B reactivation after transplantation is very high. Antiviral prophylaxis is therefore recommended. Short-term lamivudine can be used for such purposes but as it has a low genetic barrier for development of resistance, it is not recommended for use if the duration of prophylaxis is more than six months. As HBV DNA is also detected in this patient, a more robust anti-viral option is preferable. Adefovir is no longer recommended by NICE. Both tenofovir and entecavir could be considered. Entecavir is a good choice here as it has little drug interaction and unlike tenofovir, has no risk of nephrotoxicity; hence it is more suitable for this patient, who may be receiving multiple medications and could develop other complications.

47.12.2 Answer 2

C. Switch efavirenz to ritonavir-boosted darunavir.
In patients treated with the combination of efavirenz, emtricitabine, and tenofovir, the two drugs that are most likely to fail are efavirenz and emtricitabine because they both have a very low genetic barrier for the development of resistance. M184V predicts resistance to both lamivudine and emtricitabine, and a switch between the two is not going to help. K103N predicts resistance to efavirenz with cross-resistance to nevirapine, although it may remain susceptible to second-generation NNRTIs such as etravirine or rilpivirine. Adding a new class of drug to a failing regimen

is not recommended. Switching the failing efavirenz to a protease inhibitor with a higher barrier of resistance is desirable, so a switch from efavirenz to ritonavir-boosted darunavir is a good choice. Although M184V reduces the susceptibility of emtricitabine, it also makes the virus less fit and most HIV physicians will leave emtricitabine or lamivudine in the regimen despite the presence of resistance.

47.12.3 Answer 3

E. Oral valganciclovir prophylaxis for at least three months.

This patient is at high risk of acquiring CMV infection from the donor kidney and at high risk of developing CMV disease due to the higher level of immunosuppression he receives. There are two general strategies used in managing post-transplant CMV infection—prophylaxis or pre-emptive anti-viral therapy (monitor viral load and treat at the first sign of infection). There are merits for each approach. However, in a high-risk patient, a prophylactic strategy is more appropriate. The duration of prophylaxis should cover the period when the level of immunosuppression is highest, usually during the first three months post-transplant. High dose of oral valaciclovir (2g thrice daily) has been used as a CMV prophylactic agent, but this has been superseded by oral valganciclovir, which is more specific for CMV and is a much better prophylactic agent than oral ganciclovir (poor bioavailability) and IV ganciclovir (which requires a prolonged IV line).

PART EIGHT

VACCINATION

CHAPTER 48

Different types of vaccines

C. Y. William Tong

48.1 The different types of vaccines

Vaccines can be classified according to their nature into the following types:

- Inactivated vaccines:
  - Whole organism;
  - Acellular extracts.
- Live attenuated vaccines.
- Toxoid vaccines.
- Subunit vaccines.
- Conjugate vaccines.
- DNA vaccines.
- Recombinant vector vaccines.

48.2 Examples of inactivated vaccines

Inactivation of the whole organism is the most basic form of vaccine produced by killing the micro-organism causing the disease using heat, chemical or radiation and presents all the antigens in the inactivated organism as a vaccine to induce immunity in the recipient. Other methods to produce an inactivated vaccine is by extracting acellular components of the organism through filtration.

Examples of inactivated bacterial vaccines currently in use include:

- Anthrax—sterile filtrate from cultures of the Sterne strain of *B. anthracis*.
- Cholera—oral inactivated vaccine with 1mg of recombinant cholera toxin B (rCTB) in a liquid suspension of four strains of killed *V. cholerae* O1, representing subtypes Inaba and Ogawa and biotypes El Tor and classical.

- Pertussis—acellular vaccine has replaced previously used whole cell vaccine.
- Typhoid—purified Vi capsular polysaccharide from S. typhi; NB: the injectable, killed, whole-cell typhoid vaccine which contains heat-inactivated, phenol-preserved S. typhi organisms is no longer in use in the UK.

Examples of inactivated viral vaccines currently in use in the UK include:

- Hepatitis A virus.
- Hepatitis E virus.
- Influenza A and B viruses.
- Japanese encephalitis virus.
- Polio viruses 1, 2, and 3 (IPV).
- Rabies virus.
- Tick-borne encephalitis virus.

48.3 Examples of live attenuated vaccines

- Bacterial vaccines:

Bacillus Calmette-Guérin (BCG) vaccine is a live attenuated vaccine against tuberculosis derived from a *Mycobacterium bovis* strain. The oral typhoid vaccine contains a live attenuated strain of S. typhi (Ty21a) in an enteric-coated capsule.

- Viral vaccines:

The measles, mumps, and rubella (MMR) vaccine contain live attenuated strains of measles, mumps, and rubella viruses, which are cultured separately and mixed before being lyophilized.

Oral polio vaccine (OPV) against polio viruses 1, 2, and 3—OPV contains live attenuated strains of poliomyelitis virus types 1, 2, and 3 grown in cell cultures. With the eradication of poliovirus type 2, bivalent OPV targeting type 1 and 3 are now in use. Because of the risk of vaccine-associated paralysis, many countries have changed polio vaccination from OPV to IPV.

Two rotavirus vaccines are available:

1. Rotarix®: a monovalent vaccine (G1P[8]) attenuated by serial cell culture passage.
2. RotaTeq®: a combination of five bovine–human reassortant rotaviruses (G1, G2, G3, G4, P1A).

The two vaccines are not known to be interchangeable and a course of vaccine started with one should not be completed with the other. Rotarix® is the vaccine currently in use in the UK.

The varicella zoster virus (VZV) vaccine against chicken pox and shingles contains live attenuated virus derived from the Oka strain of VZV (Varilrix® and Varivax®). The shingles vaccine is for the prevention of zoster (Zostavax®). It contains a live attenuated virus derived from the Oka/Merck strain of VZV, at a significantly higher dose than the varicella vaccine.

The yellow fever vaccine is a live attenuated preparation of the 17D strain of yellow fever virus grown in specific pathogen-free embryonated chick eggs.

48.4 Comparing inactivated vaccines to live attenuated vaccines

The best example of a head-to-head comparison is OPV versus IPV (see Table 48.1).

Table 48.1 Comparison of the advantages and disadvantages of oral and inactivated polio vaccines.

OPV	IPV
Live vaccines carry the risk of reversion to virulence resulting in vaccine-associated paralytic polio (VAPP)	No risk of reversion to virulence
Contraindicated in immunocompromised patients	Not contraindicated in immunocompromised patients
The vaccine strain can be transmissible and passively immunize contacts. However, this could also result in transmission of circulating vaccine-derived polioviruses (cVDPV)	Non-transmissible
Mimic real-life infection with replication of the organism	No replication of organism. Based on direct antigenic challenge
Act directly on site of infection to induce local immunity (IgA), hence can stop transmission of wild type viruses during outbreak	No local immunity induced, cannot prevent transmission
Easy to administer. Mass immunization possible	Need expertise and facilities for injection
Cheaper to produce	More expensive
Need cold chain to prevent loss of vaccine viability	Cold chain less important
Susceptible to interference with cocirculating viral infections (non-polio enteroviruses)	Not affected by interference

48.5 Examples of subunit vaccines

Examples of subunit vaccines include:

- Hepatitis B vaccine: recombinant HBsAg in yeast
- Human papillomavirus vaccine: VP1 subunit virus like particle. There are two manufacturers, one produces a bivalent vaccine (Cervarix®: HPV 16, 18) and another a quadrivalent vaccine (Gardasil®: HPV 6, 11,16, 18).

These subunit vaccines present the antigen in the natural conformation of the native particles, thereby mimicking the natural antigenic state of the organism during the infection process.

48.6 Toxoid vaccines

Toxoid vaccines are vaccines based on toxins produced by bacteria.

Diphtheria vaccine is a cell-free purified toxin extracted from a strain of *C. diphtheriae* and converted to toxoid with formaldehyde. It is absorbed on to an adjuvant such as aluminium phosphate or aluminium hydroxide to improve immunogenicity.

Tetanus vaccine is a cell-free purified toxin extracted from a strain of *C. tetani* and converted to toxoid with formaldehyde

48.7 Conjugated vaccines

Polysaccharide coatings on some bacteria are not immunogenic to the immature immune systems of infants and younger children. By conjugating bacterial polysaccharide to proteins, the immunogenicity can be enhanced. Examples are:

Haemophilus influenza type b (Hib): capsular polysaccharide of the Hib bacteria is conjugated to a
   protein. In the UK, The Hib vaccines in use are conjugated with either a non-toxic variant of
   diphtheria toxin (CRM197) or tetanus toxoid.

Meningococcal disease (Men C and quadrivalent ACWY conjugate vaccine): capsular
   polysaccharide linked to protein. However, MenB vaccine is not a conjugated vaccine. It is a
   four-component protein vaccine made by recombinant technology.

Pneumococcal disease: Pneumococcal conjugate vaccine (PCV) contains polysaccharide from
   thirteen common capsular types (PCV13) and are conjugated to protein (CRM197) using similar
   manufacturing technology to that used for (Hib). Pneumococcal polysaccharide vaccine (PPV)
   is non-conjugated and contains purified capsular polysaccharide from each of twenty-three
   capsular types of pneumococcus (PPV23) and used in adults older than sixty-five years of age.

48.8 The latest innovations in vaccines

- DNA vaccines: When DNA of an organism is introduced into the body, some cells take up that
  DNA and express the encoded antigen on cell surfaces. This can then stimulate the immune system
  to produce an immune response. They are still in experimental stages but hold great promise.
- Recombinant vector vaccines: An attenuated virus or bacterium (vector) is used to introduce
  microbial DNA to cells of the body. Examples of vectors that have been used include
  adenovirus and vaccinia. They are thought to be more effective as they mimic natural infection
  and can induce both B and T cell response.

48.9 Combining vaccines

Many vaccines are given in combination to avoid multiple injections. There is no issue with the
immune system being exposed to multiple antigens at one time.
   Examples of combination vaccines include:

- DTaP/IPV/Hib/Hepatitis B.
- Hib/MenC.
- MMR.
- Td/IPV.
- Hepatitis A and B.
- Hepatitis A and typhoid.

48.10 Further reading

Public Health England. *The Green Book. Immunization against Infectious Disease.* https://www.gov.
uk/government/collections/immunisation-against-infectious-disease-the-green-book.   Updated
September 2014.

48.11 Assessment questions

48.11.1 Question 1

A child with a severe anaphylactic history of egg allergy presents to a vaccination clinic for advice
regarding the type of vaccine he could receive.

Which routine vaccine would you advise the parents to seek alternative?

A. 4CMenB.

B. DTaP/IPV/Hib.

C. Influenza vaccine.

D. MMR.

E. Rotavirus.

48.11.2 Question 2

A varicella-zoster virus (VZV)-susceptible healthcare worker on the oncology ward receives a dose of varicella vaccine through occupational health. She presents two weeks later with a number of vesicular rashes on the injection site and also some on her body. She is otherwise very well.

What is the *most* appropriate immediate management?

A. Administer varicella zoster immunoglobulin.

B. Advise her to avoid patient contact until all lesions have crusted over.

C. Commence treatment with aciclovir.

D. Reassure that this is normal vaccine reaction.

E. Take a blood sample for VZV, IgG, and IgM.

48.11.3 Question 3

A twenty-five-year-old patient with acute myeloid leukaemia has a successful stem cell transplant (SCT) and is in remission at twelve months post-transplant. There is no evidence of graft-versus-host-disease (GVHD). Immunization against some common infections is being considered.

What vaccine is recommended for him?

A. Intranasal influenza vaccine.

B. Measles, mumps, rubella vaccine (MMR).

C. Oral polio vaccine (OPV).

D. Pneumococcal polysaccharide vaccine (PPV23).

E. Zoster vaccine.

48.12 Answers and discussion

48.12.1 Answer 1

C. Influenza vaccine.

Most influenza vaccines are cultured in embryonated eggs and can have variable ovalbumin contents. The routine intranasal live attenuated influenza vaccine recommended for children contains up to 1.2 µg/ml of ovalbumin. It is safe for use in most children with egg allergy, but in patients with a history of anaphylaxis, an alternative inactivated vaccine with a low ovalbumin content (< 0.12 µg/ml) is recommended. MMR vaccines are also produced in eggs but are considered safe for children with anaphylactic reaction to food containing eggs. No egg-free MMR alternative is available. None of the other routine childhood vaccines contain eggs. Yellow fever vaccine is an egg-containing vaccine and needs special guidance if it is to be used in a patient with previous anaphylactic reaction to egg.

48.12.2 Answer 2

B. Advise her to avoid patient contact until all lesions have crusted over.

About 20% of VZV vaccine recipients have minor injection site complaints, such as pain, swelling, or redness; < 5% develop a localized or generalized varicella-like rash five to twenty-six days after vaccination, usually only two to five lesions and may be maculopapular rather than vesicular. A rash two weeks after a varicella vaccine may not have been caused by the vaccine. If the rash were caused by the vaccine, the risk of transmission is very small. In either case, contact with susceptible individuals with a high risk of complications should be avoided. Hence, she should be advised to stay away from patient contact till lesions have crusted over. The vaccine strain is sensitive to aciclovir. Unless it is a severe breakthrough infection, treatment is not warranted. VZIG is not indicated. To investigate if the lesion is caused by vaccine strain or wild type virus, a sample from the rash should be taken for characterization of the virus. Serology is not helpful in differentiating the two.

48.12.3 Answer 3

D. Pneumococcal polysaccharide vaccine (PPV23).

Vaccination against some common infections is recommended after successful stem cell transplantation. The recommended vaccinations include pneumococcal, Hib, tetanus, diphtheria, inactivated polio, and inactivated influenza vaccines. Other inactivated vaccines such as meningococcal, pertussis, and hepatitis A and B should also be considered. Live vaccines such as BCG, OPV, intranasal influenza vaccines, rotavirus, and zoster vaccines are contraindicated. MMR and varicella vaccination could be considered in children and seronegative adults twenty-four months after SCT if there is no GVHD.

CHAPTER 49

Vaccination schedules

Gee Yen Shin

49.1 Pathogens covered by the 2016–2017 United Kingdom Immunisation Schedule

The vaccines included in the current UK Immunisation Schedule offer protection against the following pathogens:

A. Viruses

- Measles
- Mumps
- Rubella
- Polio
- Human Papilloma Virus (certain serotypes)
- Rotavirus
- Influenza virus (flu A and B)
- Varicella zoster virus (shingles)
- Hepatitis B virus

B. Bacteria

- *Corynebacterium diphtheriae* (Diphtheria)
- *Clostridium tetani* (Tetanus)
- *Bordetella pertussis* (Pertussis)
- *Haemophilus influenzae* type B (Hib)

- *Neisseria meningitidis* (Meningococcal disease—certain serotypes)
- *Streptococcus pneumoniae* (Pneumococcal disease—certain serotypes)

The UK Immunisation Schedule has evolved over several decades and reflects changes in vaccine development and commercial availability, national and sometimes international disease epidemiology, and the latest expert opinion. It is designed to offer optimal protection against infectious diseases of childhood to infants and children at the most appropriate age.

The most up-to-date information about the UK Immunisation Schedule is available on the online version of the Department of Health publication commonly known as the 'Green Book': *Immunisation Against Infectious Disease Handbook* (see Further reading.

Various chapters of the online version are updated at regular intervals; thus, it is very important to refer to the online version of the Green Book on the website for current guidance.

Changes to the UK Immunisation Schedule are made on the recommendation of the independent Joint Committee on Vaccines and Immunisation (JCVI).

49.2 Combined vaccines in the UK Immunisation Schedule offering protection against multiple pathogens (species)

Several of the UK Immunisation Schedule vaccines are combined vaccines:

- Measles, mumps, and rubella (MMR).
- Hexavalent diphtheria, tetanus, acellular pertussis, inactivated polio virus, Haemophilus influenza type b, hepatitis B (DTaP/IPV/Hib/HepB).
- Diphtheria, tetanus, acellular pertussis, inactivated polio, and *Haemophilus influenzae* (DTaP/IPV/Hib).
- Diphtheria, tetanus, acellular pertussis, inactivated polio (DTaP/IPV).
- Tetanus, diphtheria, and inactivated polio (Td/IPV).
- Inactivated influenza vaccine: influenza A H1N1, H3N2, influenza B.
- Live attenuated intranasal influenza vaccine: influenza A H1N1, H3N2, influenza B.

In the UK, vaccines against single pathogens covered by the MMR vaccine are not recommended and not available in the National Health Service (NHS). There has been some limited demand for single-target vaccines, e.g. measles, due to misguided and unfounded concerns about the alleged risks of autism following MMR.

49.3 Vaccines a UK infant should receive by the age of twelve months

The age of twelve months is one of the key age stages in the UK Immunisation Schedule. As per the current (2016) DH Green Book, by the age of twelve months, all UK children should receive:

> Three doses of diphtheria, tetanus, polio, pertussis, and Hib-containing vaccines. Two doses of PCV (*pneumococcal* conjugate vaccine). Two doses of Men B (*Meningococcal B*) vaccine.

From late 2017 onwards, the immunisation schedule has changed such that infants will also receive three doses of a hepatitis B vaccine by the age of twelve months.

The Green Book provides a summary of what vaccines should have been received at several different key age stages.

49.4 The practical advantages of delivering combined vaccines

There are several practical advantages to delivering the immunisation schedule in the form of combined vaccines:

● Discomfort/Distress

Giving combined vaccine is less uncomfortable for the patient. Most vaccines are delivered as an intramuscular injection, which is uncomfortable/painful and can cause distress, especially to infants. Given that the same desired effect can be achieved from a combined vaccine against three or even four pathogens in a single injection, it could be considered unethical to administer three or four separate monovalent vaccines instead, which would cause three or four times as much patient discomfort and/or distress.

● Logistics/Efficiency

It is more efficient from a holistic healthcare system point of view to administer any combined vaccine compared to several monovalent vaccines. The vaccinator would have to administer multiple single-pathogen injections when one would suffice. This also complicates supply chains and simple things like having to record multiple batch numbers, rather than just one.

● Vaccine uptake and coverage

Combined vaccines are likely to be more acceptable to patients and the parents of infants as the same protection can be achieved with one injection at one time. From a public health perspective, national authorities can be reassured that with one injection, the vaccines are gaining protection against multiple pathogens.

Giving multivalent vaccines increases the chance of the immunisation schedule being completed and maximizing overall vaccine uptake and thus herd immunity in the population.

49.5 UK Immunisation Schedule vaccines offering protection against a single pathogen

Strictly speaking, the shingles vaccine, which contains a high dose of varicella-zoster virus (VZV) is the only vaccine in the immunisation schedule that offers protection against one pathogen (and one strain) only, i.e. VZV.

The shingles vaccine is unique because it is given to reduce the risk of reactivation of latent VZV in previously infected individuals. All the other vaccines in the UK Immunisation Schedule are designed to prevent primary infection.

Although monovalent hepatitis B virus vaccines have been available for many years, in terms of the routine childhood immunisation programme, infants will mainly receive the hexavalent DTaP/IPV/Hib/HepB vaccine.

49.6 Vaccinations for children with no reliable immunisation history

Various groups of children will have no reliable history of immunisation, e.g. children from war-torn countries, or hard-to-reach groups, and thus it is recommended to presume they are not adequately immunised and that they should receive the full UK Immunisation Schedule recommendation for children.

At the time of writing, the Green Book recommendation suggests that the risk of harm from leaving any such child susceptible to potentially serious communicable diseases far outweighs any risk of inadvertently immunizing an already immune child. In this case, all that would happen is a boosting of the immune response to the target pathogens, which is very likely to be beneficial.

49.7 Interruptions to the UK Immunisation Schedule

Generally speaking, if the immunisation schedule is interrupted, there is no reason that it should be started again from scratch. As per current Green Book guidance, 'If any course of immunisation is interrupted, it should be resumed and completed as soon as possible. There is generally no need to start any course of immunisation again, as immunological memory from the priming dose(s) is likely to be maintained.'

49.8 Live attenuated UK Immunisation Schedule vaccines

The following vaccines are live attenuated virus vaccines:

- MMR.
- Rotavirus.
- Live attenuated intranasal influenza vaccine (LAIV).
- VZV (shingles).

49.9 Other countries with national immunisation schedules

Most developed countries have their own detailed immunisation schedules. Examples include the US, Australia, New Zealand, and member states of the European Union. National immunisation schedules are influenced by many factors, including public health infrastructure, primary care provision, and local epidemiology of vaccine-preventable diseases.

Developing countries will have immunisation schedules tailored to local epidemiology of infectious diseases and socio-economic circumstances.

The World Health Organization (WHO) monitors the immunisation schedules of member states. It may be useful to know something about other countries' immunisation schedules when faced with patients who were born and/or grew up in other countries.

49.10 Recommended vaccines for pregnant women

Due to a national pertussis outbreak in 2012, which affected predominantly young infants, it was recommended that pregnant women should receive a vaccine against pertussis during pregnancy to boost immunity with the aim of providing passive immunity to newborn babies and young infants. The current recommendation is for pregnant women to receive DTaP/IPV vaccine between sixteen and thirty-two weeks gestation.

In addition, once evidence showed that pregnant women were at increased risk of harm from influenza A in 2010, it is recommended that pregnant women receive the seasonal inactivated influenza vaccine.

DTaP/IPV and inactivated influenza vaccine can be given at the same time.

49.11 Further reading

Public Health England. *The Green Book. Immunization against Infectious Disease*. https://www.gov.uk/government/collections/immunisation-against-infectious-disease-the-green-book. Updated September 2014.

World Health Organization. Immunization, Vaccines and Biologicals. http://www.who.int/immunization/monitoring_surveillance/data/en/. Updated June 2018.

49.12 Assessment questions

49.12.1 Question 1

Young children in the UK receive immunisation according to the UK childhood immunisation schedule.

Which of the following vaccine is not part of this schedule?
A. Inactivated influenza vaccine.
B. Live attenuated influenza vaccine (LAIV).
C. Measles/mumps/rubella (MMR) vaccine.
D. Meningococcal B vaccine.
E. Rotavirus vaccine.

49.12.2 Question 2

A one-year-old girl receives systemic prednisolone for nephrotic syndrome at a dose of 1 mg/kg/day for more than one month. Her immunisation scheduled is discussed.

Which of the following vaccines is contraindicated?
A. DTaP/IPV/Hib vaccine.
B. Meningococcal B vaccine.
C. Inactivated influenza vaccine.
D. Measles/mumps/rubella (MMR) vaccine.
E. Pneumococcal conjugate vaccine.

49.12.3 Question 3

Some vaccines in the UK are used selectively and not offered universally.

Which of the following vaccines are *not* universally offered to all children (excluding those with contraindication)?
A. Hepatitis A vaccine.
B. Live attenuated influenza vaccine.
C. Measles/mumps/rubella (MMR) vaccine.
D. Meningococcal B vaccine.
E. Pneumococcal conjugate vaccine.

49.13 Answers and discussion

49.13.1 Answer 1

A. Inactivated influenza vaccine.

Children who are not in clinical risk groups, aged between two years and seventeen years of age should receive the LAIV, not the inactivated influenza vaccine. The inactivated influenza vaccine is recommended for adults in risk groups, e.g. chronic lung or heart disease and all adults over the sixty-five years of age.

LAIV is recommended for children because there is evidence it provides better protection against influenza in this a group compared to the inactivated flu vaccine. In the UK, it is recommended that all healthcare workers with patient contact should receive the inactivated influenza vaccine for the relevant flu season.

49.13.2 Answer 2

D. Measles/mumps/rubella (MMR) vaccine.

MMR is a live attenuated virus vaccine. Live vaccines may replicate in severely immunocompromised patients. They are contraindicated in patients receiving systemic high-dose steroids, until at least three months after treatment has stopped. This would include children who receive prednisolone, orally or rectally, at a daily dose (or its equivalent) of 2mg/kg/day for at least one week, or 1mg/kg/day for one month. For adults, an equivalent dose is harder to define but immunosuppression should be considered in those who receive at least 40mg of prednisolone per day for more than one week Other examples of patients in whom live vaccines are contraindicated include patients who are currently being treated with cancer chemotherapy (or within six months of completion of the same), patients who have received a solid organ transplant who remain on immunosuppressive therapy, patients with a severe primary immunodeficiency. This is not an exhaustive list, please see DH Green Book chapter 6 for more details.

49.13.3 Answer 3

A. Hepatitis A vaccine.

In the UK, hepatitis A vaccine is not part of the routine immunisation schedule. However, as per Green Book advice, hepatitis A vaccine is recommended for children over the age of one year who are travelling to '... areas of moderate or high endemicity, such as the Indian subcontinent, for prolonged periods, particularly if sanitation and food hygiene is likely to be poor.'

Further information is available in Chapter 17. Current country-specific travel advice may be sought on the National Travel Health Network and Centre (NaTHaC)/Travel Health Pro website: https://travelhealthpro.org.uk/

Vaccination of specific groups

Gee Yen Shin

50.1 Groups requiring special consideration for vaccination

While the UK immunisation schedule is a national immunisation policy for the general population, several groups of patients and persons require a different approach to be taken. For example, some groups of patients cannot safely receive certain vaccine because they may be allergic (anaphylaxis) to some vaccine components and some patients cannot receive, e.g. live attenuated vaccines because they are severely immunocompromised.

Other patients require additional vaccines to protect them from vaccine preventable diseases because they are immunocompromised in some way, e.g. asplenia.

The following groups require special consideration:

- Pregnant women;
- Severely immunocompromised patients;
- Asplenic patients or those with dysfunctional spleens;
- Severe allergy to vaccine components;
- healthcare workers (HCWs);
- Patients with certain chronic medical conditions;
- Morbid obesity; and
- Persons travelling abroad, especially to developing countries.

50.2 Vaccinating pregnant women

In general, giving vaccines to pregnant women is not recommended due to the potential risk of medicines and vaccines harming the foetus. Specifically, live attenuated vaccines should not be given to pregnant women. It is relatively safer to give inactivated/killed vaccines to pregnant women, but most vaccines can and should be postponed until after delivery.

However, in the UK it is recommended that pregnant women receive two particular vaccines during pregnancy in order to protect the mother and foetus from avoidable harm. These are the inactivated influenza vaccine and a vaccine against *Bordetella pertussis* infection. For these two vaccines, the benefits of vaccination for the pregnant women and the foetus or newborn baby outweigh any theoretical risks of harm.

50.3 Vaccines severely immunocompromised patients should avoid

Severely immunocompromised patients should not receive live attenuated vaccines due to a risk of uncontrolled viral replication resulting in clinical disease.

Patients who are considered to be severely immunocompromised include:

- Severe primary immunodeficiency, e.g. severe combined immunodeficiency;
- Patients receiving cancer chemotherapy and those within six months of completing chemotherapy;
- Patients who have received a solid organ transplant and are on immunosuppressive therapy;
- Patients who have received a bone marrow transplant until twelve months after all immunosuppressive therapy has stopped; and
- Patients receiving high-dose systemic corticosteroids until at least three months after treatment ends.

This list is not exhaustive. The Green Book gives a detailed list of severely immunocompromised patients:

Please note that severely immunocompromised patients should receive all inactivated vaccines in the UK Immunisation Schedule. A list of live attenuated vaccines can be found in Chapter 49 of this book and the Green Book (see Further reading).

50.4 Vaccines for mildly immunocompromised patients

Patients who are mildly immunocompromised are at increased risk of morbidity and mortality from infectious diseases including vaccine preventable diseases. They should be immunised as per the UK Immunisation Schedule as long as there are no other contraindications.

50.5 Immunisation for friends/family of immunocompromised individuals

Yes. Household and close contacts of immunocompromised patients should be fully immunised as per the UK Immunisation Schedule to minimise the risk that such patients would be exposed to vaccine preventable diseases in their close contacts, e.g. household contacts. In addition, these close contacts should be immunised against varicella zoster virus (VZV) and seasonal influenza with the inactivated influenza vaccine.

Household contacts of severely immunocompromised patients eligible to receive the live attenuate influenza vaccine should be given the inactivated influenza vaccine instead.

50.6 Vaccines for patients with HIV infection

Patients with HIV infection are at increased risk of morbidity and mortality from vaccine preventable diseases. They should receive all inactivated vaccines in the UK Immunisation Schedule.

Certain live attenuated vaccines like MMR and VZV vaccine may be given to HIV-infected patients who are not severely immunocompromised as determined by their CD4 cell count. Chapter 6 of the Green Book has a reference table giving threshold CD4 counts by age group that can guide decision-making in relation to live attenuated vaccines and is updated as new evidence appears.

There is growing evidence of a risk of dissemination of Bacillus Calmette-Guérin (BCG), a vaccine against TB, in HIV-infected patients. BCG is not currently recommended in this group.

50.7 Additional vaccines for asplenic/splenic dysfunction patients

The spleen is a part of the mononuclear phagocyte system, also known as the reticulo-endothelial system, a component of the immune system. Patients without a spleen or a dysfunctional spleen are vulnerable to infection by encapsulated bacteria.

Asplenic patients are particularly vulnerable to three bacterial species:

1. Streptococcus pneumoniae.
2. Haemophilus influenzae B.
3. Neisseria meningitides.

Therefore, it is recommended that this group of patients receive vaccines against *S. pneumoniae; H. influenzae* and Meningococcus A, C, W, Y, and B. In addition, the Green Book recommends that asplenic patients also receive the seasonal influenza vaccine due to the significant risk of post-influenza secondary bacterial infection, e.g. *Streptococcus pneumoniae.*

50.8 Precautions for vaccine/vaccine component allergies

Certain vaccines may be contraindicated in individuals with confirmed severe allergic reaction, i.e. anaphylaxis to any vaccine or vaccine component(s).

As with any other prescription medicine, it is very important to take a careful allergy history before administering any vaccine. Patients who have anaphylactic reactions to certain ingredients, e.g. chicken egg proteins, must not be given vaccines which contain that material(s). In the example of severe allergy to egg protein, the standard seasonal influenza vaccine, which is produced by inoculating chicken eggs with influenza virus, is contraindicated.

Any person who has had a confirmed anaphylactic reaction to any vaccine must not receive any more doses of that vaccine.

50.9 Influenza vaccine for those with severe egg allergy

There is one ovalbumin-free inactivated seasonal influenza vaccine available (Optaflu). This can be given to persons over eighteen years of age, regardless of egg allergy status.

Chapter 19 of the Green Book (influenza immunisation) covers egg allergy in great technical detail, which may change from year to year due to variations in the vaccines each year. This includes data on thresholds of vaccine albumin content below which other seasonal inactivated influenza vaccines may be considered safe to use.

50.10 Special immunisation considerations for healthcare workers (HCWs)

HCWs with direct patient contact have a duty of care to their patients to not pose a risk to those they have responsibility for. For example, the UK medical regulator the General Medical Council (GMC) has guidelines in 'Good Medical Practice 2013' which state that healthcare workers:

> ... should be immunised against common serious communicable diseases (unless otherwise contraindicated).

Registered medical practitioners have a moral and professional duty to ensure that they do not put their patients at risk due to their own health, e.g. infectious diseases. This is consistent with the Hippocratic principle of 'primum non nocere'—'first, do no harm'.

Healthcare providers, e.g. NHS trusts also have a duty of care to their patients and they should ensure that clinical staff are immunised against vaccine preventable diseases as per the UK Immunisation Schedule (interested readers are referred to Chapter 49 of this book).

New staff undergo occupational health clearance to assess completeness of immunization and therefore whether it is safe for these employees to commence work in clinical areas. Most NHS trusts will offer their staff the vaccines which have been omitted in the past or need boosting.

A specific example of an occupational vaccine programme is the annual campaign to encourage NHS HCWs to have the seasonal influenza vaccination in order to protect patients, staff, and the families of NHS staff each autumn and winter.

HCWs susceptible to varicella zoster virus (VZV) should receive live attenuated VZV vaccine if there are no contraindications.

50.11 Underlying medical conditions requiring seasonal influenza vaccine

Certain groups are at increased risk of morbidity and mortality from influenza infection. These include adults and children over six months of age with:

- Chronic lung disease;
- Chronic liver disease;
- Chronic heart disease;
- Chronic renal impairment or renal failure;
- Recipients of renal transplants;
- Diabetes mellitus;
- Morbid obesity (BMI >40 kg/m^2); and/or
- Pregnant women.

This list is not exhaustive. Please see the current Green Book online for further details (see Further reading).

It is recommended that all those over the age of sixty-five years should receive seasonal flu vaccine.

50.12 Special considerations for HCWs

Clinical staff who perform exposure-prone procedures (EPP) e.g. most surgeons, obstetricians, and gynaecologists, are, by definition, routinely at risk of exposure to patients' blood and tissues. They are, like other HCWs, required to have been immunised against hepatitis B virus (HBV) infection. However, EPP workers who are HBV vaccine non-responders are not barred from EPP work. EPP workers would only be barred from EPP work if they are HBV surface antigen positive. Guidance in relation to HBV-infected EPP workers is determined by the UK Advisory Panel for Healthcare Workers Infected with Bloodborne Viruses.

50.13 Other groups who should receive hepatitis B vaccination

The UK is introducing hepatitis B virus vaccine into the routine childhood immunisation programme from late 2017 onwards. It will take several years for this to lead to population-level herd immunity. A number of groups of patients are recommended to receive HBV vaccine because they are at increased risk of exposure to, or harm from, HBV infection, such as:

- Chronic liver disease e.g. cirrhosis
- Chronic kidney disease including dialysis patients
- Haemophiliac patients (administered with precaution for bleeding disorders)
- Babies born to mothers with chronic HBV infection
- Healthcare workers who are at risk of coming into contact with patients' blood, blood-stained body fluids or tissues, for example through sharps injury or being injured/bitten.
- Household contacts of patients with hepatitis B infection
- Persons who inject drugs
- Staff working in prisons with regular prisoner contact

This list is not exhaustive. Please see the Green Book chapter on hepatitis B (chapter 18) for further details.

50.14 Additional vaccines for medical microbiology and/or virology laboratory staff

In addition to the general considerations for HCWs, laboratory workers who routinely handle and/or may be exposed to the following specific pathogens specific pathogens in the lab should receive vaccines against:

- Hepatitis A.
- Hepatitis B.
- Cholera.
- Meningococcus ACYW135.
- Typhoid.
- BCG—for staff handling autopsy specimens as well as in TB labs/sections.

In addition, those working in specialist virology labs who may work with the following pathogens should be immunised against:

- Japanese Encephalitis
- Yellow Fever
- Smallpox

50.15 Vaccines for people planning to travel abroad

Travelling abroad, especially to developing countries requires special consideration for travel-related vaccines. The additional vaccine requirements are driven by which countries are to be visited. A detailed discussion of this sizeable topic is outside the scope of this chapter. Immunisation of travellers will be considered under the relevant disease chapters of this book.

50.16 Further reading

British HIV Association. *Guidelines on the Use of Vaccines in HIV-Positive Adults 2015* (London, 2015). http://www.bhiva.org/documents/Guidelines/Vaccination/2015-Vaccination-Guidelines.pdf

Public Health England. *The Green Book. Immunization against Infectious Disease*. https://www.gov.uk/government/collections/immunisation-against-infectious-disease-the-green-book. Updated September 2014.

UK Advisory Panel for Healthcare Workers Infected with Bloodborne Viruses: https://www.gov.uk/government/groups/uk-advisory-panel-for-healthcare-workers-infected-with-bloodborne-viruses

UK National Travel Health Network and Centre (NaTHNaC). *Travel Health Pro*. Travel health information. Available at http://travelhealthpro.org.uk/

50.17 Assessment questions

50.17.1 Question 1

Which of the following vaccines is *specifically* recommended for pregnant women in the UK?
A. Hepatitis B vaccine.
B. Inactivated influenza vaccine.
C. Live attenuated influenza vaccine (LAIV).
D. Measles mumps rubella vaccine (MMR).
E. Vaccine against *Streptococcus pneumoniae*.

50.17.2 Question 2

Which of the following patient groups require special consideration of their immunisation needs?
A. Patients who drink alcohol every week.
B. Patients who suffer from hay fever.
C. Patients with hypercholesterolaemia.
D. Solid organ transplant recipients on maintenance immunosuppressive therapy.
E. Solid tumour cancer survivors more than a year after chemotherapy has finished.

50.17.3 Question 3

Who is *ultimately* responsible for ensuring that healthcare workers in a healthcare organization such as NHS trusts are fully immunised as appropriate for their professional role?
A. Local health and safety committee.
B. Occupational health departments.
C. The healthcare provider, e.g. NHS trust.
D. The local Infection Control Doctor
E. UK General Medical Council.

50.18 Answers and discussion

50.18.1 Answer 1

B. Inactivated influenza vaccine.
It is recommended that pregnant women receive the seasonal inactivated influenza vaccine because of the increased risk of harm during pregnancy. Hepatitis B vaccine is indicated for newborn babies of mothers who have chronic hepatitis B virus infection, not pregnant women themselves. Live attenuated vaccines like LAIV and MMR should not be given to pregnant women due to the potential risk of viral infection and harm. However, pregnant women who are found to be or known to be susceptible to rubella virus infection should be offered MMR post-partum. Routine antenatal screening for Rubella immunity ceased to be recommended in the UK in 2016. Discussion of this change in policy is outside the scope of this chapter.

50.18.2 Answer 2

D. Solid organ transplant recipients on maintenance immunosuppressive therapy.
Transplant recipients on immunosuppressive therapy should not receive live attenuated vaccines due to the risk of viral infection becoming established in a vulnerable host. In addition, their household contacts should be fully immunized as per the UK Immunisation Schedule to reduce the risk of immunosuppressed patients being unnecessarily exposed to vaccine preventable diseases. Regular alcohol consumption would not be an indication for seasonal influenza immunisation per se. However, if the alcohol consumption was excessive and sustained over a long period, sufficient to lead to cirrhosis, then seasonal influenza immunisation would be recommended. Patients with hay fever should follow the normal vaccination schedule.

50.18.3 Answer 3

C. The healthcare provider, e.g. NHS trust.
Ultimately, the healthcare provider organization like an NHS trust bears corporate responsibility for providing a safe environment for patients and staff. In this context, this means that clinical staff should not pose a risk to their patients or their colleagues from vaccine preventable diseases. Equally, employees of healthcare providers should be offered protection from vaccine preventable diseases they may encounter at work by appropriate immunisation.

In the UK, the relevant workplace legislation includes the Health and Safety at Work Act 1974 and the Control of Substances Hazardous to Health (COSHH) regulations 2002. Under COSHH, the term 'substances' includes biological agents, i.e. infectious pathogens.

Infection control doctors working with their infection prevention and control team as well as the occupational health department ensure optimal immunisation of employees against vaccine preventable diseases. However, they probably won't bear ultimate legal responsibility for any avoidable harm due to vaccine preventable diseases unless they have been negligent in some fashion.

CHAPTER 51

Post-exposure prophylaxis

C. Y. William Tong and Jayshree Dave

51.1 Post-exposure prophylaxis (PEP)

Post-exposure prophylaxis (PEP) is a treatment administered to an individual to prevent the development of infection or reduce the severity of illness after a potential or documented exposure to a microorganism. This may primarily be for the protection of the exposed individual concern, or in the case of a pregnant woman, for protecting the foetus in utero. PEP may also be useful in public health to reduce the risk of secondary spread of infection.

51.2 Information needed to assess an exposure

A good history is required in order to make a proper assessment of the risk. The following questions should be asked:

A. Which infection is suspected and is the source infectious?

It is straight forward if the diagnosis of the source of exposure is already known, e.g. known HIV, established diagnosis of tuberculosis. However, in many cases, the diagnosis of the source may not be certain, e.g. needle stick injury involving a needle of unknown origin, bitten by a stray dog, exposed to a child with a non-specific rash. In such cases, a risk assessment is required to assess the likelihood that the source may be infectious. Knowledge of local epidemiology or recent outbreaks in a particular locality may help in such risk assessment.

B. What is the nature of the exposure?

Knowledge of the mode of transmission of a microorganism is important to establish if there is any risk of transmission through the exposure (Table 51.1) In the case of mother-to-child transmission, PEP to the neonate born to a mother with an infection is effective if the mode of transmission is predominately perinatal, e.g. hepatitis B. If the mode of transmission is transplacental, it is too late to administer PEP to the baby after delivery. Instead, the expected mother should be given prophylaxis during pregnancy to prevent infection, e.g. chicken pox, or given antivirals to reduce infectivity, e.g. maternal hepatitis B with a high viral load when transplacental infection may occur. In HIV, where transmission can occur both transplacentally and perinatally, antiretroviral therapy (ART) needs to be given during pregnancy and often during labour as well as to the baby after birth.

Table 51.1 Examples of infections where PEP could be used and the mode of transmission.

Mode of transmission	Examples of exposure
Aerosols	Chicken pox or disseminated zoster, measles, pulmonary or laryngeal tuberculosis
Bites	Rabies, tetanus
Blood borne	Hepatitis B, HIV
Direct contact	Zoster (shingles)
Droplets	Anthrax, diphtheria, influenza, invasive group A streptococcal disease, invasive meningococcal disease, pertussis, plague
Enteric	Hepatitis A
Mother to child	Chicken pox, hepatitis B, HIV

C. Is the exposure significant?

In the case of airborne or droplet transmission, it is important to know how long the exposed individual was in contact with the source. Living in the same household, sharing a room or cubicle for more than fifteen minutes, or direct person-to-person contact in the form of a fact-to-face conversation is generally considered as significant enough to warrant advising prophylaxis for conditions such as chicken pox or influenza. In the case of blood-borne viruses, contact of high-risk body fluid with an open wound or mucosa is considered as significant, but not contact of body fluid with intact skin. Some infections are infectious before the onset of illness, e.g. chicken pox is infectious two days before and measles four days before the onset of rash.

D. How long ago was the exposure?

In general, the earlier the onset of PEP, the more likely it is for the prophylaxis to be effective. In many cases, this is dictated by the incubation period of the infectious agents and how fast the prophylaxis becomes effective. For example, varicella zoster virus has an incubation period ranging from ten to twenty-one days (mean fourteen to sixteen days), and therefore the window for varicella-zoster immunoglobulin (VZIG) to work as prophylaxis is about ten days from the point of contact. In the case of measles, which has a shorter incubation period of seven to eighteen days (mean ten days), vaccination with MMR is recommended within three days of contact (if no contraindication) and immunoglobulin (Ig) up to six days (for immunocompromised and pregnant women) after contact.

E. What factors made the exposed individual vulnerable?

The individual has to be susceptible to the infection. Previous history of infection is useful, but as presentation of many infections are non-specific, such history may not be reliable. For example, it is recognized that a history of chicken pox is reliable for individuals born in the UK but not for individuals born abroad. Documented history of vaccination is also useful, e.g. documented two doses of MMR is recognized as a reliable evidence of immunity to measles and rubella. If there is no definite history of prior infection or immunity, a test of immunity such as measles or Varicella IgG is the best course of action. This result should be available within the period in which the recommended prophylaxis is effective.

In many cases, normal healthy but susceptible individuals do not have a significant illness even if transmission occurred. However, those who are immunocompromised or pregnant could have a severe infection or could pass on the infection to the foetus. Examples of immunodeficiency include:

- Severe primary immunodeficiency such as severe combined immunodeficiency (SCID), Wiskott-Aldrich syndromes;
- Current treatment for malignant disease with chemotherapy or radiotherapy, and for at least six months after completion of treatment;
- Transplant recipients (solid organ or stem cell) who are on immunosuppressive treatment and in stem cell transplant, until at least twelve months after finishing all immunosuppressive treatment (longer if presence of graft-versus host disease, GVHD);

- Recipients of systemic high-dose steroids until at least three months after cessation of treatment. (In children, 2mg/kg/day for more than one week, or 1mg/kg/day for more than one month; in adults, 40mg/day of prednisolone for more than one week);
- Other types of immunosuppressive drugs (e.g. azathioprine, ciclosporin, methotrexate, cyclophosphamide, leflunomide and newer cytokine inhibitors such as anti-TNF-α monoclonal antibodies); and
- HIV infection with low CD4 count.

51.3 Specific immunoglobulins for PEP

Hyperimmune immunoglobulin is available for hepatitis B virus (HBIG), varicella-zoster virus (VZIG), rabies virus (HRIG), and *Clostridium tetani* (HTIG). For some common infections, there are sufficient specific antibodies in normal human immunoglobulins (HNIg) or intravenous immunoglobulins (IVIg) to provide protection. Thus, HNIg or IVIg can be used in the prophylaxis against infections such as measles or hepatitis A. However, as epidemiology of infections changes, the amount of viral specific antibodies in HNIg may change. In some infections, such as rubella, it has not been proven that passive antibody is effective in either preventing infection or reducing transmission to the foetus in pregnant women. It is therefore not recommended.

Table 51.2 Examples of use of active and passive immunization as PEP.

Infective organisms	Availability of Ig as PEP - Y/N (indication)	Availability of vaccine as PEP - Y/N (indication)	Combined active and passive immunization
Clostridium tetani	Y - HTIG (imi 250 IU, or 500 IU if more than twenty-four hours since injury or risk of heavy contamination or following burns)	Y* (if partial or unimmunized or immunization status not known or uncertain)	Vaccine* (if immunosuppressed or for individuals with uncertain immunization status) + HTIG if tetanus-prone wound
Corynebacterium diphtheriae	N* - only used in suspected cases	Y (if partial or unimmunized)	Vaccine + antibiotics
Hepatitis A virus	Y – HNIG (within fourteen days of contact)	Y (within fourteen days of contact)	Vaccine + HNIG if more than fifty years of age, or with chronic liver disease, otherwise vaccine preferred
Hepatitis B virus	Y – HBIG (within ninety-six hours of contact)	Y (forty-eight hours to seven days)	Vaccine + HBIG if high risk
Influenza A and B viruses	N	Y (if unimmunized)	Vaccine or antiviral
Measles virus	Y (within six days of contact)	Y (within three days of contact)	Vaccine for immunocompetent and non-pregnant contact only
Rabies virus	Y (HRIG to the wound ASAP)	Y (ASAP after exposure)	Vaccine + HRIG (to the wound)
Varicella-zoster virus	Y- VZIG (within ten days of contact)	Y (within five days of contact)	Vaccine for immunocompetent and non-pregnant contact only

* = see Green book for detail

51.4 Vaccines used as PEP

In many cases, active immunization, if given early enough, can provide adequate post-exposure prophylaxis. In high risk situations, combined active and passive immunization can be used. When simultaneous active and passive immunization is given, it is important that the vaccine and the immunoglobulin are given in different parts of the body, as the antigen and antibody will cancel out each other when mixed. If the vaccine is a live-attenuated rather than inactivated vaccine, it is contraindicated in immunocompromised or pregnant patients. In such situations, only immunoglobulins can be used (Table 51.2)

51.5 Treating exposed individuals with antimicrobials

Antimicrobials can be used as prophylaxis after exposure in some infections (Table 51.3)

VZIG is the main PEP strategy used after exposure to varicella-zoster virus, but increasingly, aciclovir prophylaxis is being used, particularly in immunosuppressed patients who missed the ten days window for receiving VZIG. The evidence for the use of aciclovir as PEP for pregnant women is limited, but extensive experience of its use during pregnancy suggested that it is safe and could be used in high risk exposure where there is no access to VZIG.

Table 51.3 Examples of infections where antimicrobials can be used as PEP.

Infective organisms (disease)	Indications	Antimicrobials recommended
Bordetella pertussis (whooping cough)	Household and close contacts	For adults: azithromycin (three days); or clarithromycin (seven days); or erythromycin (seven days); or co-trimoxazole (seven days). See Green Book for other age groups and for pregnancy
HIV	Sexual or parenteral exposure	Tenofovir + emtricitabine + raltegravir (four weeks); or tenofovir + (emtricitabine or lamivudine) + (lopinavir or atazanavir) + ritonavir (four weeks). This needs to be discussed with the HIV team if index patient is on antiretrovirals
Influenza A and B viruses	Exposed individuals who are at high risk of complications of influenza	Oseltamivir or zanamivir (ten days)
Meningococcal disease	Household and close contacts	Ciprofloxacin (single dose); rifampicin (two days); azithromycin (single dose); or ceftriaxone (single dose)
Invasive group A Streptococcus	Close contacts with symptoms; or mother and baby if either develops invasive disease in the neonatal period	Ten days of Pen V; amoxicillin; or clindamycin; or three days of azithromycin; or three days for pharyngeal carriage
Mycobacterium tuberculosis	Based upon tuberculin skin test, and chest x-ray findings interferon assay	Isoniazid and rifampicin for three months (Consult BTS guidelines)
Varicella-zoster virus	Immunosuppressed individuals who missed the window for VZIG	Aciclovir from day ten of contact till day twenty-one

* = see Green Book for detail.

51.6 Follow-up for exposed individuals

It is important to follow-up the exposed individual to ensure that the infection has been prevented. As breakthrough infection is possible, it is important for the exposed contacts to remain in appropriate isolation until the end of the incubation period, so that there is no secondary chain of transmission in the healthcare setting. Also note that the use of PEP could render the infection asymptomatic and sometimes could lead to a prolonged incubation period and delayed onset of disease.

51.7 Further reading

Bader, M. S., McKinsey, D. A., 'Postexposure Prophylaxis for Common Infectious Diseases', *American Family Physician*, 88/1 (2013), 25–32. http://www.aafp.org/afp/2013/0701/p25.html

National Institute for Health and Care Excellence. Meningitis: Bacterial Meningitis and Meningococcal Disease. Updated March 2016. http://cks.nice.org.uk/meningitis-bacterial-meningitis-and-meningococcal-disease

Public Health England. *The Green Book. Immunization against Infectious Disease.* https://www.gov.uk/government/collections/immunisation-against-infectious-disease-the-green-book. Updated September 2014.

Public Health England. Guidance for Issuing Varicella-Zoster Immunoglobulin (VZIG). Updated August 2017. https://www.gov.uk/government/uploads/system/uploads/attachment_data/file/617518/VZIG_gudiance.pdf

Public Health England. Guidelines on the Management of Rabies Exposure. Updated April 2016. https://www.gov.uk/government/uploads/system/uploads/attachment_data/file/520305/PHE_clinical_rabies_service_April_2016.pdf

Public Health England. Guidance for Public Health Management of Meningococcal Disease in the UK. Updated February 2017. https://www.gov.uk/government/collections/meningococcal-disease-guidance-data-and-analysis

Public Health England. Guidelines for Public Health Management of Pertussis. Updated June 2018. https://www.gov.uk/government/collections/pertussis-guidance-data-and-analysis

Public Health England. National Measles Guidelines. Updated August 2017. https://www.gov.uk/government/uploads/system/uploads/attachment_data/file/637338/PHE_Measles_guidance_August_2017.pdf

Riddell, A., Kennedy, I., Tong, C. Y., 'Management of Sharps Injuries in the Healthcare Setting', *British Medical Journal*, 351 (2015), h3733. doi: https://doi.org/10.1136/bmj.h3733

Steer, J. A., Lamagni, T., Healy, B., Morgan, M., Dryden, M., Rao, B., et al., 'Guidelines for Prevention and Control of Group A Streptococcal Infection in Acute Healthcare and Maternity Settings in the UK', *Journal of Infection*, 64 (2012), 1–18.

51.8 Assessment questions

51.8.1 Question 1

A woman who is twenty-eight weeks pregnant is exposed to her two-year old-child who developed chickenpox two days ago. She has no previous history of chickenpox. Her booking blood is retrieved for varicella-zoster virus (VZV) IgG testing, and the results show VZV IgG = 90 mIU/ml.

What is the most appropriate management of this pregnant woman?

A. A five-day course of aciclovir.

B. Immunization with an inactivated chicken pox vaccine.

C. Intramuscular injection of VZIG.

D. Post-natal immunization with live attenuated chicken pox vaccine.

E. Reassurance as she is immune.

51.8.2 Question 2

A medical student on elective in Thailand was bitten by a stray dog. It was an unprovoked attack. He was not previously immunized against rabies and receives a dose of cell culture-based rabies vaccine locally immediately after the incident. He returned to the UK two days later and presents to the emergency department for his wound to be examined. On examination, a partially healing bite wound is present in his right leg.

What is the most appropriate management of this medical student?

A. Administer rabies immunoglobulin to the wound and continue second dose of rabies vaccination.

B. Reassurance as he has already received appropriate PEP.

C. Reassurance as Thailand is not an endemic area for rabies.

D. Start a course of co-amoxiclav.

E. Start rabies vaccination from scratch as the vaccine dose he received in Thailand may not be reliable.

51.8.3 Question 3

An un-booked pregnant woman presented to the labour ward in advanced labour. The midwife took a blood sample and sent to the laboratory for urgent testing.

What test is the most urgent to inform immediate action before delivery?

A. Hepatitis B surface antigen (HBsAg).

B. Herpes simplex virus IgG.

C. HIV antigen/antibody test.

D. Rubella IgG.

E. Syphilis serology.

51.9 Answers and discussion

51.9.1 Answer 1

C. Intramuscular injection of VZIG.

Chicken pox could be a serious illness in pregnant women. Fatality due to fulminant varicella pneumonia has been reported in late second to early third trimester (twenty-seven to thirty-two weeks). The risk of congenital varicella syndrome is < 1% in the first twelve weeks and around 2% between thirteen and twenty weeks of pregnancy. Risk of congenital varicella syndrome in the foetus is much lower after twenty weeks, but severe and fatal neonatal infection could occur following maternal varicella one week before to one week after delivery. PEP in the form VZIG should be given to susceptible and exposed pregnant women, primarily to protect the woman from severe disease, but also to protect the foetus. The current vaccine for VZV is a live attenuated vaccine and is contraindicated in pregnancy. Aciclovir could be used in pregnancy (though not licensed) if VZIG is not available or the window missed. However, the course should cover the duration of the incubation period, and a five-day course is not long enough.

   To qualify for VZIG, the patient has to be proven to be susceptible. Current PHE guidelines recommend an immunity cut-off of 100 mIU/ml for pregnant women and a higher threshold of 150 mIU/ml for immunosuppressed patients. The level of 90 mIU/ml in this patient indicates susceptibility. VZIG (1g in adult) should be given intramuscularly within ten days of contact.

51.9.2 Answer 2

A. Administer rabies immunoglobulin to the wound and continue second dose of rabies vaccination.

The incubation period for rabies is typically one to three months but may vary from less than one week to more than two years. Due to the potentially long incubation period for rabies there is no time limit for giving PEP. However, if the exposure is more than one year ago, HRIG is not generally indicated. The risk of rabies is high as South East Asia is an endemic area for rabies, the wound as described is not minor (category III), and he is not previously immunized. In this case, a five-dose course of rabies vaccine together with HRIG is recommended. Most vaccines used globally are now derived from primate or avian diploid cell culture and are compatible with the UK vaccines. The first dose of cell culture-based vaccine received in Thailand can be accepted as the first dose in a 0, 3, 7, 14, 28–30 days schedule.

The total antibody level induced by active immunization is much greater than by passive immunization. Hence, HRIG is not given more than seven days after vaccination or to an individual who is already partially or previously immunized. HRIG should be given at the site of the wound. If this is difficult or the wound has completely healed, then this can be given by intramuscular injection in the anterolateral thigh.

51.9.3 Answer 3

C. HIV antigen/antibody test.

Infection screening of pregnant women usually takes place during antenatal booking in the first trimester. In the UK, this consists of HIV antigen/antibody, hepatitis B surface antigen, and syphilis serology. Rubella screening used to be part of the antenatal screening but this has ceased since April 2016. Herpes simplex serology is not useful unless there is documented genital herpes in the mother and it is not clear if the infection is primary or reactivation. Syphilis is transmitted transplacentally. PEP is therefore not feasible although the baby can be treated if transmission to the baby is confirmed. Both HIV and hepatitis B results need to be known as soon as possible in order to manage the newborn appropriately. UK guidelines require the administration of hepatitis B vaccine to babies born to infected mother within twenty-four hours of birth. HBIG should be used simultaneously if the mother is known to have high infectivity or the infectivity status is unknown. The HIV status is the most urgent information required as this affect the mode of delivery (vaginal or Caesarean section), the use of ART during labour and PEP to the newborn. Hence, the HIV test is the most urgent test required.

PART NINE

THE MANAGEMENT OF HIV INFECTION

CHAPTER 52

Epidemiology and natural history of HIV

Palwasha Khan, Sarah Parry and Chloe Orkin

CONTENTS

52.1 HIV and its origins

The human immunodeficiency virus (HIV) is a member of the genus *Lentivirus*, a subgroup of retrovirus (*Retroviridae*), that causes HIV infection, which, if untreated, results in acquired immunodeficiency syndrome (AIDS) and death. It was first described in 1981 during an epidemic of a previously unknown immunodeficiency syndrome in the US. The term HIV was accepted in 1986. HIV is thought to originate from simian immune deficiency virus (SIV).

52.2 The difference between HIV-1 and HIV-2

HIV-1 was discovered first, with the epidemic of AIDS in the US in 1981. In 1986, a related virus subsequently known as HIV-2, was identified in West Africa. The viruses differ in several aspects; HIV-1 is found worldwide, whereas HIV-2 is predominantly found in West Africa. HIV-1 is a more virulent and rapidly progressive virus; HIV-2 tends to be present in lower viral quantities and progresses more slowly.

52.3 The global burden of HIV and the global response to the HIV pandemic

The number of people living with HIV (PLWH) rose from an estimated 9.0 million in 1990 to 36.9 million in 2014, due in part to a substantial improvement in survival rates as a result of effective anti-retroviral treatment. By 2014, annual new HIV infections had dropped to 2.0 million, down from 3.1 million in 2000, representing a decline of about 35%, although there remain an estimated 5600 people newly infected with HIV every day.

It is estimated that without the global response that was mounted in 2000, notably the 'Combatting of HIV/AIDS' (the 6th Millennium Development Goal, which focused on halting and reversing trends for HIV by the end of 2015) there would have been six million new infections in 2013 alone. The main driver of progress has been widespread roll-out of antiretroviral treatment (ART) and behavioural change interventions, resulting in increased condom use, fewer multiple sexual partnerships, and delayed sexual debut.

HIV-related deaths peaked in 2004–2005, and deaths fell by 24% between 2000 and 2014 from 1.2 million (0.98–1.6 million) in 2014 compared to 1.6 million (1.3–2.1 million) in 2000 (Figure 52.1). The drop in AIDS-related mortality has been even steeper among children aged under fifteen years of age due to the enormous progress made with prevention of mother-to-child transmission (PMTCT). This has been largely due to the rapid expansion of use of antiretroviral treatment for PMTCT of HIV and the expansion of paediatric HIV treatment. Elimination of mother-to-child transmission is now a realistic goal and the World Health Organization (WHO) is leading the way, with elimination of MTCT a reality in many countries.

By mid-2015, 15.8 million PLWH were receiving ART; of those, 11.4 million were living in the WHO African Region. In contrast in 2000, only about 11,000 people in the region were receiving ART. As ART coverage increases, survival increases and so will HIV prevalence, with bigger demands on the health systems responsible for providing care. On January 1st 2016, the MDGs were

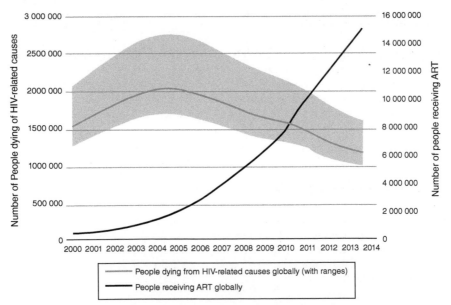

Figure 52.1 Number of people dying from HIV-related causes annually and numbers of people receiving ART globally, 2000–2014.

Reproduced with permission from World Health Organization. *Global health sector response to HIV, 2000-2015: focus on innovations in Africa*. Geneva, Switzerland: World Health Organization. © 2016 World Health Organization. Available at: http://www.who.int/hiv/pub/progressreports/2015-progress-report/en

replaced by the Sustainable Development Goals (SDGs) with the aim to end the AIDS epidemic by 2030.

52.4 The different modes of HIV transmission

HIV is transmitted in human body fluids by three major routes:

1. *Sexual*: via vaginal, rectal, or penile mucosa from semen or vaginal fluid;
2. *Parenteral*: through sharing needles, syringes, or via blood products;
3. *Mother-child*: through pregnancy (in utero), during labour, or through breastfeeding.

Heterosexual transmission is the main mode of transmission globally. The following equation describes the components which determine the epidemic dynamics of sexual HIV transmission:

$$R_0 = C \times \beta \times D$$

R_0 the basic reproductive number, describes the epidemic potential of an infectious agent in a specific population. When, on average, one infected person infects more than one other person, $R_0 > 1$, epidemic spread will occur. If $R_0 < 1$, i.e. on average, one infected person does not infect more than one other person, transmission of infectious agent will not result in an epidemic, and if maintained may result in elimination of the infectious agent from the population.

C, is the exposure rate of susceptible individuals to infectious partners, such as rate of sexual partner change in the population.

β, is the probability of HIV transmission given exposure, e.g. for one episode of unprotected receptive anal intercourse (with ejaculation) the probability of transmission is $\sim$ 1 in 65 (1.5%).

D, is the duration of infectious period.

52.5 Groups at greater risk of acquiring HIV

There are two broad types of HIV epidemics: (1) *generalized*, which affects men, women, and children in a population, and (2) *concentrated*, which affects specific population groups. These specific groups are known as 'key populations', groups who are most at risk of HIV. In most settings outside of sub-Saharan Africa, HIV disproportionately affects injecting drug users, men who have sex with men (MSM), transgender people, and sex workers, compared to the general population. Some of the factors that have contributed to the HIV epidemic in sub-Saharan African are:

- Prevalence of concurrent sexual partnerships;
- Inadequately controlled sexually transmitted infections, such as genital herpes simplex, which increases risk of transmission per sexual intercourse act;
- Lack of male circumcision;
- Underlying social, cultural, and economic factors; and
- Lack of political will to address the emerging epidemic.

52.6 How HIV affects the immune system and its difference from AIDS

HIV belongs to a group of viruses called 'retroviruses'. The virus attaches to and enters CD4-positive lymphocytes, which are a type of white blood cell that coordinate the body's immune response and defence against infections. By attacking the immune system, HIV gradually causes damage, making an individual susceptible to a variety of so-called 'opportunistic' infections and malignancies that would not normally cause disease in an immunocompetent person. AIDS occurs when CD4-positive lymphocyte numbers fall significantly (usually to < 200 cells/μl), leading to profound immunodeficiency. AIDS is defined by a set of opportunistic conditions such as *Pneumocystis jiroveci (carinii)* pneumonia (PCP) and tuberculosis. AIDS is the final stage of HIV infection. You cannot catch AIDS—it is the HIV infection that can be transmitted.

52.7 Factors influencing HIV disease progression

Progression rates vary according to the interaction between the virus and host (the patient), and environmental factors.

52.7.1 Viral factors

- Changes in virus phenotype and genotype:
  - Switching of the co-receptor usage from CCR5 to CXCR4 in late HIV infection;
  - Viral mutations which alter viral fitness and thus pathogenicity;
  - Viral mutations which alter drug susceptibility, rendering some drugs (or even classes of drugs) ineffective.

52.7.2 Host factors

More rapid progression may be seen in:
- Women;
- Older age;
- Co-infection: hepatitis B, hepatitis C, and tuberculosis co-infection may alter the immune system;
- Certain HLA types and gene mutations;
- Poor premorbid nutritional state; and
- Depression.

52.7.3 Environmental factors

- Drug use and social deprivation are associated with risk of more rapid progression.

52.8 Stages of disease occurring in untreated HIV

Two major classification systems are currently in use for tracking and monitoring the HIV epidemic. The US Centers for Disease Control and Prevention (CDC) developed a staging system for HIV, most recently revised in 1993, based on CD4 cell counts and clinical features (Table 52.1). AIDS was defined as all HIV-infected individuals with CD4 counts < 200 cells/μL (or CD4 percentage < 14%) plus all those with certain HIV-related conditions and symptoms (Table 52.1; all those in categories A3, B3, and C1–C3). The CDC staging system is often used in clinical and epidemiological research.

52.8.1 Category A

- Asymptomatic HIV infection;
- Primary HIV infection;
- Persistent generalized lymphadenopathy (PGL).

Table 52.1 CDC classification system of HIV disease (Revised, 1993).

CD4 (count/μL)	Clinical categories		
	A Asymptomatic HIV, Primary HIV, or PGL	B Symptomatic Conditions, not A or C	C AIDS-Indicator Conditions
≥ 500	A1	B1	C1
200–499	A2	B2	C2
< 200	A3	B3	C3

PGL = Persistent generalized lymphadenopathy.

52.8.2 Category B: Symptomatic Conditions

- Bacillary angiomatosis;
- Candidiasis: oral, or recurrent vulvovaginal;
- Cervical dysplasia or carcinoma *in situ*;
- Constitutional symptoms (e.g. fever, or persistent diarrhoea);
- Herpes zoster (shingles), involving two or more episodes or at least one dermatome;
- Idiopathic thrombocytopenic purpura (ITP);
- Listeriosis;
- Oral hairy leucoplakia;
- Pelvic inflammatory disease;
- Peripheral neuropathy.

52.8.3 Category C: AIDS-defining conditions

- Bacterial pneumonia (two or more episodes in twelve months);
- Candidiasis: pulmonary or oesophageal;
- Cervical cancer;
- Coccidioidomycosis;
- Cryptococcosis;
- Cryptosporidiosis;
- Cytomegalovirus (CMV);
- Herpes simplex: chronic (duration over one month), pulmonary or oesophageal;
- Histoplasmosis (extrapulmonary);
- HIV encephalopathy;
- Isosporiasis;
- Kaposi's sarcoma (KS);
- Lymphoma;
- *Mycobacterium avium* complex (MAC);
- *Mycobacterium tuberculosis*;
- *Pneumocystis jiroveci* pneumonia (PCP);
- Progressive multifocal leukoencephalopathy (PML);
- *Salmonella* septicaemia (recurrent);
- Wasting syndrome due to HIV.

HIV-wasting syndrome is defined by the CDC as involuntary weight loss (> 10% of baseline body weight), plus either unexplained chronic diarrhoea (two or more loose stools per day for one or more months) or chronic weakness and unexplained fever for one or more months.

The second classification system is the World Health Organization (WHO) clinical staging system for HIV infection and disease, developed in 1990 and revised in 2007 (Table 52.2). The WHO staging system is based on clinical findings and does not require a CD4 count, and therefore is used in many resource-limited settings in which CD4 testing is not available. Stages are determined by clinical conditions or symptoms, which guide the diagnosis and management of HIV and AIDS.

52.9 The natural history of untreated HIV infection

As demonstrated by the staging systems, the course of untreated HIV infection is characterized by progressive loss of immune function, allowing the development of bacterial and viral infections, opportunistic infections, and malignancies.

- Primary infection: An acute retroviral illness (similar to influenza or infectious mononucleosis) occurs in approximately half of patients, between two to five weeks post-infection. This is known as a 'seroconversion illness'. Symptoms include fever, malaise, diarrhoea, sore throat, nausea, and a widespread maculopapular rash. During this time, the virus rapidly disseminates throughout the body. The patient usually has a very high viral load and a rapid drop in CD4 cells can be seen.
- Asymptomatic stage: Primary stage viraemia reduces, allowing some recovery of CD4 count (usually to > 500 cells/μL). Patients are usually asymptomatic but may have minor clinical symptoms such as PGL and some skin disorders, such as seborrhoeic dermatitis and oral ulceration.
- Symptomatic stage: As the CD4 count drops below 500 cells/μL, patients may develop mild to moderate symptoms such as diarrhoea, weight loss, fevers, and recurrent bacterial infections. With a CD4 count between 50–200 cells/μL (usually with an associated rise in HIV viral load), AIDS-defining illnesses can develop, such as PCP, KS, and lymphoma. Conditions associated with very severe immunodeficiency are seen with a CD4 count < 50 cells/μL, such as CMV retinitis, disseminated mycobacterial infections, PML, and AIDS-related dementia.

Patients progress through these stages at different rates. On average, without treatment, it takes eight to ten years from HIV acquisition to AIDS. However, in the current era, a person living with HIV can assume a normal life expectancy if they are taking antiretroviral therapy, responding to treatment, and accessing care. Each individual's life expectancy will vary depending on how early in the natural history of disease their HIV was diagnosed, comorbid conditions, and lifestyle factors.

52.10 How antiretroviral therapy impacts the natural history of HIV

Antiretroviral therapy (ART) is commenced for various reasons. The primary aim is the prevention of the mortality and morbidity associated with chronic untreated HIV infection. ART works in various ways to inhibit viral replication, thereby achieving virological suppression and allowing for the recovery of immune functioning. It does not clear HIV completely but reduces the amount of HIV in the body to a level where the immune system can function, although some immune dysfunction may still exist. A further aim of ART is to reduce the transmission of HIV, both sexually and mother-to-child, thus reducing the incidence of new HIV infections.

The term 'elite controllers' refers to a rare group of people living with HIV, who are naturally able to control viral replication, keeping HIV at clinically undetectable levels without

Table 52.2 WHO clinical staging of HIV/AIDS for adults and adolescents.

Clinical stage	Clinical conditions or symptoms
Primary HIV infection	• Asymptomatic • Acute retroviral syndrome/illness
Clinical stage 1 (Asymptomatic)	• Asymptomatic • Persistent generalized lymphadenopathy
Clinical stage 2 (Mild symptoms)	• Moderate unexplained weight loss (< 10% of presumed or measured body weight) • Recurrent respiratory tract infections (sinusitis, tonsillitis, otitis media, and pharyngitis) • Herpes zoster • Angular cheilitis • Recurrent oral ulceration • Papular pruritic eruptions • Seborrhoeic dermatitis • Fungal nail infections
Clinical stage 3 (Moderate symptoms)	• Unexplained severe weight loss (> 10% of presumed or measured body weight) • Unexplained chronic diarrhoea for more than one month • Unexplained persistent fever (> 37.6°C, intermittent or constant, for more than one month) • Persistent oral candidiasis • Oral hairy leukoplakia • Pulmonary tuberculosis (current) • Severe bacterial infections (such as pneumonia, empyema, pyomyositis, bone or joint infection, meningitis, or bacteraemia) • Acute necrotizing ulcerative stomatitis, gingivitis, or periodontitis • Unexplained anaemia (haemoglobin < 8 g/dL), neutropenia (neutrophils < 0.5 x 10^9/L) or chronic thrombocytopenia (platelets < 50 x 10^9/L)
Clinical stage 4 (Severe symptoms)	• HIV-wasting syndrome • *Pneumocystis* pneumonia • Recurrent severe bacterial pneumonia • Chronic herpes simplex infection (orolabial, genital, or anorectal for more than one month, or visceral herpes at any site) • Oesophageal candidiasis (or candidiasis of trachea, bronchi, or lungs) • Extrapulmonary tuberculosis • Kaposi's sarcoma • Cytomegalovirus infection (retinitis or infection of other organs) • Central nervous system toxoplasmosis • HIV encephalopathy • Extrapulmonary cryptococcosis, including meningitis • Disseminated non-tuberculosis mycobacteria infection • Progressive multifocal leukoencephalopathy • Chronic cryptosporidiosis (with diarrhoea) • Chronic isosporiasis • Disseminated mycosis (histoplasmosis, coccidiomycosis, or penicilliosis) • Recurrent non-typhoidal *Salmonella* bacteraemia • Lymphoma (cerebral or B-cell non-Hodgkin), or other solid HIV-associated tumours • Invasive cervical carcinoma • Atypical disseminated leishmaniasis • Symptomatic HIV-associated nephropathy or symptomatic HIV-associated cardiomyopathy • Reactivation of American trypanosomiasis (meningoencephalitis or myocarditis)

ART. Long-term non-progressors are HIV-infected individuals who maintain a CD4 cell count > 500 without ART, despite a detectable viral load. Both situations are likely due to host genetic traits conferring greater resistance to HIV and/or a more robust immune response.

52.11 Assessment questions

52.11.1 Question 1

A situation report on HIV in the UK published in 2015 by Public Health England stated that 70% of all people living with (diagnosed and undiagnosed) HIV (72,800/103,700) had an undetectable viral load (less than 200 copies/UL).

How many percent off the ambitious 90-90-90 UNAIDS target is the UK with respect to the target for viral suppression?
A. 3%.
B. 5%.
C. 10%.
D. 12%.
E. 20%.

52.11.2 Question 2

A thirty-six-year-old man with HIV infection is seen in your clinic. He wants to start a family with his HIV-negative wife but is worried about transmitting HIV to her.

Which of the following strategies is *inappropriate* in the discussion?
A. Advise against child-bearing due to risk of HIV transmission.
B. Antiretroviral therapy for the HIV-infected patient, to achieve virological suppression.
C. Pre-exposure prophylaxis (PrEP) use in the female partner.
D. Sperm washing with intrauterine insemination.
E. The need to screen both partners for STIs and treat if found.

52.11.3 Question 3

A twenty-eight-year-man is seen in the GU department with a fever, sore throat, and widespread rash. His last negative HIV test was two months ago. He has had multiple episodes of unprotected receptive anal sex since then. A sexual health screen is performed and his HIV test was reported as HIV p24 antigen positive, HIV antibody negative.

What is the most appropriate advice and management?
A. Advise the patient that a second confirmatory test is required before the diagnosis of HIV can be made.
B. Advise the patient that his HIV test was indeterminate and ask for a repeat test in four weeks.
C. Diagnose primary HIV infection and consider immediate ART.
D. Diagnose primary HIV infection and reassure the patient that he is unlikely to require treatment for HIV until his CD4 count drops to below 350.
E. Reassure the patient that it is a false positive result as HIV antibody is negative.

52.12 Answers and discussion

52.12.1 Answer 1

A. 3%.
In 2014, the UN Programme on HIV/AIDS (UNAIDS) announced ambitious new global targets which build on its 'Getting to Zero' strategy that aim to end the HIV epidemic by 2030.

The UNAIDS 'Fast-Track' 90-90-90 targets for 2020 are that:
- 90% of people living with HIV will know their HIV status
- 90% of people diagnosed with HIV will receive antiretroviral treatment
- 90% of people on treatment will have suppressed viral loads.

According to the UNAIDS 90-90-90, 73% $[0.9^3 = 0.729]$ of all people living with (diagnosed and undiagnosed) HIV should be virally suppressed. Therefore, the UK is only 3% points short of the target.

52.12.2 Answer 2

A. Advise against child-bearing due to risk of HIV transmission.

In 2011, a landmark study, HIV Prevention Trials Network (HPTN) 052, showed early initiation of antiretroviral treatment in people living with HIV with a CD4 count between 350 and 550, reduced HIV transmission to HIV-negative partners by 96%.

This finding has been substantiated in number of follow-up studies, which has led to the idea that treatment as prevention could be used as part of a 'test and treat' strategy—increasing testing and treatment coverage to decrease community viral load and reduce the rate of new HIV infections although this strategy is highly dependent upon HIV-positive individuals adhering to treatment for life.

The more recent PARTNER study has provided the strongest evidence that the risk of HIV transmission is negligible when an HIV-positive person has an undetectable viral load. The study population was comprised of both heterosexual and homosexual individuals and included those not using condoms. Data on 58,000 episodes of condomless sex, including anal sex, were analysed and there were no transmissions (phylogenetically linked) to the positive partner. There was also no evidence that the presence of sexually transmitted infections or viral load blips (VL above level of detectability but less than 200 copies/ml) increased the risk of transmission.

52.12.3 Answer 3

C. Diagnose primary HIV infection and consider immediate ART.

Primary HIV infection (PHI) is HIV infection that is diagnosed within six months of the estimated time of HIV transmission. It can be diagnosed based on clinical history (e.g. previous negative test within six months) and laboratory results (e.g. p24 antigen positive, antibody negative, and avidity index testing). There is now substantial evidence from clinical trials, most recently the START study, that immediate initiation of ART is of clinical benefit to all individuals diagnosed with HIV. In the context of PHI, the 2015 BHIVA treatment guidelines suggest prioritizing early ART initiation particularly in any patient presenting with neurological involvement, an AIDS-defining illness, low initial CD4 count (< 350cells/μL), high plasma viral load (> 100,000 copies/ml), and short-test interval (PHI diagnosed within twelve weeks of a previous negative test). These situations are associated with increased morbidity and very rapid disease progression compared to others without these features during PHI.

Although patients with PHI may be in a particularly fragile psychological state, they should be assessed by an HIV specialist within two weeks of diagnosis for assessment and consideration of immediate ART. The patient should be informed that early ART is associated with preservation of immune function and CD4 cell count, reduction in the morbidity associated with high viraemia and rapid CD4 cell depletion seen during acute infection, and reduction in the risk of HIV transmission to others at a time of very high viral load (and thus higher risk of transmission). In addition, commencing ART in PHI may limit the development of the viral reservoir (latent pool of infected cells) which is the current barrier to HIV remission or cure; this is an on-going area of research.

CHAPTER 53

Laboratory diagnosis and monitoring of HIV infection

Anna Jeffery-Smith and C. Y. William Tong

53.1 Diagnosing HIV in the laboratory

In the majority of UK laboratories initial testing for HIV is now performed using a fourth generation test, which is a combination test for antibody to HIV and p24 antigen. These tests should be able to detect antibody to both HIV-1 and HIV-2. In addition, due to the heterogeneity of the virus they should be able to reliably detect antibody to the main circulating subtypes of HIV-1, i.e. group M (Major), O (Outlier), and N (non-M, non-O). The p24 antigen is an HIV capsid protein which is produced in large quantities during initial infection, prior to seroconversion. The sensitivity and specificity of fourth generation tests is typically > 99%. However, all positive results need further confirmation tests, as discussed below.

Third generation laboratory assays only test for the presence of antibody to HIV. Though it includes the detection of IgM (which is not included in second generation assays), they do not detect early infection with isolated HIV antigen prior to seroconversion.

Point-of-care testing for HIV is performed in the clinic or at bedside. Like laboratory based assays these tests can be either third or fourth generation. The sensitivity and specificity of point-of-care tests is considered lower than that of laboratory tests, and all positive results require confirmation with a laboratory assay.

53.2 Defining the window period

The window period is the length of time following infection with HIV until the appearance of laboratory markers of HIV infection in the blood. This period varies depending on which marker, i.e. antibody or antigen, is being tested for.

The window period for fourth-generation tests is between eleven days and one month. Patients being counselled prior to this testing should be advised that a negative result does not cover risk exposures in the preceding month. These patients should be advised to have repeat testing if they have any further exposure risks in the preceding month prior to testing. For third-generation tests the window period is up to three months, correlating with the amount of time it may take for antibodies to HIV to develop.

53.3 Laboratory confirmation of HIV infection

Laboratories have specific standard operating procedures (SOP) for the confirmation of diagnosis of HIV, depending on which assays are available. Methods include:

- Repeat testing on the original sample clot with the same assay;
- Performing a different laboratory assay on the same sample—for example an additional third- or fourth-generation assay;
- A repeat sample from the patient on the same assay;
- All HIV infections should be confirmed with a laboratory assay that can differentiate between HIV-1 and HIV-2 antibodies, as these infections require different therapy and monitoring; and
- Testing for HIV-1 RNA.

53.4 Other tests used to diagnose infection in patients with equivocal serology

Equivocal or indeterminate HIV serology occurs when an initial laboratory test is positive, but this is not confirmed by the additional serological testing undertaken in the laboratory. A repeat serum sample from the patient should be sought for repeat serological testing to confirm that there is no mix up of identity. Line blot assays use a range of different antigens from HIV-1 and HIV-2 and can be used to identify which specific antibodies are present in a patient's blood causing a reactive result in the initial screening assay.

In addition, testing for the presence of HIV RNA in plasma can be performed. Routine laboratory testing for HIV RNA is designed to detect HIV-1. This testing will not detect HIV-2 RNA, which requires separate testing.

53.5 Baseline laboratory tests for patients diagnosed with HIV

Baseline laboratory testing for patients newly diagnosed with HIV infection can be separated into HIV related tests, testing related to other infectious agents, and a metabolic/biochemical screen (Table 53.1).

53.6 HIV resistance testing

- At baseline (time of diagnosis).
- At the commencement of antiretroviral therapy (ART) if there is a delay, and this testing was not done at baseline or there is a high risk of super infection with resistant virus or exposure to ART based on the patient history.
- Suboptimal viral load response to therapy initiation ($<1 \log^{10}$ drop in four weeks).

Table 53.1 Recommended baseline laboratory testing in a newly diagnosed HIV patient.

HIV-related tests	Other infectious agents	Metabolic/biochemical tests
Confirmation of HIV-1/HIV-2 status	Hepatitis A IgG[2]	Full blood count
Testing for primary HIV infection – avidity RITA	Hepatitis B surface antigen and core antibody[2]	Renal profile
HIV-1 (or HIV-2) plasma viral load	Hepatitis C IgG	Liver profile
Baseline genotypic resistance test	STI screen: syphilis serology, NAAT for gonorrhoea and chlamydia	Bone profile
CD4+ T cell count	Measles and varicella IgG[2,3]	Dipstick urinalysis
(Viral tropism test)[1]	Rubella IgG[4]	Urine protein/creatinine ratio if protein positive in the urine dipstick
	Interferon gamma release assay[5]	HLA-B*57:01[7]
	Parasitic infections screen[6]	

[1] Not normally recommended at baseline, only in the rare occasion when a CCR5 inhibitor is being considered as first-line therapy.
[2] Vaccine-preventable diseases.
[3] If no history of previous infection, test, or vaccination.
[4] In women with child-bearing potential if no previous history of test or vaccination.
[5] As per BHIVA tuberculosis guideline.
[6] If persistent eosinophilia and relevant travel history.
[7] If abacavir therapy being considered.
NAAT: Nucleic Acid Amplification Test
RITA: Recent Infection Testing Algorithm
STI: Sexually Transmitted Infection

- Virological failure—viral load > 200 copies/ml on two samples while on ART.
- At each episode of virological failure to guide further regimens; all previous resistance profiles should be considered in patients with previous virological failures.
- On CSF samples if CSF viral load is detectable on therapy.
- In pregnant women: prior to initiation of ART and repeated if detectable viral load at week thirty-six of pregnancy.
- Tropism testing should be requested prior to the commencement of a CCR5 co-receptor antagonist and if there is virological failure on this therapy to check for tropism switch.

53.7 Laboratory monitoring for HIV-infected pregnant women

Women newly diagnosed with HIV in pregnancy should undertake the same baseline testing as other patients newly diagnosed with HIV. In addition, HIV resistance testing should be performed prior to commencing ART, unless the diagnosis occurs in late pregnancy. For late presenting women ART should be commenced based on epidemiological data promptly and adapted in response to the results of any identified resistance mutations.

Following commencement of ART a viral load should be repeated within two to four weeks, at least once every trimester, at thirty-six weeks, and at the time of delivery.

53.8 Laboratory tests for children born to HIV-infected mothers

HIV nucleic acid testing (RNA or proviral DNA) testing should be undertaken at the following time points:

- Within the first forty-eight hours after birth and prior to discharge from hospital.
- Two weeks following completion of anti-retroviral prophylaxis (six weeks of age).
- Two months following completion of anti-retroviral prophylaxis (twelve weeks of age).
- Monthly if breastfeeding is taking place to detect late transmission of HIV.

HIV antibody testing should be undertaken at eighteen months for loss of maternal antibody. This can take up to two years.

The gold standard molecular test for detection of HIV infection in infants is HIV DNA PCR on peripheral blood lymphocytes. Recent studies have demonstrated that HIV RNA PCR on plasma has a similar sensitivity, but the requirement for a larger volume sample for RNA testing can result in the sample needing to be diluted, and therefore result in an increase in the lower limit of detection.

Infant molecular testing should be compared with maternal viral samples when examining for mother-to-child transmission. It is important to ensure that maternal RNA or DNA can be amplified with the PCR primers being used to test the infant's blood. If maternal virus is not detected with initial primers, different primers should be tested. If maternal virus does not amplify with multiple sets of primers, the infant's results should be reviewed with caution, and clinical and serological markers reviewed.

Maternal ART with agents that can cross the placenta can reduce the detection of HIV RNA in the infant where transmission has taken place in utero. The risk is highest in mother's commencing ART late in pregnancy. In such high risk situations, additional HIV DNA PCR should be undertaken when the infant is two to three weeks of age.

In addition, ART in the neonatal period can delay the detection of both HIV DNA and RNA in the infant. As a result, molecular testing following cessation of neonatal ART prophylaxis should be performed as detailed.

53.9 Elite controllers

'Elite controller' is the term given to patients who are HIV seropositive, but have no detectable HIV RNA and have maintained CD4 counts in the absence of ART. Studies following up outcomes in 'elite controllers' have shown that they appear to have a pro-inflammatory state compared with HIV-negative patients, and HIV-positive patients with controlled viral loads on ART. Research is ongoing to understand the processes contributing to this immune control, but there are indications that patients with suppressed virus secondary to ART have fewer hospital admissions and lower levels of cardiovascular and psychiatric complications than 'elite controllers'.

53.10 Further reading

British HIV Association. *Guidelines for the Routine Investigation and Monitoring of Adult HIV-1-Positive Individuals 2016* (London, 2016). http://www.bhiva.org/documents/Guidelines/Monitoring/2016-BHIVA-Monitoring-Guidelines.pdf

British HIV Association. *Guidelines for the Management of HIV Infection in Pregnant Women 2012 (2014 interim review)* (London, 2014). http://www.bhiva.org/documents/Guidelines/Pregnancy/2012/BHIVA-Pregnancy-guidelines-update-2014.pdf

53.11 Assessment questions

53.11.1 Question 1

A 22-year-old man presents to the sexual health clinic with a history of unprotected receptive anal sex with a male partner one week ago. He has subsequently been informed by the partner that he was recently diagnosed with HIV. A routine sexual health check and blood tests are performed. Results of an HIV antigen/antibody (fourth-generation) are negative.

What is the most appropriate next investigation?
A. HIV RNA testing of a plasma sample immediately.
B. No further testing required.
C. Perform HIV point-of-care test in one week.
D. Repeat fourth-generation HIV serology test in three weeks.
E. Send the serum sample for Western blot confirmation.

53.11.2 Question 2

A patient diagnosed with HIV six months ago is reviewed in the clinic. He has been on antiretroviral therapy (ART) for four weeks with tenofovir, emtricitabine, and efavirenz. No antiretroviral resistance mutations are detected on the baseline resistance test. Blood tests show the following results (Table 53.2):

Table 53.2 Investigation results for a patient diagnosed with HIV six months ago who is reviewed in the clinic.

	Pre-treatment	Four weeks after starting ART
CD4 count (/μl)	25	50
Plasma HIV viral load (log^{10} copies/ml)	5.5	5.1

What is the most appropriate action to be taken at the end of this clinic appointment?
A. Change the ART regimen to include an integrase inhibitor.
B. Intensify by adding a protease inhibitor.
C. Repeat HIV resistance testing on the second viral load sample.
D. Request tropism testing.
E. Review in clinic in three months with repeat HIV viral load and CD4 T cell count.

53.11.3 Question 3

A 48-year-man attends for review in the HIV clinic. He has been on therapy with tenofovir, emtricitabine, darunavir, and ritonavir for the last eighteen months. There have been no problems with adherence to therapy or side effects during this time and no episode of virological failure.

Blood tests from this period are shown in Table 53.3:

What is the most appropriate outcome of the clinic appointment?
A. Repeat HIV viral load and CD4 count in twelve months.
B. Repeat HIV viral load and CD4 count in six months.
C. Repeat HIV viral load and CD4 count in nine months.
D. Repeat HIV viral load in twelve months, no need to repeat CD4.
E. Repeat HIV viral load in three months, no need to repeat CD4.

Table 53.3 Blood test for a 48-year-man who attends for review in the HIV clinic.

	Pre-treatment	Four weeks after starting ART	Six months after starting ART	Eighteen months after starting ART
CD4 count (/μl)	300	Not tested	550	970
Plasma HIV viral load (log^{10} copies/ml)	4.6	3.4	Not detected	Not detected

53.12 Answers and discussion

53.12.1 Answer 1

D. Repeat fourth-generation HIV serology test in three weeks.
As the risk exposure is one week prior to the laboratory testing this patient is within the window period. He should be advised to have a further test four weeks after the risk exposure, i.e. in three weeks' time, as a fourth-generation laboratory test is being used. The patient should also be counselled regarding barrier contraception to reduce the risk of sexually transmitted infections and regarding the use of post-exposure prophylaxis. Post-exposure prophylaxis must be administered within seventy-two hours of the risk of exposure in order to be effective.

53.2 Answer 2

C. Repeat HIV resistance testing on the second viral load sample.
This patient has had a suboptimal response to ART with less than a 1 $\log^{10}$ copies/ml drop in viral load over the four weeks since commencing ART. Patient adherence to therapy should be checked and a repeat HIV resistance test should be performed to guide changes to therapy.

The detection of genotypic resistance in the majority of laboratories is currently performed by the Sanger sequencing method. This method is able to detect mutant quasispecies present as 20–25% of the virus population. Mutations present at lower levels will not be detected and may be unmasked by the use of ART, allowing viruses harbouring the resistant mutation to become the dominant population in the face of selection pressure. Repeating the resistance testing in situations such as this where there has been inadequate response to therapy will reveal the ART resistance mutations in the new dominant populations. Next-generation sequencing techniques are able to detect quasispecies populations present at much lower levels, and therefore, are more comprehensive in detailing the genetic mutations associated with resistance phenotypes present.

53.3 Answer 3

D. Repeat HIV viral load in twelve months, no need to repeat CD4.
The patient has had an undetectable viral load for over twelve months on a protease inhibitor (PI)-based ARV regimen. He is tolerating therapy well with no previous evidence of virological failure or rebound. Current guidance recommends that patients established on PI based therapy with undetectable viral loads can have routine viral load testing at intervals of up to twelve months. The patient does not require further CD4 cell count testing as he has had a CD4 count > 350/ μl on two occasions a year apart with the suppressed viral load.

If there is a detectable viral load or evidence of virological failure on subsequent HIV viral load testing this should be confirmed with a further sample from the patient. The CD4 count should be repeated if there is evidence of treatment failure or new HIV related symptoms.

In addition to these HIV specific tests it is vital that patients attending for routine follow up in the HIV clinic should have a review of their medications including adherence, adverse effects and any concerns regarding their medications. A full medication history should be sought including recreational drug use to identify potential drug–drug interactions and possible risk behaviour putting the patient at risk of further infections. This history will direct further testing including hepatitis virus screening and STI screening as necessary.

Patients should have at least annual review of their full blood count, renal function, liver function, urinalysis for protein, glucose and blood, lipid profile, and diabetic assessment as guided by their previous results and medications.

CHAPTER 54

Therapeutic options for HIV infection

Subathira Dakshina, Palwasha Khan, and Chloe Orkin

CONTENTS

54.1 The aims of treating HIV infection

Treatment of HIV infection has seen dramatic developments since the start of the epidemic over thirty-five years ago. Since the advent of highly active antiretroviral therapy (HAART), HIV infection has gone from being a terminal illness with the inevitable development of AIDS to a now-treatable chronic condition with infected individuals living a 'normal' and healthy lifestyle when tested early and engaged in care. Antiretroviral therapy (ART) has become simpler with minimal pill burden and fewer side effects. In the UK ART can only be prescribed by a HIV specialist ensuring the patient is engaged in care and under regular monitoring and follow up.

HIV infection affects the immune system through depletion of CD4 T-lymphocytes. There are several goals and aims of treating HIV infection.

54.1.2 Viral suppression and immune reconstitution

The main function of ART is to prevent HIV viral replication, which in turn reduces viral load (VL) and depletion of CD4 cells thereby preventing the development of AIDS and eventual mortality.

54.1.2 Pro-inflammatory state

HIV infection induces a pro-inflammatory state, which is associated with several conditions especially in late presenters. Common conditions include cardiovascular disease including cardiomyopathy, increased risk of venous thromboembolism due to a hypercoagulable state, HIV-associated nephropathy, disorders of the central nervous system, bone disorders, various dermatological conditions, and acceleration of ageing. Timely initiation of ART can help reduce and reverse such conditions.

54.1.3 Treatment as prevention

Studies demonstrate early initiation of ART and maintaining a suppressed VL minimizes the risk of onward sexual transmission of HIV. Though barrier protection is always advised in serodiscordant couples, recent studies support the reduced risk of transmission in virologically suppressed serodiscordant sexual couples, which has led to changes in post- and pre-exposure prophylaxis guidelines and enabling serodiscordant couples to conceive naturally.

54.1.4 Preventing mother-to-child transmission

All HIV positive women should be initiated on ART and virologically suppressed ideally prior to conception. It is now routine practice in the UK and many parts of the world to perform HIV testing during pregnancy. If tested positive during pregnancy ART should be initiated and, depending on the stage of pregnancy and the VL, a Caesarean section may be necessary and the neonate may require prophylactic ART.

54.2 Starting antiretroviral therapy

ART should be initiated in all HIV-positive individuals regardless of CD4 count for all the reasons stated. Policy writers internationally and locally have adopted these changes in their ART guidelines following evidence from recent landmark studies, such as the START study.

Several factors can affect timing of ART initiation:

- Concurrent opportunistic infections (see 54.8.2 Opportunistic infections);
- Comorbidities;
- Patient choice and lifestyle; and
- Availability and supply of ART drugs in resource-limited settings.

54.3 Drug classes available and their modes of action

Antiretroviral drugs are classified according to the mode of inhibition in the viral lifecycle (Table 54.1). Key targets for drugs are to inhibit HIV entry into a CD4 T lymphocyte cell, inhibit transcription of HIV RNA into DNA and prevent HIV replication and budding. Commonly used drugs from the different classes are found on AIDSmap chart; see Further reading for more information.

54.3.1 Nucleoside/nucleotide reverse transcriptase inhibitor (NRTI)

NRTIs act as competitive substrate inhibitors of the enzyme reverse transcriptase which transcribes viral RNA into DNA thereby preventing viral replication. Commonly prescribed examples include tenofovir, emtricitabine, abacavir, lamivudine, and zidovudine.

54.3.2 Non-nucleoside reverse transcriptase inhibitor (NNRTI)

These are non-competitive inhibitors of reverse transcriptase by binding to an allosteric site of the enzyme. HIV-2 is naturally resistant to NNRTIs. Commonly prescribed examples include efavirenz, nevirapine, etravirine, and rilpivirine.

54.3.3 Protease inhibitors (PI)

PIs inhibit the protease enzyme preventing the cleavage of essential proteins (gag proteins) necessary for viral maturation and budding from the host cell membrane. Commonly prescribed

Table 54.1 Classification of antiretroviral drugs according to the mode of inhibition in the viral lifecycle.

Part of lifecycle	Function	Examples of antiviral for this target
Attachment	gp120 binds to CD4 receptor and CCR5 co-receptor	CCR5 antagonist (e.g. maraviroc)
Fusion	HIV envelope fuses with cell membrane of CD4 positive cells	Fusion inhibitor (e.g. enfuvirtide)
Reverse transcription	Reverse transcriptase converts HIV RNA into HIV DNA	NNRTI (e.g. efavirenz, nevirapine, rilpivirine, etravirine) NRTI (e.g. tenofovir, lamivudine, abacavir, emtricitabine)
Integration	Integrase inserts HIV DNA into cellular DNA	Integrase inhibitors (e.g. raltegravir, dolutegravir, elvitegravir)
Protein synthesis, processing, and assembly	Long-chain HIV proteins are processed into individual components which are assembled to form new virions	Protease inhibitors (e.g. daraunavir, atazanavir, lopinavir)
Budding	Release of mature virions to infect further cells	None at present

examples include atazanavir, darunavir, and lopinavir (all are prescribed with boosting ritonavir or darunavir, and ataznavir can be boosted with cobicistat).

54.3.4 Fusion inhibitors

These drugs inhibit the entry of HIV into the host cell by interfering with the binding and fusion of the virus to the cell membrane through the co-receptor CCR5. However, the virus can switch the presentation of the co-receptor from CCR5 to CXCR4. CCR5 antagonists will be ineffective if there is a switch in the tropism from CCR5 to CXCR4. A tropism assay is crucial if this class of drug is to be considered. A commonly prescribed example is maraviroc.

54.3.5 Integrase strand transfer inhibitors (INSTI)

These drugs inhibit the viral enzyme integrase which is essential for integration of viral DNA into the host cell DNA. Commonly prescribed examples include raltegravir and dolutegravir (elvitegravir with cobicistat).

54.4 Different classes of drugs used in combination

Combination ART or HAART was a significant milestone in the history of HIV infection. HAART is made up of three active drugs consisting of a backbone of two NRTIs and a third agent. The following HAART regimens are examples based on the British HIV Association (BHIVA) guidelines (Table 54.2) and are similar to international prescribing standards.

54.4.1 The nucleotide backbone

The backbone consists of two NRTIs which often come as a dual fixed dose combination. Commonly used backbone combinations are tenofovir disoproxil fumarate (TDF) + emtricitabine

Table 54.2 Recommendations for choice of first line ART regimen (BHIVA guidelines).

	Preferred	Alternative
NRTI backbone	tenofovir + emtricitabine*	abacavir + lamivudine***

Third agent	NNRTI – rilpivirine**
	PI – atazanavir/r or darunavir/r or
	    ataznavir/cobicistat or darunavir/
	    cobicistat
	INSTI – raltegravir, elvitegravir, with
	    cobicistat or dolutegravir
		NNRTI – efavirenz

* TDF should only be prescribed if Creatinine Clearance is above >70ml/min.
** Recommended if baseline viral load (VL) < 100,000
***Recommended only if baseline VL < 100,000 except when initiated in combination with dolutegravir, in which case abacavir/lamivudine can be used at any baseline VL. Abacavir is contraindicated if HLA-B*57:01 positive.

(Truvada), tenofovir alafenamide (TAF) + emtricitabine (Descovy), abacavir + lamivudine (Kivexa) or Zidovudine + lamivudine (Combivir).

54.4.2 The third agent

Ritonavir-boosted PIs, NNRTIs, or INSTIs are the recommended choice as the third agent in first-line treatment. NNRTIs are not commonly prescribed in second-line or salvage regimen due to the accumulation of drug-resistant mutations.

The choice of ART regimen is dependent on an array of factors and should ideally be tailored to individual patients and in accordance with local and national guidelines.

The following factors must be considered when initiating ART:

- Patient choice—are they ready to start, single tablet regimen versus multiple pills;
- ART-naïve or ART-experienced patient;
- If HIV VL is > 100,000 Truvada is recommended, whereas Kivexa is advised in VL < 100,000 (but can be given with dolutegravir);
- Drug resistance: transmitted or acquired;
- Hypersensitivity and allergies: HLAB5701-positive individuals are susceptible to abacavir hypersensitivity;
- Concurrent opportunistic infections: may delay initiation of ART;
- Side effects: nausea, vomiting, and diarrhoea are commonly seen on initiation of ART which normally settles within a few days. Patient should be monitored for unwanted side effects such as skin rash and hepatitis.
- Co-morbidities: avoid TDF-based regimen in underlying renal pathology (creatinine clearance < 70ml/min) and efavirenz in individuals with co-existing mental health disorders;
- Polypharmacy and drug-drug interactions: thorough drug history including over-the-counter medications and herbal remedies must be reviewed;
- Drug availability and cost-effectiveness;
- Social history: work-life patterns, dietary requirements.

54.5 Preparing and monitoring patients for treatment

All patients must be appropriately counselled prior to initiation of ART and the process should be an informed discussion in a multidisciplinary manner involving the patient, clinician, HIV pharmacists and additional allied professionals depending on the patient's need at the time.

Until further advances are available, at present ART will need to be taken for life and it is paramount that the individual is ready to start and adhere to the therapy. Perceptual barriers, such as personal beliefs and preferences, along with logistical barriers, such as limitations in resources, must be considered.

Baseline investigations before initiating ART:

- CD4 and HIV VL;
- HIV viral genotype resistance assay;
- Full blood count;
- Renal function including urine protein:creatinine ratio;
- Liver function;
- HLA B*57:01 and
- Exclude active opportunistic infections such as TB.

Two weeks post-ART initiation 'safety blood tests' are performed monitoring renal, liver and bone marrow function. Response to treatment is assessed after one month when a VL is performed. A two-log viral load drop would be expected at this stage and by six months the patient should be virologically suppressed (undetectable VL).

Once established on ART and virologically suppressed VL can be measured every six months and CD4 count once a year (frequency of testing will depend on patient adherence and clinical outcomes). Adherence should be discussed at every visit and if the patient has a VL blip/re-bound adherence support should be offered and a HIV resistance assay performed.

Therapeutic drug monitoring of individual ART drugs is not routinely recommended but may be of help if poor adherence or drug-drug interactions is suspected when a patient is virologically failing.

54.6 Drug adherence and drug resistance

The vast majority of ART regimens are oral pills and are mostly once-daily formularies with a few that need to be taken twice a day. Due to pharmacodynamics ART needs to be taken daily and at the same time to maintain appropriate therapeutic plasma drug levels. Poor adherence can lead to viraemia, viral mutation, drug resistance, virological failure and ultimately life-threatening immunosuppression.

Virologically failing patients will need a HIV resistance assay to determine the resistance profile. Alternative ART regimen will need to be commenced depending on the resistance profile and following discussions in a multidisciplinary HIV resistance meeting. At this point adherence support is essential which can be in the form of in-depth discussion with a healthcare professional or pharmacist or organisations offering peer support. Where there is a risk of frequent prolonged treatment interruptions PI-based ART regimen is often prescribed as first line as it is associated with less frequent selection for drug resistance.

54.7 Switching or stopping treatment

Once commenced on ART patients are expected to remain on the therapy for life and it is not recommended to stop or interrupt ART. In certain circumstances ART regimen or a particular drug within the regimen may need to be stopped or switched. For instance, if there are unwanted side effects or to minimize drug-drug interactions in the setting of concurrent illnesses. In such situations, if a patient is on an NNRTI regimen with an NRTI backbone replace all drugs with a PI based therapy such as darunavir/ritonavir for 4 weeks then stop. This will help prevent development of

NNRTI mutations in view to their prolonged half-life. Replacement therapy is not needed when stopping a PI-based regimen.

54.8 Consideration of special circumstances

54.8.1 Primary HIV infection

The WHO definition of primary HIV infection is the time from HIV acquisition to the development and appearance of HIV antibody or viral products (HIV p24 antigen or HIV RNA) in the system circulation. Current UK guidelines recommend all individuals with suspected or diagnosed primary HIV infection are reviewed by an HIV specialist and offered immediate ART.

54.8.2 Opportunistic infections

The BHIVA and WHO recommend in severely immunocompromised (CD4 <200) individuals presenting with an AIDS defining infection, or with a serious bacterial infection to start ART within two weeks of initiation of specific antimicrobial treatment. This is to reduce and prevent to the occurrence of immune reconstitution inflammatory syndrome (IRIS)—a paradoxical clinical deterioration after ART initiation due to an exaggerated inflammatory reaction from a re-invigorated immune system. It can present as an unmasking of a latent or sub-clinical opportunistic infection or clinical deterioration of a previously diagnosed and treated infection.

54.8.3 Viral hepatitis co-infection

HIV-positive patients co-infected with hepatitis B virus (HBV) should be treated with fully suppressive ART inclusive of drugs active against HBV regardless of CD4 cell count. Tenofovir and emtricitabine combination is the recommended NRTI backbone. Hepatitis C virus (HCV) co-infected patients should be assessed for HCV treatment regardless of CD4 count. If CD4 cell count permits treatment of HCV before commencing ART is an option to minimize drug-drug interaction or if there are concerns over adherence.

54.8.4 Pregnancy

All pregnant women are tested for HIV as part of their antenatal care. Those who conceive on an effective ART should continue with the regimen. Treatment-naïve women should ideally be commenced on ART and suppress their VL prior to conception. If ART naïve and pregnant ART should be commenced by 24 weeks of pregnancy with standard ART regimens. In late-presenting women not on treatment ART should be commenced without delay and in settings of high VL >100,000 quadruple therapy consisting of raltegravir is advised. A stat dose of nevirapine along with zidovudine/lamivudine and raltegravir is recommended in women diagnosed with HIV at labour.

54.8.5 Ageing

People are living longer with HIV and co-morbidities associated with old age are more common in the ageing HIV population. Standard ART regimens are recommended in older people living with HIV and routine screening for cardiovascular, metabolic, renal, and neurocognitive impairment is necessary and modifiable risk factors and life style measures (such as smoking cessation) should be advised. Occasionally ART drugs may need to be adjusted for instance, studies recommend avoiding abacavir in individuals with high cardiovascular disease markers and TDF should be avoided in those with renal impairment or bone disorders.

54.8.6 Drug-drug interactions

ART drugs are metabolized through the liver using the cytochrome P450 pathways and hence, drug-drug interactions are very common. It is paramount to take a thorough drug history before commencing ART and at every follow-up visit and it is important to inform patients to advice encounters with other healthcare professionals (such as their GP and dentists) of their ART drug history. A very useful website for checking drug interactions is www.hiv-druginteractions.org.

54.9 Further reading

Interested readers are referred to the websites here for further information about current guidelines and information about HIV and AIDS.
- www.BHIVA.org/currentguidelines
- www.aidsmap.org
- http://www.aidsmap.com/resources/Antiretroviral-drugs-chart/page/1412453/)
- www.hiv-druginteractions.org

54.10 Assessment questions

54.10.1 Question 1

A forty-nine-year-old man is newly diagnosed through routine sexual health screening to have HIV infection. He has a background history of hypertension on treatment and is a smoker with a twenty-pack year history. He consumes twenty-five units alcohol per week and uses intranasal crystal meth intermittently. He has not disclosed his HIV status to his regular male partner.

Investigations:

CD4 cell count	448/μl
HIV-1 viral load	97,000 copies/ml
Hepatitis B surface antigen	negative
Hepatitis B core antibody	Positive

What is the most appropriate next step in management?
A. Delay ART until drug, alcohol and smoking addressed and patient has disclosed to the partner.
B. Commence ART with Kivexa and a PI, offer support with smoking, alcohol, and drug use.
C. Commence ART with Truvada and a PI, offer support with smoking, alcohol, and drug use.
D. Commence ART with Truvada and an NNRTI, offer support with smoking, alcohol, and drug use.
E. Commerce ART with Truvada and a PI and advise GP to monitor blood pressure and address smoking, alcohol, and drug use.

54.10.2 Question 2

A forty-year-old lady, originally from sub-Saharan Africa and diagnosed HIV-positive six years ago, presents to the antenatal clinic for screening test. She has stopped taking Truvada/efavirenz six months ago due to marriage break-up. There is a history of gastritis with occasional omeprazole use.

Investigations:

CD4 cell count	350/ μl
HIV-1 viral load	30,000 copies/ml
HIV-1 genotypic resistance assay	Evidence of drug resistance to NNRTIs

What is the most appropriate next step in management?
A. Delay ART until patient feels ready to start.
B. Restart Truvada/efavirenz.

C. Start Kivexa/atazanavir and offer adherence support.

D. Start Truvada and atazanavir/ritonavir, continue omeprazole, and offer adherence support.

E. Start Truvada and darunavir/ritonavir, switch omeprazole to ranitidine, and offer adherence support.

54.10.3 Question 3

A thirty-year-old man is diagnosed HIV-positive following a diagnosis of pulmonary TB one week ago. He has a history of depression but is off antidepressants.

Investigations:	
CD4	100/ μl
HIV-1 viral load	70,000 copies/ml

What is the most appropriate next step in management?

A. Complete two months of TB treatment, then commence ART with Truvada+PI.

B. Start standard TB treatment and start ART two weeks later with Truvada+PI.

C. Treat TB with standard TB treatment but switch rifampicin to rifabutin and start Truvada+PI based-regimen.

D. Treat TB with standard therapy and commence Truvada/efavirenz two weeks post-TB treatment initiation.

E. Treat TB with standard treatment and commence ART after two weeks with Triumeq (Abaca vir+lamivudine+dolutegravir).

54.11 Answers and discussion

54.11.1 Answer 1

C. Commence ART with Truvada and a PI, offer support with smoking, alcohol, and drug use.
This is a complex older patient with multiple comorbidities and potential risk of poor adherence. Ideally ART should not be delayed in this patient as it will:

- Avoid further immunosuppression;
- Avoid comorbidities associated with ageing HIV population; and
- Prevent onward transmission.

It is important to involve the patient in discussions on ART initiation and support with adherence offering appropriate service to help with smoking cessation, and drug and alcohol use. The patient should be supported through the process of disclosure to his partner.

In view of HBV status and likely increased cardiovascular risk factor, Truvada would be the appropriate backbone and with the potential risk of poor adherence, a PI would be a suitable third agent.

54.11.2 Answer 2

E. Start Truvada and darunavir/ritonavir, switch omeprazole to ranitidine, and offer adherence support.
It is important to identify and address the issues surrounding her poor adherence. Counselling and peer support may be of benefit here. In view of the resistance pattern, the patient will need to be started on a PI-based regimen and can continue on Truvada. Due to drug-drug interactions between PIs and proton pump inhibitors it would be advisable to start this patient on ritonavir-boosted darunavir and switch the omeprazole to ranitidine.

54.11.3 Answer 3

E. Treat TB with standard treatment and commence ART after two weeks with Triumeq
(Abacavir + lamivudine + dolutegravir).

Current guidelines advise commencing ART after about two weeks of initiating TB treatment.
Reducing drug-drug interactions is key when considering ART in the contact of TB drugs. Option
C was the choice before newer drugs were available, but with the advent of INSTI tests such as
dolutegravir, option E is the most appropriate choice in this scenario.

CHAPTER 55

Opportunistic infections in HIV Infection

Elizabeth Williams

CONTENTS

55.1 Defining opportunistic infection (OI)?

An infection is defined as opportunistic when it affects those with severe immunosuppression, i.e. takes an opportunity to cause disease in a host with a weakened immune system. In people living with HIV it mainly affects those with a CD4 count < 200 although it is not impossible in those with CD4 count > 200. The CD4 percentage is also important as those with a CD4% < 14 are also more likely to have an OI. The lower the CD4 count the higher the risk of OIs, and some OIs are seen much more commonly with very low CD4 counts, e.g. cryptococcal meningitis in those with CD4 count of < 100.

Before the introduction of antiretroviral therapy OIs were much more common than they are now, with previously up to 80% of those with AIDS having pneumocystis pneumonia (PCP). Since the introduction of antiretrovirals (ARVs) the rates of OIs has reduced greatly but unfortunately there are people who are still diagnosed late with an OI at diagnosis. Those with poor adherence or difficulty accessing ARVs are also more likely to be affected.

In the UK in 2014, 40% of people diagnosed with HIV had a CD4 count of <350 which is defined as a late diagnosis (and 22% had a CD4 count of <200 which is defined as a very late diagnosis). In comparison to someone diagnosed with HIV early, those who are diagnosed late have a 10 times higher risk of dying in the year after they are diagnosed. This highlights the need for routine HIV testing so that people are diagnosed early to reduce the incidence of OIs further.

55.2 Common OIs in people living with HIV

The most common OIs seen in the UK are pneumocystis pneumonia (PCP), central nervous system (CNS) toxoplasmosis, cryptococcal meningitis, cytomegalovirus (CMV) retinitis, *Mycobacterium avium intracellulare* (MAI) infection and candidiasis.

55.3 Reducing the risk of OI

All those with HIV and a CD4 count ≤ 200, or with a CD4% < 14 should be given prophylaxis against PCP. Prophylaxis should also be recommended for those with oral candidiasis or a previous AIDs –defining illness. The options are co-trimoxazole 480mg od or 960mg 3x/week (960mg once daily can be given although does not confer any greater protection and has increased risk of side effects), dapsone 50mg once daily, or pentamidine nebulisers 300mg once every 4 weeks. Co-trimoxazole 480mg once a day is the preferred option unless there is a contraindication such as allergy, as it also offers some protection against toxoplasmosis and some diarrhoeal diseases. If pyrimethamine is added to dapsone this also reduces the risk of toxoplasmosis infection. Pentamidine nebulisers are less effective when used in those with very low CD4 counts or who have previously had PCP. Pentamidine nebulisers do not reduce the risk of any other OIs and do not aerate the lungs equally therefore if PCP does occur it is more likely to be at the lung apices. Prophylaxis can be stopped once CD4 count is consistently >200 for at least 3 months with an undetectable viral load. Patients should be advised not to eat raw meat and to avoid cat litter if possible to reduce the risk of toxoplasmosis. For patients with a CD4 count < 50, dilated fundoscopy should be done every 3 months to monitor for evidence of CMV retinitis.

55.4 Pneumocystis pneumonia (PCP)

Pneumocystis pneumonia was previously known as *Pneumocystis carinii* pneumonia, hence the acronym PCP. It is caused by a fungus which is now renamed as *Pneumocystis jiroveci*. It typically presents with shortness of breath, especially on exertion, cough and fever, frequently these symptoms have been present for weeks or months, although less commonly symptoms can be of acute onset. On examination patients are tachypnoeic, often with mild fever and mildly low oxygen saturations which often reduce further after exertion Measuring oxygen saturation before and after exertion is a useful test as low oxygen saturation is common finding in PCP and fairly rare in other conditions. Useful investigations are chest x-ray to rule out bacterial pneumonia as cause of symptoms or secondary infection on top of PCP and for pneumothoraces. Chest X-ray appearances for PCP are variable and a normal chest x-ray does not rule out PCP. Classic x-ray changes are described as bilateral diffuse symmetric interstitial infiltrates that are usually characteristically central. Other investigations include arterial blood gas for PaO_2, induced sputum looking for *Pneumocystis jiroveci* using Grocott methenamine silver stain, although commonly bronchoscopy and bronchoalveolar lavage samples are needed. Bronchoscopy may not be possible if the patient is not stable enough. *Pneumocystis jiroveci* can be found up to 7-10 days after treatment has been started therefore if PCP is clinically suspected treatment should not be delayed whilst further investigations are carried out and microscopy is awaited. Cases are classified as mild to moderate and moderate to severe depending on PaO_2 or oxygen saturations (SpO_2), with a PaO_2 of <9.3kPa or SpO_2 of <92% indicating moderate to severe infection. First line treatment is co-trimoxazole given for 21days. For mild to moderate disease, this can be given orally at a dose of 90mg/kg/day in 2-4 divided doses, and in moderate to severe disease IV 120mg/kg/day for first 3 days then reducing to 90mg/kg/day in 2-4 divided doses. Those with moderate to severe infection should also be treated with prednisolone; 40mg bd for first 5 days, 40mg od for next 5 days and then 20mg od for the remaining 11 days. Second line treatment regimens include clindamycin/primaquine, IV pentamidine, trimethoprim/ dapsone or atovaquone. These should only be used if there is known sulpha allergy, patient experiences toxicity on co-trimoxazole or there is likely treatment failure (ie no clinical response after at least 5 days of first line therapy). If there has been no response, other differentials should be considered in case of incorrect diagnosis. Pneumothoraces and respiratory failure are possible complications, intensive care may be needed.

55.5 Toxoplasmosis

Toxoplasma gondii is a feline parasite. Asymptomatic primary infection occurs due to exposure to cat faeces or eating contaminated meat. This is very common in the general population and varies widely from country to country. Clinical disease only occurs in those with a suppressed immune system causing single or multiple brain abscesses therefore presentation with features of a space occupying lesion which vary depending on the area(s) of the brain affected. May also be symptoms of raised intracranial pressure such as headache, nausea and vomiting. Seizures, confusion and reduced Glasgow coma score can also occur. Focal neurological signs will depend on the location of the lesion(s). A contrast enhanced CT head scan (Figures 55.1 and 55.2) showing ring enhancing lesion(s) with surrounding oedema is essential for diagnosis. MRI head with gadolinium contrast is also useful though often not possible as first imaging but is useful for comparison with follow up scans to monitor for response. If there is significant doubt of the diagnosis then brain biopsy can be done but this is rarely performed unless there has been no improvement in clinical features or MRI head scan after 2 weeks of treatment. For this reason it is important that steroids are not given unless necessary as this will affect the follow up MRI images. First line treatment is with

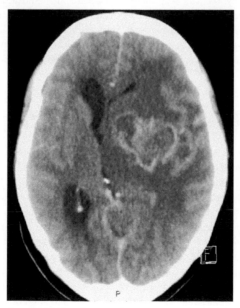

Figure 55.1 Contrast-enhanced CT head image showing ring enhancing lesion in the left lentiform nucleus and thalamus.

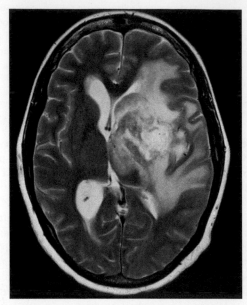

Figure 55.2 MRI head image showing same lesion with surrounding oedema.

sulphadiazine (15mg/kg/day four times daily) plus pyrimethamine (200mg stat and then 75mg once daily) given with folinic acid (15-30mg once daily) orally for six weeks. Alternative regimes include clindamycin and pyrimethamine, trimethoprim and sulphamethoxazole or atovaquone with sulphadiazone or pyrimethamine. Sulphadiazine can cause crystal uropathy and renal dysfunction so it is important that patients are well hydrated. Secondary prophylaxis is needed after the initial 6 weeks of treatment and is usually with the same medications as the initial treatment but at lower doses. Antiepileptics such as levetiracetam or sodium valproate should be given if patient has seizures.

55.6 Cryptococcal meningitis

Cryptococcal meningitis is caused by the encapsulated yeast *Cryptococcus neoformans*. Clinical disease can occur at multiple body sites including skin and lungs but meningitis is the most common and serious. It often presents with severe headache, nausea, vomiting, fever, confusion, reduced consciousness level. Reabsorption of cerebrospinal fluid is reduced leading to raised intracranial pressure therefore on examination patient may have papilloedema, reduced GCS and signs of meningism. Lumbar puncture is extremely important for diagnosis and to reduce intracranial pressure which will reduce symptoms. A markedly raised opening pressure is common. If it is greater than 25cm H_2O then it is advisable to aim for a closing pressure of <20cm H_2O or half the opening pressure if the opening pressure is <40cm H_2O. Cerebrospinal fluid (CSF) samples should be sent for white cell count and differential, India ink staining and cryptococcal antigen, as well as others investigations to rule out differentials. Serum cryptococcal antigen can also be done as well as blood cultures. However, a positive result in blood cannot determine the site of infection. Treatment is with IV liposomal amphotericin B (4mg/kg/day) and flucytosine (100mg/kg/day) for 2 weeks followed by high dose fluconazole (400mg od for first 10 weeks and then 200mg od) as maintenance therapy. Daily lumbar punctures may be needed when patient first started on treatment. If difficult to manage a lumbar drain or a shunt may be required. Patients with cryptococcal meningitis may experience immune reconstitution inflammatory syndrome (IRIS) when antiretrovirals are started so some clinicians are cautious about starting antiretrovirals early but in the UK the advice is to start within the first two weeks of *cryptococcus* treatment.

55.7 Cytomegalovirus (CMV)

Cytomegalovirus is a human beta herpes virus. Seroprevalance is high in the general population, but particularly high in men who have sex with men (MSM). Clinical disease can occur at various sites, including the GI tract, lungs and nervous system, but 75% of cases affect the retina causing reduction in visual acuity and if left untreated can lead to blindness. Dilated fundoscopy shows typical lesions ('pizza-pie' appearance of the fundus) due to necrotizing retinitis. Serum CMV DNA quantitative level is a useful test for monitoring response, but a high CMV titre does not necessarily indicate end organ disease. Ophthalmology review is important for diagnosis and management. Treatment is with oral valganciclovir 900mg bd for 2-4 weeks and then halved to 900mg od as maintenance treatment, usually needed until CD4 >100 and VL <40. Intravitreal anti-CMV treatment injections may also be needed, and this would be guided by ophthalmology. Other treatment options are IV ganciclovir, foscarnet or cidofovir.

55.8 *Mycobacterium avium-intracellulare (MAI)?*

Also known as *Mycobacterium avium* complex and is a group of common environmental organisms. Unlike *Mycobacterium tuberculosis*, it is not transmitted from one person to another. Disseminated *Mycobacterium avium-intracellulare* can cause multiple non-specific symptoms such as weight loss, fevers, night sweats, lethargy and diarrhoea typically in people with CD4 counts <50. They may have lymphadenopathy and/or hepatomegaly and splenomegaly. Diagnosis is made on mycobacterial culture from blood, bone marrow or tissues such as lymph node or liver. 98% of cases of disseminated *Mycobacterium avium* complex can be diagnosed if 2 sets of mycobacterial blood cultures are taken. First line treatment is with clarithromycin or azithromycin plus ethambutol. Sometimes rifabutin is added in some cases especially if CD4 <25, patients are very symptomatic or blood tests such as ALP, albumin, haemoglobin, are particularly abnormal. Duration of therapy is governed by clinical response to treatment and improvement in CD4 count and viral load suppression e.g. viral load undetectable and CD4 >100 for at least 3 months. Some patients may be on MAI treatment lifelong

55.9 Is candida an OI?

Candidiasis is infection with candida species, most commonly *Candida albicans*. Most often it causes oral candidiasis with white plaques on the palate, buccal mucosa, gums and/or tongue, or vulvo-vaginal candidiasis. Less commonly than in women it can cause symptoms in male genitalia causing balanitis. These can occur in immunocompetent individuals but more likely in those who are immune-compromised and can be more severe. In immunocompromised individuals candidiasis can also occur at other body sites, in particular the oesophagus and this is an AIDS-defining diagnosis. Cases are usually diagnosed clinically due to typical lesions on direct visualisation or endoscopy, and from history but samples can be taken for microscopy or culture. Culture is needed if speciation is required which is useful if it is not responding to treatment for *Candida albicans* or to look for other candida species eg *C. krusei* or *C. glabrata*. Topical nystatin can be used for oral candidiasis. Oral or IV fluconazole (50-100mg od for 7-14 days) can be used for oral, genital and oesophageal candidiasis and itraconazole can be used if no response with fluconazole. Fluconazole is always ineffective in treating *C. krusei* as it is resistant. Invasive candidiasis should be treated with IV treatment. Vulvo-vaginal candidiasis and balanitis due to candidal infection can be treated with topical clotrimazole in the form of clotrimazole cream or pessary. Routine prophylaxis for mucosal candidiasis is not recommended.

It is not recommended to prescribe prophylaxis for mucosal candidiasis routinely.

55.10 Starting antiretrovirals

As the immune system improves when antiretrovirals are started there is a risk that patients can have IRIS which can be severe and sometimes fatal therefore there are differing opinions about the optimal timing of starting antiretroviral (ARV) therapy. Some advise starting antiretrovirals within the first 2 weeks of treatment initiation of an OI, due to concern about risk of other OIs, while others advise waiting until at least 2 weeks of OI treatment has been given to reduce the risk of IRIS. There have been many studies into this but the settings and patient groups are not necessarily generalizable. There has been particular concern about timing of antiretroviral initiation in patients with crypotococcal meningitis as some studies have shown a higher mortality with early initiation especially if patients have severe disease, and some advise to delay antiretroviral initiation until after 5 weeks. However, the British HIV association (BHIVA) guidelines advise to start antiretrovirals within the first 2 weeks of OI treatment initiation for all OIs. If a patient is already on antiretrovirals and had been taking, these should be continued.

55.11 Further reading

British HIV Association and British Infection Association Guidelines for the Treatment of Opportunistic Infection in HIV-seropositive Individuals 2011 http://www.bhiva.org/documents/Guidelines/OI/hiv_v12_is2_Iss2Press_Text.pdf.
There is a very useful downloadable smartphone app.
Public Health England. HIV new diagnoses, treatment and care in the UK: 2015 report. October 2015, https://www.gov.uk/government/uploads/system/uploads/attachment_data/file/469405/HIV_new_diagnoses_treatment_and_care_2015_report20102015.pdf
Phair J et al. The risk of *Pneumocystis carinii* pneumonia among men infected with human immunodeficiency virus type 1. Multicenter AIDS Cohort Study Group. N Engl J Med 1990; 322: 161–165.
Nelson M et al. British HIV Association and British Infection Association Guidelines for the Treatment of Opportunistic Infection in HIV-seropositive Individuals 2011. HIV Medicine (2011), 12 (Suppl. 2), 1–140.
Loyse A et al. Histopathology of the arachnoid granulations and brain in HIV-associated cryptococcal meningitis: correlation with cerebrospinal fluid pressure. AIDS 2010; 24: 405-10.
Dockrell DH et al. Candidiasis section of the updated guidelines: consultation version (2018) (British HIV Association and British Infection Association Guidelines for the Treatment of Opportunistic Infection in HIV-seropositive Individuals 2011).
Lawn S et al. Optimum time to start antiretroviral therapy during HIV-associated opportunistic infections Curr Opin Infect Dis. 2011; 24: 34–42.

Boulware DR et al. Timing of Antiretroviral Therapy after Diagnosis of Cryptococcal Meningitis. COAT trial team. N Engl J Med. 2014; 370: 2487–2498.

Waters L et al. BHIVA guidelines for the treatment of HIV-1 positive adults with ART 2015 (2016 interim update). August 2016.

55.12 Assessment question

52.12.1 Question 1

A 37 year old man presented with night sweats, fevers, diarrhoea and weight loss for the preceding 5 months. A point of care HIV test was positive. Baseline blood tests showed he was mildly anaemic, with low serum albumin, and his CD4 count was 21 cells/mm3. Standard blood cultures showed no growth but mycobacterial blood cultures grew Mycobacterium avium. He was commenced on treatment with clarithromycin, ethambutol and rifabutin, and then started on antiretrovirals a week later.

How long should he continue clarithromycin, ethambutol and rifabutin?
A. Symptom free for 3 months.
B. Viral load undetectable and CD4 >200 for at least 3 months.
C. Viral load undetectable and CD4 >200 for at least 6 months.
D. Viral load undetectable and CD4 >100 for at least 3 months.
E. Viral load undetectable and CD4 >100 for at least 6 months.

55.13 Answer and discussion

52.13.1 Answer 1

D. Viral load undetectable and CD4 >100 for at least 3 months.

MAI treatment can be very prolonged and some patients may be on MAI treatment lifelong as their CD4 count never improves significantly. It is also important that MAI treatment is not stopped before a full clinical response has been seen even if viral load is fully suppressed and CD4 count greater than 100. If treatment is stopped too early patients are at risk of symptoms returning.

PART TEN

TRAVEL AND GEOGRAPHICAL HEALTH

Geographical pattern of infectious diseases and infection prevention for travellers

Desmond Hsu and Zahir Osman Eltahir Babiker

CONTENTS

56.1 Geo-climatic considerations for the spread of infectious diseases

Infectious diseases are transmitted either directly from person to person via direct contact or droplet exposure, or indirectly through a vector organism (mosquito or tick) or a non-biological physical vehicle (soil or water). Vector-borne infectious diseases are highly influenced by climate factors such as temperature, precipitation, altitude, sunshine duration, and wind. Therefore, climate change is a major threat for the emergence and re-emergence of infectious diseases, e.g. re-emergence of dengue fever in some parts of southern Europe.

The natural reservoirs of infectious diseases are either humans (anthroponoses) or animals (zoonoses). Population movement due to travel or civil unrest risks introducing non-immune populations to regions that are endemic for certain infectious diseases. By contrast, global trade contributes to the movement of animals or arthropods across the world and this poses a major risk for introducing infectious diseases to previously non-endemic settings, e.g. rats on board commercial ships and the global spread of hantaviruses; international trade in used car tyres and the risk of introducing flavivirus-infected mosquitoes into non-endemic settings; and the contribution of migratory birds to the introduction and the spread of West Nile virus in the United States.

56.2 The importance of pre-travel consultations

The unprecedented growth of international travel facilitates the swift movement of pathogens by travellers from one region to another. The main determinants of travel-related infections are destination country, activities undertaken during travel, and pre-existing morbidities. Therefore, the pre-travel consultation aims to assess potential health hazards associated with the trip, give advice on appropriate preventative measures, and educate the traveller about their own health.

Attitudes towards seeking pre-travel health advice vary by the type of traveller. For example, those visiting friends and relatives (VFRs) in their country of origin are less likely to seek pre-travel health advice compared to tourists and therefore stand a higher chance of presenting with preventable infections such as malaria.

56.3 Aspects of a pre-travel consultation

The key aspects of a pre-travel consultation include:

- comprehensive risk assessment based on the demographic and clinical background of the traveller as well as the region of travel and itinerary.
- delivery of targeted and personalized health messages.
- provision of specific recommendations regarding chemoprophylaxis and/or vaccination.

Assessment of the health background of travellers includes the following:

- significant medical history (over sixty years of age, recent illness or surgery, chronic illness, pregnancy or breastfeeding status if female of childbearing age, mental health problems, seizure disorder, immunocompromised status, disability).
- current medications.
- immunization history.
- allergies (drugs, vaccines, eggs, latex).

High-risk travellers include:

- immunocompromised individuals.
- travellers with pre-existing comorbidities.
- pregnant and breastfeeding women.
- elderly travellers (over sixty years of age).
- VFRs.

Assessment of the traveller's itinerary includes the following:

- destination: countries and regions to be visited, including order if more than one.
- setting: urban versus rural locations; high versus low altitude settings.
- season of travel: rainy versus dry season.
- duration of travel: dates and length of stay in different places.
- time to departure: it is important to ascertain this as it is likely impact on the feasibility of administration of some pre-travel vaccines and may limit the choices for antimalarial prophylactic drugs.
- purpose of travel: leisure, work, VFR, pilgrimage, medical tourism.
- accommodation: type of shelter, sanitary facilities, use of insecticide-treated nets (ITNs), and air-conditioning systems.

- modes of transportation: backpacking, public or private transport, and use of animals as means of transport.
- planned activities: participation in wedding/funeral events, trekking, cycling, safari tour, freshwater sports, healthcare/relief work, animal rides or any other form of animal contact.

56.4 Health messages during a pre-travel consultation

Targeted pre-travel advice aims to prevent specific communicable as well as non-communicable travel-associated diseases.

Prevention of communicable diseases:

- safe food and water consumption: eating freshly cooked meals, drinking bottled water.
- use of personal protective measures to reduce the risk of vector-borne infections: avoidance of outdoor exposure during vector feeding times, wearing full-length loose-fitting garments, use of ITNs, use of DEET (N,N-diethyl-meta-toluamide)-based insect repellents, inspection during and after high-risk activities for ticks and tick bites and taking appropriate measures for tick removal if bitten.
- safe sexual practices: avoidance of risky sexual behaviour, use of barrier contraceptive methods.
- avoidance of percutaneous blood exposure: tattoos, piercings, acupuncture, and injecting drug misuse.
- avoidance of animal contact; especially in countries where rabies is prevalent.
- vector avoidance as appropriate: avoidance of freshwater exposure in certain regions (schistosomiasis), avoidance of walking barefoot on soil and beaches (hookworms).

Prevention of non-communicable diseases:

- prevention of deep venous thrombosis, altitude sickness, and heat stroke as appropriate.
- prevention of road traffic collisions and other personal injuries.

56.5 Recommended chemoprophylaxis

56.5.1 Malaria

Antimalarial prophylaxis should be recommended for travellers intending to visit sub-Saharan Africa, parts of the Middle East, large areas of South and South East Asia, and areas of Central and South America. Up-to-date epidemiology and advice on malaria prophylaxis can be found on the National Travel Health Network and Centre (NaTHNaC) website http://www.nathnac.net or Travax website www.travax.nhs.uk, which is maintained by Health Protection Scotland (HPS).

56.5.2 Traveller's diarrhoea

The risk for developing traveller's diarrhoea can be reduced by adopting good hygienic practices. High-risk travellers for diarrhoeal illnesses include:

- patients with severe inflammatory bowel disease.
- patients with advanced cardiac or renal disease who may be particularly sensitive to changes in fluid balance.
- severely immunocompromised patients.

Prophylactic antibiotics for high-risk patients should be used for the full duration of the trip. Further risk-benefit assessment should be carried out if the duration of the trip exceeds three weeks. Ciprofloxacin is the prophylactic antibiotic of choice but attention should be paid to potential drug interactions and contraindications.

'Stand-by' antibiotics may be prescribed to travellers heading to high-risk areas who are not eligible for prophylactic antibiotics and who may not have immediate access to medical assistance should the need arise. A three-day course of ciprofloxacin would be appropriate for such travellers. Children and pregnant or breastfeeding women as well as travellers to countries with high rates of fluoroquinolone resistance can be prescribed a short course of azithromycin instead.

56.6 Recommended vaccinations

Up-to-date information on the epidemiology of infectious diseases and the likely risk of exposure in the country(ies) that the traveller is planning to visit is available from NaTHNaC or Travax websites. Examples of vaccines that are usually prescribed to UK travellers are outlined in Table 56.1.

Table 56.1 Examples of commonly prescribed vaccines to UK travellers.

Type of Vaccine	Explanation	Examples
Routine	Vaccines recommended in the UK, regardless of travel	Diphtheria, MMR (measles, mumps, and rubella), Polio, Tetanus, BCG (at-risk children)
Required	Vaccines that are mandatory for entering certain territories	Yellow fever: a requirement for entry into some South American and African countries; Meningococcal meningitis (ACWY vaccine): a requirement for travellers to Saudi Arabia visiting Mecca for Hajj or Umrah
Recommended	Vaccines that may be recommended based on risk assessment	Cholera, Hepatitis A, Hepatitis B, Japanese encephalitis, Meningococcal meningitis (ACWY vaccine), Rabies, Tick-borne encephalitis, BCG, Typhoid, Yellow fever

56.7 Post-exposure prophylaxis

Post-exposure prophylaxis (PEP) can be provided against HIV, hepatitis B, hepatitis A, measles, varicella zoster virus (VZV), tetanus, and rabies. In-depth discussion of PEP for HIV, HBV, VZV, measles, and tetanus is presented elsewhere in this book.

56.8 Management of animal bites

General measures:

1. immediately wash the wound for several minutes with soap and running water.
2. apply a disinfectant to the wound.
3. apply a simple dressing to protect the wound.

4. seek immediate medical attention for risk assessing rabies and tetanus and whether antibiotics should be given.

5. where possible, suturing of the wound should be delayed until risk assessments have been made.

Rabies-specific risk assessments should include:

- date of exposure.
- location: gives a clue to the prevalence of rabies in the country or region.
- type of animal: bat, primate, rodent or other terrestrial mammals.
- other characteristics of the animal: domesticated, displaying signs of rabies.
- type of the exposure: bite, scratch, lick, etc.
- immune status of the traveller: rabies vaccination history, immune competence of the traveller.

56.9 Further reading and useful resources

Chen, L. H., Hochberg, N. S., Magill, A., 'The Pre-Travel Consultation', in G. W. Brunette, ed., CDC Health Information for International Travel (Oxford, 2016), 16–138. Available from: http://wwwnc.cdc.gov/travel/yellowbook/2016/the-pre-travel-consultation/the-pre-travel-consultation

Freedman, D., Chen, L., Kozarsky, P., 'Medical Considerations before International Travel. New England Journal of Medicine, 375/3 (2016), 247–260.

Public Health England. Guidelines on Rabies Post-Exposure Treatment. Updated April 2016. https://www.gov.uk/government/uploads/system/uploads/attachment_data/file/520305/PHE_clinical_rabies_service_April_2016.pdf

Hill, D., Ericsson, C., Pearson, R., Keystone, J. S., Freedman, D. O., Kozarsky, P. E., et al., 'The Practice of Travel Medicine: Guidelines by the Infectious Diseases Society of America', Clinical Infectious Diseases, 43/12 (2006), 1499–1539.

Ramsay, M. The Green Book. Immunisation against Infectious Disease (London, 2006). Available from: https://www.gov.uk/government/collections/immunisation-against-infectious-disease-the-green-book#the-green-book

56.10 Assessment questions

56.10.1 Question 1

A thirty-four-year-old man attends the infectious diseases' outpatients clinic to seek advice on Yellow fever vaccination before travelling to Mombasa for a two-week holiday. His itinerary includes flying to Nairobi in three weeks' time, followed by taking an overnight train to Mombasa. He previously saw a general practitioner who gave him appropriate advice on other pre-travel vaccinations and chemoprophylaxis. He has chronic HIV infection and had been taking tenofovir, emtricitabine, and ritonavir-boosted darunavir. He does not have any food or drug allergies.

Investigations:

CD4 count	143×10^6/L (430–1690)
HIV viral load	<40 copies/mL

What is the most appropriate advice on Yellow fever (YF) vaccination?

A. Administer YF vaccination.

B. Advise alternative destination.

C. Advise delaying holiday.
D. Issue an exemption certificate.
E. Repeat HIV surrogate markers.

56.10.2 Question 2

A twenty-five-year-old man attends the emergency department two days after returning from a two-week holiday to Thailand because he had been bitten by a cat on the last day of his holiday. He had received three doses of rabies vaccine two years previously and is up to date with routine immunizations.

On examination, he is afebrile and haemodynamically stable. He has a puncture wound and a small laceration on his right calf.

What is the most appropriate next step in management?
A. Flucloxacillin.
B. Human rabies immunoglobulin.
C. No further action.
D. Observe the cat.
E. Rabies vaccine.

56.10.3 Question 3

A thirty-six-year-old woman attends the travel clinic to seek advice on the use of antibiotics to prevent travel-associated diarrhoea. She is planning a two-week holiday to Thailand. She has Crohn's disease and has been taking azathioprine.

What is the most appropriate antimicrobial prophylaxis for this patient?
A. Azithromycin.
B. Ciprofloxacin.
C. Doxycycline.
D. Rifaximin.
E. Tinidazole.

56.11 Answers and discussion

56.11.1 Answer 1

D. Issue an exemption certificate

YF vaccine is contraindicated in HIV-infected individuals with CD4 counts $< 200 \times 10^6$/L because of increased risk of disseminated diseases caused by the live-attenuated vaccine strain. Although YF is endemic in Kenya, the risk of exposure is low in Nairobi and Mombasa and therefore vaccination is generally not recommended for these cities. Although the stretch of land between Nairobi and Mombasa has YF activity, the risk of YF exposure remains low in this scenario because *Aedes aegypti* is a daytime biting mosquito and our patient is planning an overnight trip to Mombasa. Options B and C risks undermining patient's autonomy and may have undesirable financial consequences. Option E doesn't present any immediate benefit to this patient's management.

56.11.2 Answer 2

E. Rabies vaccine

This patient had a high-risk bite in a high-risk country for rabies. He needs basic wound care and two further doses of rabies vaccines as he has already received a full course of primary pre-exposure rabies vaccinations.

56.11.3 Answer 3

A. Azithromycin

Azithromycin would be the preferred agent for this high-risk immunocompromised traveller mainly because fluoroquinolone-resistant campylobacter is a leading cause of traveller's diarrhoea in South and Southeast Asia. Furthermore, azithromycin is active against all the other major causes of traveller's diarrhoea. Malaria chemoprophylaxis with doxycycline has been shown to be effective against enterotoxigenic *Escherichia coli* and *Campylobacter spp*, but not *Salmonella spp*. Rifaximin is not effective in the treatment of invasive enteric pathogens.

CHAPTER 57

Malaria

Angelina Jayakumar and Zahir Osman Eltahir Babiker

CONTENTS

57.1 Defining malaria

Malaria is a tropical parasitic infection of the red blood cells caused by the protozoal species *Plasmodium falciparum*, *P. vivax*, *P. ovale*, *P. malariae*, and *P. knowlesi*. It is transmitted through the bite of the female *Anopheles* mosquito. The average incubation period is twelve to fourteen days. Congenital and blood-borne transmissions can also occur.

P. falciparum and *P. vivax* account for most human infections but almost all deaths are caused by *P. falciparum*, with children under five years of age bearing the brunt of morbidity and mortality in endemic countries. *P. falciparum* is dominant in sub-Saharan Africa whereas *P. vivax* predominates in Southeast Asia and the Western Pacific. *P. ovalae* and *P. malaria* are less common and are mainly found in sub-Saharan Africa. *P. knowlesi* primarily causes malaria in macaques and is geographically restricted to southeast Asia.

57.2 How malaria parasites cause disease

While taking a blood meal, the female anopheline mosquito injects motile sporozoites into the bloodstream. Within half an hour, the sporozoites invade the hepatocytes and start dividing to form tissue schizonts. In *P. vivax* and *P. ovale*, some of the sporozoites that reach the liver develop into hypnozoites and stay dormant within the hepatocytes for months to years after the original infection. The schizonts eventually rupture releasing daughter merozoites into the bloodstream.

The merozoites develop within the red blood cells into ring forms, trophozoites, and eventually mature schizont. This part of the life cycle takes twenty-four hours for *P. knowlesi*; forty-eight hours for *P. falciparum*, *P. vivax*, *P. ovale*; and seventy-two hours for *P. malariae*. In *P. vivax* and *P. ovale*, some of the sporozoites that reach the liver develop into hypnozoites and stay dormant within the hepatocytes for months to years after the original infection.

The hallmark of malaria pathogenesis is parasite sequestration in major organs leading to cytoadherence, endothelial injury, coagulopathy, vascular leakage, pro-inflammatory cytokine production, and tissue inflammation.

57.3 The main features of imported malaria in the United Kingdom

Malaria is the most frequently imported tropical disease in the UK with an annual case load of around 2000. *P. falciparum* is the predominant imported species, and failure to take chemoprophylaxis is the commonest risk factor. Malaria has been mostly imported by patients visiting friends and relatives (VFRs) in their countries of origin and the West African diaspora has been disproportionately affected by it in the UK. While malaria mortality is low in the UK, inter-regional variations have been observed and these appear to be dependent on the level of local expertise in the recognition and management of imported malaria.

The July–September period, which coincides with school summer holidays in the UK, represents the peak season of presentation of imported malaria. A later seasonal peak in *P. falciparum* mortality has been observed during October–December and this might be explained by misdiagnosis of malaria (e.g. viral illness) and predominance of 'winter travellers' (e.g. tourists enticed by last-minute cheap winter holiday packages to Africa).

In view of the UK's ageing population, it is worth noting that patients older than sixty-five years of age have a high risk of dying from imported malaria. This vulnerability is most likely due to pre-existing comorbidities and a greater risk for adverse drug-drug interactions.

The majority of patients with vivax malaria are of South Asian heritage. The June–September period is associated with a higher risk for acquiring *P. vivax*. Patients arriving from South Asia during the October–March season tend to have a longer latency period compared to those arriving from April to September.

57.4 Clinical manifestations of malaria

Symptoms can be non-specific and can include chills, sweating, malaise, myalgia, arthralgia, abdominal pain, diarrhoea, vomiting, anorexia, cough, and headache. Fever is a common finding, especially in the early course of illness but some patients may be afebrile at the time of clinical assessment. Physical examination may be unremarkable, but anaemia, mild jaundice, and splenomegaly may be found.

57.5 Diagnosing malaria

The key laboratory investigation for malaria is the examination of three thick and thin blood smears over twenty-four to forty-eight hours, ideally by an experienced microscopist. Out of hours, this is not always possible, and rapid diagnostic tests (RDTs) are now commonly used in conjunction with smears. RDTs use monoclonal or polyclonal antibodies directed against particular antigens, e.g. histidine rich protein 2 or parasite lactate dehydrogenase. RDTs may only be used in addition to blood smears, and do not replace traditional microscopy in confirming the diagnosis. The proportion of parasitized red blood cells on thin films should be estimated in cases of falciparum malaria, in order to assess disease severity.

Other important investigations include full blood count, coagulation profile, liver and kidney function tests, blood glucose, human immunodeficiency virus (HIV) testing, and a pregnancy test in women of childbearing age.

57.6 Managing severe falciparum malaria

In all patients with clinically suspected or confirmed falciparum malaria, it is important to differentiate between uncomplicated and complicated (severe) malaria, as this dictates management. Features of severe falciparum malaria consist of:

- impaired consciousness or seizures (cerebral malaria).
- acute respiratory distress syndrome (ARDS) or pulmonary oedema.
- shock (blood pressure < 90/60 mmHg).
- acidosis (pH 7.3).
- renal impairment (oliguria < 0.4 ml/kg bodyweight per hour or serum creatinine > 265 µmol/L).
- haemoglobinuria (without glucose-6-pyruvate dehydrogenase [G6PD] deficiency).
- spontaneous bleeding/disseminated intravascular coagulation.
- hypoglycaemia (plasma glucose < 2.2 mmol/L).
- severe anaemia (haemoglobin < 80 g/L).
- parasitaemia > 10% (> 2% parasitaemia is associated with increased risk of developing severe disease and warrants parenteral therapy).

Severe falciparum malaria is a medical emergency requiring urgent parenteral antimalarial therapy, supportive care, and close monitoring for life-threatening complications. It should prompt early critical care review in the event of deterioration.

Resuscitation should be managed carefully as lactic acidosis is thought to be a result of microvascular obstruction due to parasitized erythrocytes rather than hypovolaemia, and aggressive fluid resuscitation may lead to over-filling. Signs of shock necessitate the administration of broad-spectrum antibiotics as severe malaria is sometimes complicated by bacterial infections, in particular by gram-negative organisms. Daily blood films can be helpful to monitor parasite density and document resolution of infection.

Intravenous artesunate is the treatment of choice for severe falciparum malaria and has been shown to be superior to intravenous quinine dihydrochloride in reducing mortality in adults and children. However, if there is difficulty in obtaining artesunate, then treatment should never be delayed while procuring it: parenteral quinine dihydrochloride should be started initially where artesunate is unavailable. Following at least twenty-four hours of parenteral artesunate, if the patient has improved, a full course of an artemisinin combination therapy (ACT) should be given. Alternatively, atovaquone plus proguanil or oral quinine sulphate plus doxycycline (substituted with clindamycin in pregnant women) could be used.

57.7 Managing uncomplicated falciparum malaria

High-risk groups and those who are clinically unwell should be admitted to hospital because of the risk of deterioration even after treatment has been instituted. Outpatient management could be considered if safe and effective local protocols are in place to risk stratify patients and to re-assess or re-admit them if needed.

The main therapeutic options for uncomplicated falciparum malaria in the UK are:

- oral artemisinin combination therapy (ACT): artemether-lumefantrine or dihydroartemisin-piperaquine for three days.

- oral atovaquone plus proguanil for three days (not suitable for those who have acquired malaria while taking it for prophylactic purposes).
- oral quinine sulphate plus doxycycline (or clindamycin in pregnant women) for seven days.

57.8 Managing non-falciparum malaria

Non-falciparum malaria can be treated with either an oral ACT or chloroquine. If it is a mixed infection with *P. falciparum*, then ACTs are the first line therapy. If *P. vivax* or *P. ovale* is present, then the dormant liver hypnozoites should be eradicated with primaquine after the initial treatment with an ACT or chloroquine. G6PD level should be checked before using primaquine as it can cause haemolysis in those who are G6PD deficient.

Chloroquine resistance has been reported in Southeast Asia, India, and parts of South America. There is also data to suggest that certain strains of *P. vivax* in Southeast Asia, and in particular Papua New Guinea, are 'primaquine tolerant' and require higher doses to clear the dormant liver stages.

57.9 Managing malaria in pregnant women

Malaria is associated with poor maternal, foetal, and perinatal outcomes and therefore pregnant travellers should be advised to avoid malaria-endemic regions if possible. Furthermore, there is little safety data on antimalarial therapy during pregnancy.

For uncomplicated falciparum malaria, artemether-lumefantrine is the treatment of choice in the second and third trimester. Quinine sulphate in conjunction with clindamycin can be used in all trimesters. Intravenous artesunate is the recommended first-line therapy for severe disease. A multidisciplinary approach is vital to provide optimal management for both mother and baby.

In non-falciparum malaria, chloroquine can be used throughout pregnancy. However, primaquine may not be used during pregnancy, and instead weekly suppressive chloroquine prophylaxis should be given. Primaquine can be given following delivery or on completion of breastfeeding.

57.10 Preventing malaria

Public health England recommends a four-step 'ABCD' approach to preventing malaria:

- **A**wareness of risk (traveller education).
- **B**ite prevention (mosquito repellents and insecticides-treated nets, loose fitting and long clothing).
- **C**hemoprophylaxis (must be appropriate for the travel destination and tailored to the traveller's needs).
- **D**iagnose promptly and treat without delay.

57.11 Further reading and useful resources

Broderick C, Nadjm B, Smith V, Blaze, M., Checkley, A., Chiodini, P. L., et al., 'Clinical, Geographical, and Temporal Risk Factors Associated with Presentation and Outcome of Vivax Malaria Imported into the United Kingdom over 27 Years: An Observational Study', British Medical Journal, 350 (2015), h1703.

Checkley A, Smith A, Smith V., Blaze, M., Bradley, D., Chiodini, P. L., et al., 'Risk Factors for Mortality from Imported Falciparum Malaria in the United Kingdom over 20 years: An Observational Study', British Medical Journal, 344 (2012), e2116.

Lalloo, D., Shingadia, D., Bell, D., Beeching, N. J., Whitty, C. J. M., Chiodini, P. L., et al., 'UK Malaria Treatment Guidelines 2016', *Journal of Infection*, 72 (2016), 635–649.

Public Health England. Guidelines for Malaria Prevention in Travellers from the UK 2017. Updated March 2018. https://assets.publishing.service.gov.uk/government/uploads/system/uploads/attachment_data/file/660051/Guidelines_for_malaria_prevention_in_travellers_from_the_UK_2017.pdf

Smith, A., Bradley, D., Smith, V., Blaze, M., Behrens, R. H., Chiodini, P. L., et al., 'Imported Malaria and High-Risk Groups: Observational Study Using UK Surveillance Data 1987–2006', British Medical Journal, 337 (2008), a120.

Whitty, C., Chiodini, P., Lalloo, D., 'Investigation and treatment of imported malaria in non-endemic countries', British Medical Journal, 346 (2013), f2900.

World Health Organization. Basic Malaria Microscopy. Part I Learner's Guide (2nd edn, Geneva, 2010). Available at http://apps.who.int/iris/bitstream/10665/44208/1/9789241547826_eng.pdf

57.12 Assessment questions

57.12.1 Question 1

A twenty-four-year-old man presents to the emergency department with fever, nausea, and muscle aches for two days. He returned ten days previously from a two-month backpacking trip to Cambodia. He initially took doxycycline for malaria prophylaxis but this was later discontinued because he developed a photosensitive rash. On examination, his temperature is 39.2 °C, heart rate 100 beats per minute, blood pressure 115/75 mmHg, peripheral oxygen saturation 99% on room air. Abdominal examination reveals a palpable splenic tip.

Investigations:	
Haemoglobin	157 g/L (130–180)
Platelets	65×10^9/L (150–400)
Malaria thick blood film:	*plasmodium species* parasites seen
Malaria thin blood film:	trophozoites with large single chromatin dots and amoeboid cytoplasm are seen inside enlarged distorted red blood cells containing pale red dots

Which plasmodium species is most likely responsible for this infection?
A. falciparum.
B. knowlesi.
C. malariae.
D. ovale.
E. vivax.

57.12.2 Question 2

A thirty-year-old woman attends the travel clinic to seek advice on appropriate malaria chemoprophylaxis. She is planning to travel to the Gambia in two weeks' time to participate in an essential five-day high-stakes business trip. She is twenty weeks pregnant.

What is the most appropriate malaria chemoprophylaxis?
A. Atovaquone plus proguanil.
B. Chloroquine plus proguanil.
C. Clindamycin.
D. Doxycycline.
E. Mefloquine.

57.12.3 Question 3

A sixty-year-old man presents to the emergency department with a two-day history of fever, muscle aches, nausea, and vomiting ten days after arriving from a one-month holiday to Nigeria. He has ischaemic heart disease and is taking atenolol, verapamil, pravastatin, and aspirin. On examination, his temperature is 39.1 °C, pulse 100 beats per minute, blood pressure 110/70 mmHg, and peripheral oxygen saturation 99% on room air.

Investigations:	
Haemoglobin	162 g/L (130–180)
Platelets	41 × 109/L (150–400)
Serum sodium	134 mmol/L (137–144)
Serum potassium	3.5 mmol/L (3.5–4.9)
Serum urea	8.5 mmol/L (2.5–7.0)
Serum creatinine	117 μmol/L (60–110)
Random plasma glucose	7.9 mmol/L
Peripheral blood film microscopy	multiple ring stages of *Plasmodium falciparum* seen (8.4% parasitaemia)

What is the most appropriate next step in management?
A. Artemether plus lumefantrine.
B. Artesunate.
C. Exchange blood transfusion.
D. Quinine dihydrochloride.
E. Quinine sulphate plus doxycycline.

57.13 Answers and discussion

57.13.1 Answer 1

E. vivax
P. vivax tends to invade younger red blood cells (RBCs) and the stippling pattern associated with it is known as Schuffner's dots. *P. falciparum* has thin delicate ring stages with two chromatin dots. The trophozoites of *P. ovale* are compact whereas those of *P. malariae* may have band forms. *P. ovale* infects young RBCs, *P. malariae* infects older RBCs, and both *P. falciparum* and *P. knowlesi* infect all age groups of RBCs. The early stages of *P. knowlesi* resemble those of *P. falciparum* whereas the late stages resemble *P. malariae*. Molecular testing can differentiate between different types of malaria parasites.

57.13.2 Answer 2

E. Mefloquine
Pregnant women should be advised to avoid travel to malaria-endemic regions where possible. If travel is unavoidable and there are no contra-indications, then mefloquine can be used throughout pregnancy (caution in first trimester).

57.13.3 Answer 3

B. Artesunate
Intravenous artesunate is the treatment of choice for severe falciparum malaria. Concomitant use of quinine and verapamil is contra-indicated because of increased risk of cardiac arrhythmias.

CHAPTER 58

Fever in returned travellers

Desmond Hsu and Zahir Osman Eltahir Babiker

CONTENTS

58.1 Fever in returned travellers

Travel-related problems have been reported in up to two-thirds of travellers to developing countries and approximately 10% of them seek medical advice during or after return from abroad. Furthermore, global migration from the developing to the developed world has increased over the past decades and these individuals may present with tropical infections soon after arrival in non-endemic settings.

Fever, with or without localizing symptoms or signs, is a common presenting symptom in returning travellers. Most unwell travellers seek medical attention within one month of return from abroad. Travellers who visit friends and relatives (VFRs) in their countries of origin are disproportionately affected by the burden of imported infections, e.g. 70% of patients with imported malaria in the United Kingdom (UK) are VFRs. While most febrile travellers have common infections such as respiratory or urinary tract infection, it is of paramount importance not to miss potentially life-threatening tropical infections.

58.2 Taking an accurate travel history

Evaluation of fever in returning travellers requires an understanding of the geographical distribution of infectious diseases, risk factors for acquisition, incubation periods, and major clinical syndromes of travel-associated infections.

The following points should be considered when assessing febrile international travellers:

A. Travel dates: the relationship between the timing of the onset of symptoms and travel dates should be assessed.

B. Geography:
  - travel destination: a detailed itinerary is required.
  - local setting: urban vs rural locations; type of accommodation, e.g. air-conditioned hotel room, outdoor camping, etc.

C. Risk factors for acquiring infectious diseases (Table 58.1):
   - purpose of travel: visiting friends and family; social gatherings (e.g. funerals and weddings); mass gatherings (e.g. Hajj pilgrimage, Kumbh Mela religious festival, Olympic games, etc.); tourism; business; voluntary work.
   - contact with unwell individuals.
   - activities while abroad (examples):
      - food consumption: street food, seafood, raw food, unpasteurized dairy products, exotic foods, bush meat, etc.
      - contact with animals: visits to game parks, farms, caves, bites or scratches by bats or terrestrial animals, visits to 'wet markets', birding events, etc.
      - bites: ticks, insects, snakes, spiders, etc.
      - use of local healthcare system: dental or surgical procedures, blood transfusion, dialysis, tattoos, acupuncture.
      - fresh or salty water exposure: water sports, visits to paddy fields, swimming, beach sports, etc.
      - risky behaviour activities: unprotected sexual intercourse, injecting drug use and sharing of needles, intoxication with alcohol or recreational drugs.

D. Medications:
   - malaria chemoprophylaxis: drug, duration, and adherence.
   - pre-departure vaccinations as well as history of routine vaccinations.
   - antibiotics taken while abroad.

Table 58.1 Examples of travel-related activities and risk of infectious diseases.

Exposure	Associated infection
Drinking unclean water	Shigellosis, salmonellosis, viral gastroenteritis, hepatitis A, hepatitis E, giardiosis, cryptosporidiosis
Contact with fresh water reservoir	Leptospirosis, schistosomiasis
Consumption of contaminated, under-cooked, or unpasteurized food	Acute gastroenteritis, brucellosis, listeriosis, toxoplasmosis
Animal bites	Rabies, cat-scratch disease, skin and soft tissue infections
Animal contact	Q-fever, anthrax, toxoplasmosis, Hantavirus infections, plague
Bird contact	Psittacosis, avian influenza
Mosquito bites	Malaria, arboviral infections (e.g. dengue, chikungunya, zika, Japanese encephalitis, Yellow fever, West Nile fever), lymphatic filariaisis
Tick bites	Spotted fevers (e.g. tick typhus, Rocky mountain spotted fever), Lyme disease, tick-borne encephalitis, Crimean-Congo haemorrhagic fever, tularaemia, babesiosis
Fly bites	African trypanosomiasis, onchocerciasis, leishmaniasis, Loa loa, sandfly fever
Other bites	*Fleas:* murine (endemic) typhus and plague *Lice:* louse-borne (epidemic) typhus *Mites:* scrub typhus *Triatomine bugs:* Chagas disease
Contaminated soil	Hookworms, Strongyloides, melioidosis, fungal infections
Unprotected sex	HIV, hepatitis C, syphilis, chlamydia, gonorrhoea
Injections, body-piercing	Hepatitis B and C, HIV

E. Significant personal medical history:
  ● age: older than sixty-five years of age
  ● immune status: HIV infection, current or recent immunosuppressive therapy, underlying malignancy, etc.
  ● pregnancy status (females of childbearing age).
  ● pre-existing morbidities.
  ● current medications (check potential for adverse drug-drug interactions).

58.3 Incubation periods of frequently imported tropical infections

Correlating the date of onset of symptoms with travel dates gives clues about the duration of the incubation period of the underlying infection. Most frequently imported tropical infections have incubation periods of twenty-one or fewer days. The following are examples of incubation periods of some of the important tropical infections:

● Twenty-one days or fewer: malaria, arthropod-borne viral infections (e.g. dengue, chikungunya), enteric fever, acute gastro-enteritis (bacterial, parasitic, viral), rickettsial infections (e.g. scrub typhus, tick typhus), acute respiratory infections (e.g. influenza, legionella, coronaviruses), melioidosis, meningococcal disease, plague, relapsing fever, brucellosis, leptospirosis, Q-fever, viral haemorrhagic fever, acute infectious mononucleosis (cytomegalovirus, Epstein-Barr virus), HIV, coccidioidomycosis, histoplasmosis.
● More than twenty-one days: malaria, viral hepatitis (A–E), amoebic liver disease, visceral leishmaniasis, rabies, tuberculosis, brucellosis, filariasis, HIV, acute schistosomiasis (Katayama fever).

58.4 Clinical and epidemiological features of travel-associated infections

Patients may present with undifferentiated fever or may have localizing symptoms and signs which may provide further clues to their underlying infection (Table 58.2). Furthermore, fever may be associated with specific gastro-intestinal, respiratory, dermatological, or neurological problems. The presence of peripheral eosinophilia may indicate an underlying worm infestation.

Recent GeoSentinel surveillance data (2007–2011) showed that malaria (primarily falciparum) was the most common febrile illness imported from sub-Saharan Africa, whereas dengue fever was the most commonly imported infection in travellers returning from Southeast Asia, Latin America, and the Caribbean. Furthermore, enteric fever was commonly associated with travel to South-Central Asia, whereas rickettsial infections (mainly tick-borne rickettsiosis) were mainly seen in travellers returning from sub-Saharan Africa. Interestingly, almost 40% of febrile retuning travellers had no specific aetiology identified.

Bacterial gastroenteritis due to *Campylobacter, Salmonella,* and *Shigella* species has been frequently documented in travellers returning from Southeast Asia, sub-Saharan Africa, the Middle East, and North Africa. Giardiasis is most common in travellers returning from the Indian sub-continent. Cosmopolitan respiratory tract infections are common among ill returning travellers, with influenza A and B accounting for nearly 10% of these infections.

Animal bites or scratches requiring rabies post-exposure prophylaxis and cutaneous larva migrans in returning travellers from Southeast Asia, sub-Saharan Africa, and Latin America and the Caribbean are the top-ranking skin problems. Neurological presentations are infrequent and

Table 58.2 Physical findings suggestive of cause of pyrexia.

Physical finding	Possible cause
Rash (maculopapular)	Arboviral infections (e.g. dengue, chikungunya), rickettsial infections, acute schistosomiasis, measles, rubella, parvovirus, acute HIV, EBV, and CMV, enteric fever (rose spots), secondary syphilis, viral haemorrhagic fever
Rash (petechial)	Meningococcal septicaemia, viral haemorrhagic fever, leptospirosis, severe sepsis
Eschar	Scrub typhus, tick typhus, Lyme disease, anthrax
Jaundice	Viral hepatitis, malaria, leptospirosis, viral haemorrhagic fever, Yellow fever
Lymphadenopathy	Plague, rickettsial infections, toxoplasmosis, HIV, tuberculosis
Hepatomegaly	Malaria, visceral leishmaniasis, liver abscess, viral hepatitis, leptospirosis, brucellosis
Splenomegaly	Malaria, visceral leishmaniasis, trypanosomiasis, brucellosis

often non-specified but notable tropical causes are ciguatera intoxication in travellers returning from the Caribbean and neurocysticercosis and tuberculosis in travellers returning from the Indian sub-continent. Other important travel-associated infections include schistosomiasis (sub-Saharan Africa), filariasis (sub-Saharan Africa), and Lyme disease (North America and continental Europe).

In the UK, a single-centre fifteen-year prospective study showed that most travellers to sub-Saharan Africa presented with classical tropical infections and that falciparum malaria has remained the commonest diagnosis despite an overall declining trend. By contrast, most travellers to Asia had non-tropical infections, but enteric fever, dengue fever, and non-falciparum malaria have been the leading tropical infections requiring hospital admission.

58.5 Requesting investigations

The choice of tests depends on the presenting clinical syndrome as well as the outcome of risk assessment for potential dangerous pathogens. It is strongly recommended to follow the most up-to-date clinical algorithms developed by Public Health England (http://www.phe.gov.uk) for triaging patients with potential dangerous pathogens, e.g. viral haemorrhagic fever, avian influenza, the Middle East respiratory syndrome coronavirus (MERS-CoV), or any other emerging pathogen. Furthermore, collection and processing of clinical samples obtained from patients with potentially dangerous pathogens should be performed in accordance with the recommendations of the Advisory Committee on Dangerous Pathogens (ACDP).

The following list provides general guidance on the type of clinical samples and tests that can be arranged to investigate fever in returning travellers with low risk for dangerous pathogens:

- full blood count, renal and liver function tests, and C-reactive protein.
- malaria parasites: thick and thin blood films and rapid malaria antigen test for all travellers arriving from endemic regions.
- peripheral blood culture (at least 20–30ml of blood per two-bottle set).
- urinalysis and mid-stream urine culture.
- HIV antigen/antibody test.
- pregnancy test (women of childbearing age).

- serum save plus EDTA-blood samples on all patients (these are useful baseline samples to obtain for further specialist testing for tropical pathogens by the reference laboratory based on the clinical syndrome and the travel destination).
- nasopharyngeal swabs or sputum for respiratory viral PCR panel as appropriate.
- stool for microscopic detection of ova, cysts, and parasites; bacterial culture; and enteric viral PCR panel as appropriate.
- chest X-ray as appropriate.
- abdominal ultrasound scan as appropriate.

58.6 Implications for infection prevention and control in healthcare settings

Obtaining relevant and accurate travel history in all patients presenting with fever is of paramount importance as this may well be a game changer in terms of clinical management. Furthermore, risk assessment for potentially dangerous pathogens must be carried out in all patients with recent travel history. Where possible, patients should be triaged in a neutral-pressure single-occupancy room and further escalation to a negative-pressure room should be considered if the patient is deemed to have high risk for dangerous pathogens after careful risk assessment. Personal equipment offering protection against direct contact with droplets and bodily fluids should be considered by healthcare workers pending further clinical and diagnostic assessments. Furthermore, laboratory staff should be forewarned if clinical samples are being sent from high-risk patients so that appropriate laboratory safety procedures can be followed.

Returning travellers who have been hospitalized in countries with high rates of antibiotic resistance should be screened for multi-drug resistant organisms, including Carbapenem-resistant *Enterobacteriaceae*. Similarly, blood-borne virus screening should be considered for returning travellers who have received haemodialysis or organ transplantation abroad.

58.7 Further reading and useful resources

Checkley, A., Chiodini, P., Dockrell, D., Bates, I., Thwaites, G. E., Booth, H. L., et al., 'Eosinophilia in returning travellers and migrants from the tropics: UK recommendations for investigation and initial management', *Journal of Infection*, 60 (2010), 1–20.

Johnston, V., Stockley, J., Dockrell, D., Warrell, D., Bailey, R., Pasvol, G., et al., 'Fever in Returned Travellers Presenting in the United Kingdom: Recommendations for Investigation and Initial Management', *Journal of Infection*, 59 (2009), 1–18.

Leder, K., Torresi, J., Libman, M. D., Cramer, J. P., Castelli, F., Schlagenhauf, P., et al. GeoSentinel Surveillance of Illness in Returned Travelers, 2007–2011', *Annals of Internal Medicine*, 158 (2013), 456–468.

Marks M, Armstrong M, Whitty C. J. M., Doherty, J. F., 'Geographical and temporal trends in imported infections from the tropics requiring inpatient care at the Hospital for Tropical Diseases, London—a 15-year study', *Transactions of the Royal Society of Tropical Medicine and Hygiene*, 110/8 (2016), 456–463.

Public Health England. *Rare and Imported Pathogens Laboratory (RIPL): Specimen Referral Guidelines and Service User Manual 2016.* Updated June 2018. https://assets.publishing.service.gov.uk/government/uploads/system/uploads/attachment_data/file/714550/SPATH039RIPL_User_Manual_May_2018.pdf.

Schlagenhauf P, Weld L, Goorhuis A, Gautret, P., Weber, R., von Sonnenburg, F., et al., 'Travel-Associated Infection Presenting in Europe (2008–12): An Analysis of EuroTravNet Longitudinal

Surveillance Data, and Evaluation of the Effect of the Pre-Travel Consultation', *Lancet Infectious Diseases*, 15 (2015), 55–64.

Thwaites, G., and Day, N., 'Approach to fever in the returning traveler', *New England Journal fo Medicine*, 376 (2017), 548–560.

58.8 Assessment questions

58.8.1 Question 1

A thirty-five-year-old man attends the emergency department with a two-week history of profuse watery diarrhoea associated with belching and flatulence. Two days previously, he returned from a two-month backpacking trip to Laos. He has previously been fit and well. He was taking atovaquone/proguanil, loperamide, and oral rehydration solution.

On examination, his temperature is 36.8 °C, pulse 100 beats per minute, and blood pressure 110/70 mmHg.

Investigations:

Haemoglobin	137 g/L (130–180)
Mean corpuscular volume	85 fL (80–96)
Serum urea	8.4 mmol/L (2.5–7.0)
Serum creatinine	90 μmol/L (60–110)
Malaria parasites	not detected

What is the most likely pathogen?
A. *Ancylostoma duodenale.*
B. *Escherichia coli.*
C. *Giardia lamblia.*
D. *Trichuris trichiura.*
E. *Vibrio cholerae.*

58.8.2 Question 2

A forty-two-year-old man presents to the emergency department having developed chills, headaches, and muscle and joint pains two days after returning from a two-week carp fishing holiday in France. On examination, his temperature is 38.5 °C, pulse 110 beats per minute, and blood pressure 105/67 mmHg.

Investigations:

Haemoglobin	145 g/L (130–180)
Platelet count	99 × 10⁹/L (150–400)
White cell count	7.9 × 10⁹/L (4.0–11.0)
Neutrophil count	6.7 × 10⁹/L (1.5–7.0)
Lymphocyte count	0.4 × 10⁹/L (1.5–4.0)
Serum sodium	131 mmol/L (137–144)
Serum potassium	3.6 mmol/L (3.5–4.9)
Serum urea	9.1 mmol/L (2.5–7.0)
Serum creatinine	188 μmol/L (60–110)
Serum total bilirubin	20 μmol/L (1–22)
Serum alanine aminotransferase	18 U/L (5–35)
Serum alkaline phosphatase	55 U/L (45–105)

What is the most likely pathogen?
A. *Coxiella burnetii*.
B. *Leptospira interrogans*.
C. *Mycobacterium marinum*.
D. *Rickettsia typhi*.
E. Sin nombre hantavirus.

58.8.3 Question 3

A forty-five-year-old woman presents to the emergency department with a three-day history of fever, painful swollen hands and ankles, and a skin rash. She returned five days previously from a one-month holiday to a plantation on the coastal region of Guyana. She did not take any malaria prophylaxis but was up to date with her routine immunizations. On examination, she is afebrile. Examination of her hands reveals tender fusiform swellings involving her fingers. Both ankles are warm to touch and have a limited range of movement. There is a blanching maculopapular rash over her torso.

Investigations	
Haemoglobin	125 g/L (115–165)
Platelet count	100×10^9/L (150–400)
White cell count	6.4×10^9/L (4.0–11.0)
Neutrophil count	3.7×10^9/L (1.5–7.0)
Lymphocyte count	0.6×10^9/L (1.5–4.0)

What is the most likely diagnosis?
A. Chikungunya.
B. Dengue fever.
C. Parvovirus infection.
D. Rubella.
E. Zika.

58.9 Answers and discussion

58.9.1 Answer 1

C. *Giardia lamblia*
Giardiasis is characterized by diarrhoea (often early morning, explosive, and greasy), abdominal pain, bloating, and flatulence. Persistent diarrhoea may lead to malabsorption and lactose intolerance.

58.9.2 Answer 2

B. *Leptospira interrogans*
Leptospirosis, acquired through exposure to rats' urine, is the most likely diagnosis in view of the fishing trip to mainland Europe. The geographical distribution of sin nombre hantavirus is restricted to North America.

58.9.3 Answer 3

A. Chikungunya
Although all the viruses listed in the question are arthritogenic, small joint arthritis is typically associated with chikungunya. The coastal regions of Guyana are considered low-risk areas for malaria.

Index

Tables and figures are indicated by an italic *t* and *f* following the page number